theclinics.com

NEUROLOGIC CLINICS

Peripheral Neuropathies

GUEST EDITOR
Yadollah Harati, MD

February 2007 • Volume 25 • Number 1

SAUNDERS

An Imprint of Elsevier, Inc.
PHILADELPHIA LONDON TORONTO MONTREAL SYDNEY TOKYO

W.B. SAUNDERS COMPANY
A Division of Elsevier Inc.

1600 John F. Kennedy Blvd., Suite 1800, Philadelphia, PA 19103-2899

http://www.theclinics.com

NEUROLOGIC CLINICS
February 2007
Editor: Donald Mumford

Volume 25, Number 1
ISSN 0733-8619
ISBN 1-4160-4337-3
978-1-4160-4337-9

Neurologic Clinics (ISSN 0733-8619) is published quarterly by Elsevier Inc., 360 Park Avenue South, New York, NY 10010–171. Months of issue are February, May, August, and November. Business and editorial offices: 1600 John F. Kennedy Blvd., Suite 1800, Philadelphia, PA 19103-2899. Customer Service Office: 6277 Sea Harbor Drive, Orlando, FL 32887–4800. Accounting and circulation offices: 6277 Sea Harbor Drive, Orlando, FL 32887-4800. Periodicals postage paid at New York, NY, and additional mailing offices. Subscription prices are $198.00 per year for US individuals, $313.00 per year for US institutions, $99.00 per year for US students, $248.00 per year for Canadian individuals, $367.00 per year for Canadian institutions, $259.00 per year for international individuals, $367.00 per year for international institutions and $132.00 for Canadian and foreign students/residents. To receive student/resident rate, orders must be accompanied by name of affiliated institution, date of term, and the *signature* of program/residency coordinator on institution letterhead. Orders will be billed at individual rate until proof of status is received. Foreign air speed delivery is included in all *Clinics* subscription prices. All prices are subject to change without notice. POSTMASTER: Send address changes to *Neurologic Clinics*, Elsevier Periodicals Customer Service, 6277 Sea Harbor Drive, Orlando, FL 32887-4800. **Customer Service: 1-800-654-2452 (US). From outside of the US, call 1-407-345-4000.**

Neurologic Clinics is also published in Spanish by Nueva Editorial Interamericana S.A., Mexico City, Mexico.

Neurologic Clinics is covered in *Current Contents/Clinical Medicine, Index Medicus, EMBASE/Excerpta Medica,* and *PsycINFO,* and *ISI/BIOMED.*

Printed in the United States of America.

GUEST EDITOR

YADOLLAH HARATI, MD, FACP, Professor of Neurology, and Director, Baylor Neuropathy Center and Muscle and Nerve Pathology Laboratory, Department of Neurology, Baylor College of Medicine, Houston, Texas

CONTRIBUTORS

JAMES W. ALBERS, MD, PhD, Professor of Neurology, Department of Neurology, University of Michigan, Ann Arbor, Michigan

TED M. BURNS, MD, Associate Professor, Department of Neurology, University of Virginia, Charlottesville, Virginia

P. JAMES B. DYCK, MD, Associate Professor, and Director of Peripheral Neuropathy Research Laboratory, Mayo Clinic College of Medicine, Rochester, Minnesota

ROY FREEMAN, MD, Professor of Neurology, Harvard Medical School, Boston; Director, Center for Autonomic and Peripheral Nerve Disorders, Beth Israel Deaconess Medical Center, Boston, Massachusetts

CLIFTON L. GOOCH, MD, Professor of Clinical Neurology, and Director, Columbia Neuropathy Research Center; Director, Electromyography Laboratory, Columbia University College of Physicians and Surgeons, New York, New York

YADOLLAH HARATI, MD, FACP, Professor of Neurology, and Director, Baylor Neuropathy Center and Muscle and Nerve Pathology Laboratory, Department of Neurology, Baylor College of Medicine, Houston, Texas

CHRISTOPHER J. KLEIN, MD, Department of Neurology, Division of Peripheral Nerve Diseases, Mayo Clinic, Rochester, Minnesota

NEERAJ KUMAR, MD, Consultant, Department of Neurology, Mayo Clinic; Assistant Professor, Mayo Clinic College of Medicine, Rochester, Minnesota

JUSTIN Y. KWAN, MD, Assistant Professor, Neuromuscular Diseases, Department of Neurology, Baylor College of Medicine, Houston, Texas

RICHARD A. LEWIS, MD, Professor and Associate Chair of Neurology, Wayne State School of Medicine, 8-D University Health Center, Detroit, Michigan

ZACHARY LONDON, MD, Lecturer, Department of Neurology, University of Michigan, Ann Arbor, Michigan

GÉRARD SAID, MD, FRCP, Chief, and Professor of Neurology, Service de Neurologie, Hôpital de Bicêtre, Universitê Paris XI, Bicêtre, France

GREGORY A. SCHAUBLIN, MD, Department of Neurology, University of Virginia, Charlottesville, Virginia

STEVEN VERNINO, MD, PhD, Department of Neurology, University of Texas Southwestern Medical Center, Dallas, Texas

LOUIS H. WEIMER, MD, Associate Clinical Professor of Neurology, and Director, Autonomic Function Laboratory, Columbia University College of Physicians and Surgeons, New York, New York

ASA J. WILBOURN, MD, EMG Laboratory, Cleveland Clinic; Clinical Professor of Neurology, Case Western Reserve University School of Medicine, Cleveland, Ohio

GIL I. WOLFE, MD, Department of Neurology, University of Texas Southwestern Medical Center, Dallas, Texas

CONTENTS

FORTHCOMING ISSUES

May 2007

Neck and Back Pain
Kerry Levin, MD, *Guest Editor*

August 2007

Dementia
Neill Graff-Radford, MD, *Guest Editor*

November 2007

Brain Tumors in Adults
Patrick Y. Wen, MD, and
David Schiff, MD, *Guest Editors*

RECENT ISSUES

November 2006

Preoperative and Perioperative Issues in Cerebrovascular Disease
José Biller, MD, *Guest Editor*

August 2006

Psychoneuroimmunology
Gregory G. Freund, MD, *Guest Editor*

May 2006

Neurology Case Studies
Randolph W. Evans, MD, *Guest Editor*

February 2006

Brain Injury and Cardiac Arrest
Romergryko G. Geocadin, MD
Guest Editor

November 2005

Sleep Disorders
Robert W. Fayle, MD, *Guest Editor*

August 2005

Otoneurology
Joseph M. Furman, MD, PhD, and
Susan L. Whitney, PhD, PT, NCS, ATC
Guest Editors

ELSEVIER
SAUNDERS

Neurol Clin 25 (2007) xi–xii

NEUROLOGIC
CLINICS

Preface

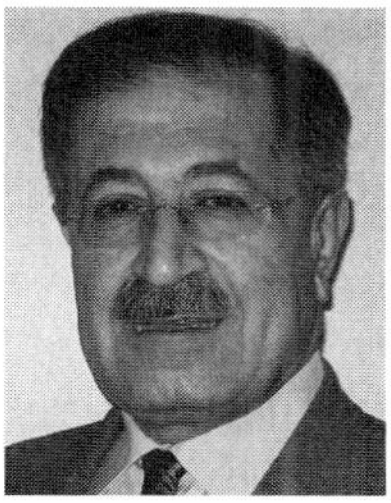

Yadollah Harati, MD, FACP
Guest Editor

In this issue of *Neurologic Clinics* several distinguished colleagues and experts in peripheral neuropathies are assembled to review a variety of neuropathies to help clinicians keep abreast of new information on the topic. Peripheral neuropathies constitute a challenging group of diseases that have many etiologies and represent one of the major causes of disability in all parts of the world. With a few exceptions, the reviews contained in this issue cover many of these etiologies and together provide a framework for diagnosis and treatment.

The importance of proper electrophysiologic studies and autoantibody testing in peripheral neuropathies is emphasized in two separate reviews. Because there is an overlap between the clinical manifestations of some neuropathies and plexus disorders, a separate review is devoted entirely to plexus disorders. Inherited, vasculitic, paraproteinemic, nutritional, toxic, immunomediated, infectious, and autonomic neuropathies are extensively covered, and when appropriate the photomicrographs are printed in color. In each review, the authors have added some of their own valuable experience in approaching the diagnosis and management of neuropathies. This issue, however, is not intended to replace the available comprehensive and excellent textbooks on peripheral neuropathies; rather, the intent is to allow the clinician, who may not have time to read or integrate all the original and recent publications, learn from the latest developments.

I am indebted to each of the authors for their scholarly contributions and for helping me achieve this goal. I also thank Donald Mumford and others at Elsevier for their patience and efficiency throughout the production of

0733-8619/07/$ - see front matter
doi:10.1016/j.ncl.2007.02.002

this issue. Finally, putting this issue together would not have been possible without the support of Gita and Ali Saberioon, to whom I extend my sincere appreciations.

Yadollah Harati, MD, FACP
Neuropathy Center and Muscle and Nerve Pathology Laboratory
Baylor College of Medicine
6550 Fannin #1801
Houston, TX 77030, USA

E-mail address: yharati@bcm.edu

ELSEVIER
SAUNDERS

Neurol Clin 25 (2007) 1–28

NEUROLOGIC
CLINICS

The Electrodiagnosis of Neuropathy: Basic Principles and Common Pitfalls

Clifton L. Gooch, MD[a,*], Louis H. Weimer, MD[b]

[a]Columbia Neuropathy Research Center, Electromyography Laboratory, Columbia University College of Physicians and Surgeons, 710 West 168th Street, New York, NY 10032, USA
[b]Autonomic Function Laboratory, Columbia University College of Physicians and Surgeons, 710 West 168th Street, New York, NY 10032, USA

Nerve conduction studies and needle electromyography (EMG) are critical tools for diagnosis and research in patients with neuropathy, but the proper performance and interpretation of these methods remain of paramount importance. In this article we review the basic principles of these techniques and their clinical application to neuropathy, with a special focus on potential sources of error and how to avoid them.

Basic principles

Sensory and motor nerve conduction studies

Nerve conduction studies measure the strength and speed of impulses propagated down the length of a peripheral nerve. During nerve conduction studies, an action potential is triggered at a specific point along the nerve using a bipolar stimulator placed on the skin surface. The intensity of stimulation is increased from zero to a level just above that needed to depolarize all the axons within the nerve (a supramaximal stimulation) to ensure full activation. The action potentials of these axons travel together down the nerve to the recording site, where they generate a summated waveform. For sensory nerve conduction studies, the recording electrodes are placed on the skin directly over the nerve (usually over a pure sensory branch) at a fixed distance from the stimulation site (Fig. 1), where they record a sensory nerve action potential (SNAP) waveform (Fig. 2). The electrical strength of the impulse, which reflects the number of axons successfully

* Corresponding author.
E-mail address: clg33@columbia.edu (C.L. Gooch).

doi:10.1016/j.ncl.2007.01.011 *neurologic.theclinics.com*

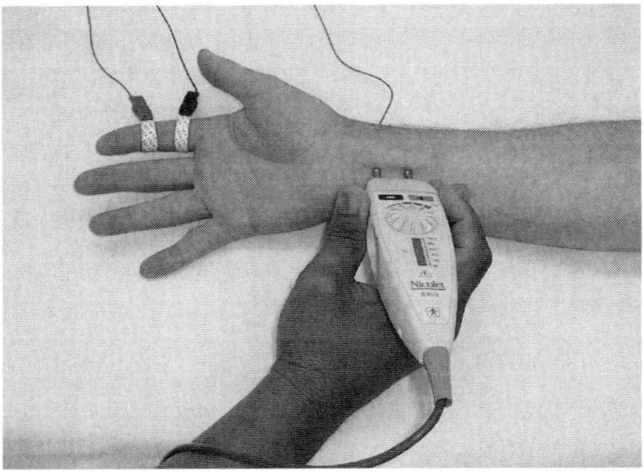

Fig. 1. Sensory nerve conduction studies of the median nerve. The bipolar stimulator is placed over the course of the median nerve at the wrist, whereas the active and reference recording electrodes are placed over the course of the median pure sensory branches in the index finger, which ensures that only sensory nerve responses are recorded. The ground electrode is placed over the dorsum of the hand.

activated (all the axons in a single nerve are activated by this technique in a normal subject), is reflected in the amplitude of the waveform, which is measured in microvolts for sensory waveforms. The speed of transmission is reflected in the latency, which is the time between stimulation of the nerve and recording of the waveform, measured in milliseconds. By also measuring the distance between the stimulating and recording sites, the latency can

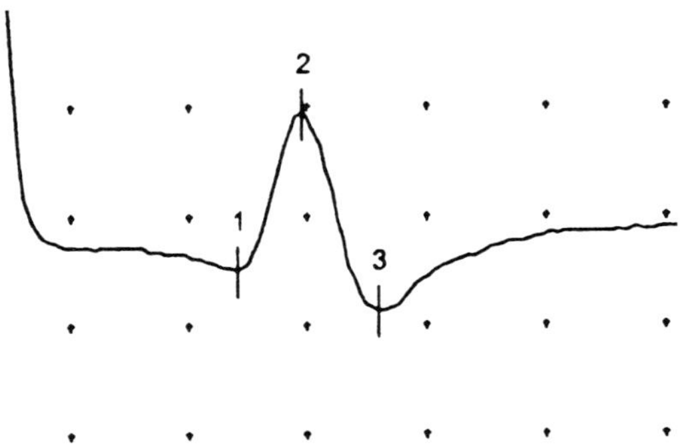

Fig. 2. SNAP generated by the setup in Fig. 1. The horizontal space between two dots (graticules) is one division and indicates time in milliseconds, which enables measurement of latency. This display value is called the sweep speed (set to 1 msec/division here). Vertical divisions indicate the strength of the potential. This display value is called the sensitivity or gain (set to 10 μV/division here). The time between the stimulus artifact and the peak of the SNAP waveform (the sensory latency) is 2.75 msec in this study, and the peak-to-peak height of the waveform (the sensory amplitude) is 13.2 μV, both of which are within the normal range for control subjects.

be used to calculate a nerve conduction velocity, another measure of conduction speed. Motor nerve conduction studies are performed in a similar fashion, except that the recording electrodes are placed over an innervated muscle (rather than the nerve itself) to ensure that a pure motor response is recorded (Fig. 3).

Each individual motor axon within a nerve supplies its own population of muscle fibers within an innervated muscle (and each axon and its muscle fibers comprise a motor unit). In a normal subject, activation of all the axons within a nerve causes depolarization of all the muscle fibers in the muscle innervated by that nerve. This summated muscle potential is then recorded as a waveform, the compound motor action potential (CMAP) (Fig. 4). The CMAP is an order of magnitude larger than the SNAP because of the high electropotency of muscle and is usually reported in millivolts rather than microvolts. Latency is not as accurate a measure of the speed of conduction in motor nerves because of the variability introduced by transmission across the neuromuscular junction to the muscle from which the response is recorded. Consequently, velocity measures are used and calculated in such a way as to factor out the effects of neuromuscular junction transmission [1–3].

The amplitude of the generated waveform and the speed of nerve conduction provide important information regarding nerve function. Waveform amplitude usually correlates best with axonal integrity, whereas conduction velocity depends highly on the degree of myelination because of the advantages provided by salutatory conduction. Consequently, loss of amplitude suggests axonal loss or dysfunction, whereas slowing of conduction velocity or latency prolongation usually implies demyelination. Focal demyelination at a single site between the simulation and recording electrodes (as with

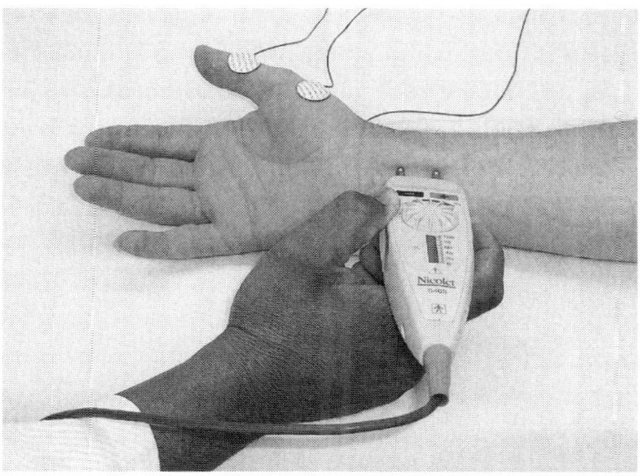

Fig. 3. Motor nerve conduction studies of the median nerve. The bipolar stimulator is placed over the course of the median nerve at the wrist, whereas the active recording electrode is placed over the median-innervated muscles in the thenar eminence, with the reference placed over a neutral distal point.

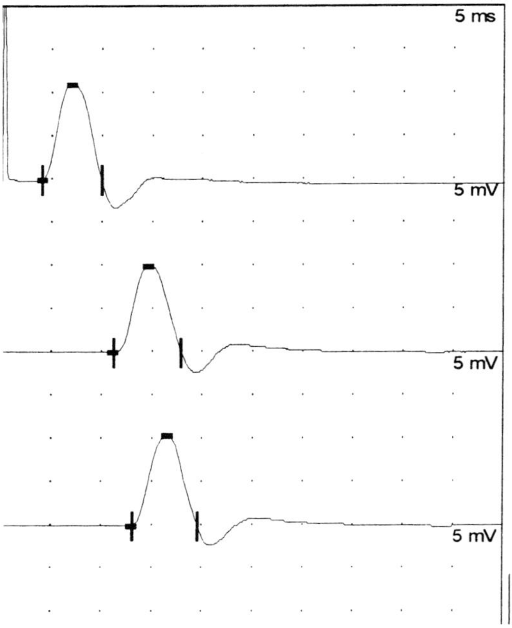

Fig. 4. CMAP. These responses were recorded from the extensor digitorum brevis muscle of the foot following stimulation of the peroneal nerve. The top waveform was recorded after stimulation at the ankle, the middle waveform after stimulation below the knee (inferolateral to the fibular head) and the bottom waveform after stimulation at the knee (in the popliteal fossa). The sweep speed is 5 msec/division and the sensitivity is 5 mV/division. These waveforms have onset latencies of 4.0, 11.1, and 13 msec, respectively (corresponding to the increasing distance between the stimulating and recording electrodes at each of the stimulation sites). Conduction velocities (calculated using latency and inter-electrode distances) are 46 m/sec for the proximal and distal segments of the nerve, whereas the amplitudes are 11.5, 10.4, and 10.2 mV, respectively, all of which are within normal limits.

entrapment neuropathy) may be severe enough to cause complete block of transmission in a substantial number of axons within the nerve, however. When this occurs, the strength of the impulse (which is the sum of the total number of activated axons within the nerve) is significantly degraded at the site of focal injury. Waveform amplitude falls as the impulse passes over the site of injury, and this loss of amplitude is proportionate to the percentage of motor axons blocked, like decreased water depth in a river downstream from a dam. This phenomenon, known as conduction block, is an important diagnostic feature of most acquired demyelinating neuropathies and is identified by comparing the waveform amplitude recorded from a nerve segment above or below a site of injury to that recorded with the injured segment between the stimulating and recording electrodes (Fig. 5).

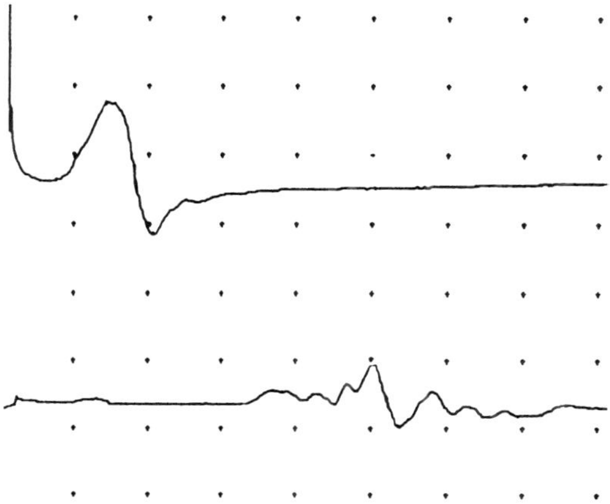

Fig. 5. Conduction block with temporal dispersion. These CMAPs were recorded from a patient with demyelinating neuropathy over the abductor hallucis muscle of the foot after stimulation of the tibial nerve at the ankle (*top waveform*) and the knee (*bottom waveform*). The sweep speed was 5 msec/division and the sensitivity was 1 mV/division. When the waveform recorded after stimulation at the ankle is compared with the waveform recorded after simulation at the knee, a dramatic 54% drop in amplitude (from 1.1 to 0.5 mV) is seen. Waveform duration also increases with concurrent increases in waveform complexity. These findings suggest demyelination of the nerve between the stimulation sites, with block of conduction in most motor axons, along with increasing variability in the range of axonal conduction times causing increased waveform duration (temporal dispersion).

The precise degree of amplitude loss needed to confirm conduction block remains controversial and may vary from nerve to nerve. For research purposes, amplitude drops of 50% over a tested nerve segment (in a properly performed study) are considered diagnostic of conduction block and strongly suggest focal demyelination or axonal ischemia [1–5]. Temporal dispersion occurs because conduction velocities differ between individual motor and sensory axons of varying size and other factors; some dispersion is normal. Over a longer distance this difference is magnified, and signals from each of the individual axons within a stimulated nerve arrive at the recording electrodes at different times. This dispersion of arrival times generates the rising and falling phases of the recorded waveform and is reflected primarily in its duration. Sensory axons demonstrate considerably more dispersion than motor axons. With loss of myelin in a nerve, temporal dispersion can increase dramatically and serves as a marker of demyelinating injury.

Late responses

Routine nerve conduction studies are limited to accessible (ie, superficially located) nerve segments in the arms and legs. Direct stimulation of the deep proximal nerves and the nerve roots is technically challenging and often unreliable. Consequently, long latency reflex tests or late responses are typically used to assess these segments. When a stimulus is delivered to the distal nerve, action potentials are propagated both proximally and distally. The impulse traveling distal to proximal up the motor axons (in a direction opposite to the normal flow, or antidromic) eventually reaches the anterior horn cell pool, depolarizing one or a few anterior horn cells. Thus activated, these anterior horn cells then each generate small action potentials that travel back down their axons to the muscle (this time in the direction paralleling the normal flow of motor impulses, or orthodromic), activating a small portion of the muscle. A recording electrode over the muscle then registers a waveform known as the F wave (so named because it was originally recorded from the intrinsic muscles of the foot) (Fig. 6). The time required for this round trip up and down the motor nerve is measured as the F wave latency.

Although pathology at any point along the nerve can prolong the F wave latency, if normal function of the distal nerve has been documented by routine motor nerve conduction studies, F wave latency prolongation must be caused by slowing in the proximal segment of the nerve or its roots. F wave testing has limited sensitivity, however; a single normal axon may generate a normal response because the single fastest response in a group of F wave is

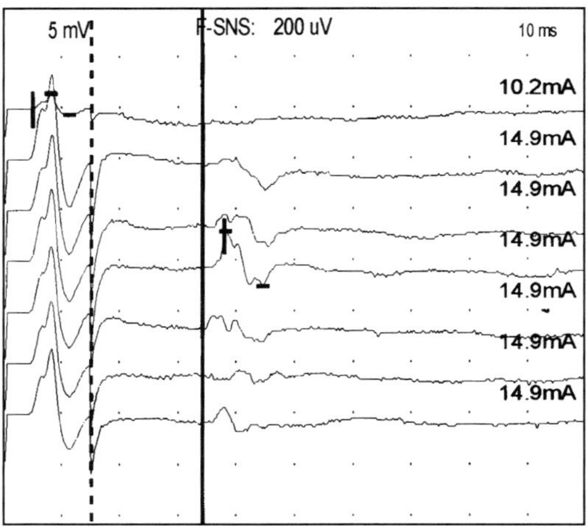

Fig. 6. F waves. This group of F waves was recorded from the thenar eminence after repeated median nerve stimulation in a patient with cervical radiculopathy. The screen is split: lower sensitivity (5 mV/division) recordings to enable display of the full initial CMAP amplitudes are to the left of the dotted line, and higher sensitivity (200 μV/division) recordings are to the right of the dotted line for clear display of the much smaller F wave responses. The sweep speed is 10 msec/division. The darker vertical line marks the onset of the earliest F wave latency in the group. This F wave latency was slightly prolonged at 34 msec because of the patient's C8 radiculopathy.

used (by convention) to measure the minimum latency and compared with normative data tables. Consequently, F wave testing is most meaningful when abnormal, and a normal F wave study does not exclude neuropathy or focal nerve injury. A different long latency response, the H reflex (named after Hoffman, who first described it in 1918) can be elicited in the legs by electrical stimulation of the IA sensory nerve afferents in the tibial nerve at the knee, triggering an ankle jerk reflex (a monosynaptic stretch reflex), with recording over the soleus muscle in the calf. H reflexes are normally recordable only from a limited number of muscles. Clinically, they aid primarily in diagnosing S1 radiculopathy and provide one of the few methods of assessing sensory and motor nerve root function [1–4,6,7].

Needle electromyography

Needle EMG plays a more limited role in the evaluation of neuropathy but remains important during initial diagnostic evaluation to exclude potential clinical mimics (eg, anterior horn cell disease, radiculopathy, myopathy). During this portion of the examination, a needle recording electrode is placed directly into the selected muscle, which is then voluntary contracted by the patient (rather than activated by electrical stimulation). Normal, full voluntary contraction of a muscle requires activation of the cortical motor strip, followed by descent of impulses down the upper motor neuron pathway and spinal cord to the anterior horn cells of each motor axon. Action potentials generated in the motor axon are propagated down the nerve to the neuromuscular junction, where electrochemical transmission activates the contraction cascade in each individual muscle fiber. A single motor axon, all of its branches, and all of its innervated muscle fibers comprise the motor unit, and the strength of a muscle contraction is determined primarily by how many motor units are simultaneously activated and how fast they are repetitively firing. The recording characteristics of the EMG needle electrode enable live recording and analysis of individual and aggregate motor unit waveforms.

During needle EMG, five core parameters are measured: insertional activity, spontaneous activity, motor unit configuration, motor unit recruitment, and the interference pattern. Increased insertional activity (the burst of activity generated by needle movement through the muscle) is a hallmark of denervation, although it also may appear with muscle fiber irritation from some myopathies. Spontaneous activity represents the spontaneous depolarization of muscle fibers while the muscle is at rest (manifested by fibrillations and positive sharp waves), without activation by their motor axons. Spontaneous activity does not occur in normal subjects and is a staple feature of active denervation caused by injury of the motor nerve or its roots, although it can, much less commonly, be caused by irritative myopathies (eg, polymyositis) (Fig. 7). Assessment of the waveform generated by motor unit activation (the motor unit action potential [MUAP]) also yields

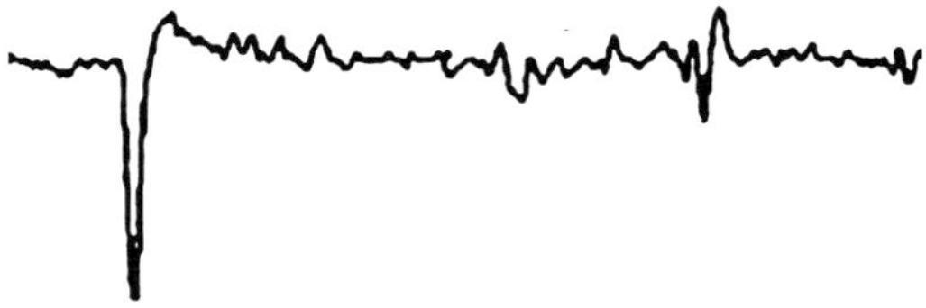

Fig. 7. Spontaneous activity. This waveform was recorded during needle EMG from the triceps muscle of a patient with cervical radiculopathy. A positive sharp wave (named after its sharp initial positive [downward] deflection) is on the left, whereas a smaller triphasic fibrillation is on the right. These markers of active denervation result from the spontaneous depolarization of denervated single muscle fibers.

important information (Fig. 8). When muscle fibers lose their innervation because of death of the motor axon supplying them, surviving motor axons in the same nerve branch to reinnervate these newly orphaned fibers in a process known as collateral reinnervation. Collateral reinnervation gradually recovers detached muscle fibers, but this process takes several months. As a consequence of collateral reinnervation, the average number of muscle fibers supplied by each axon increases, which creates larger MUAP waveforms that have longer duration, higher amplitude, and increased complexity (neurogenic MUAPs). These neurogenic MUAPs are markers of chronic motor axon injury (Fig. 9). When enough motor axons are lost or fail to transmit their action potential to the muscle, visible gaps appear in the interference pattern of overlapping MUAP waveforms normally generated when all the motor units in a muscle fire together during maximal voluntary contraction. This phenomenon is known as an incomplete interference pattern (Fig. 10). Loss or failure of the motor axons also alters the rate at which additional motor units are activated (or recruited) as voluntary contraction is ramped up from zero to maximum, which produces an

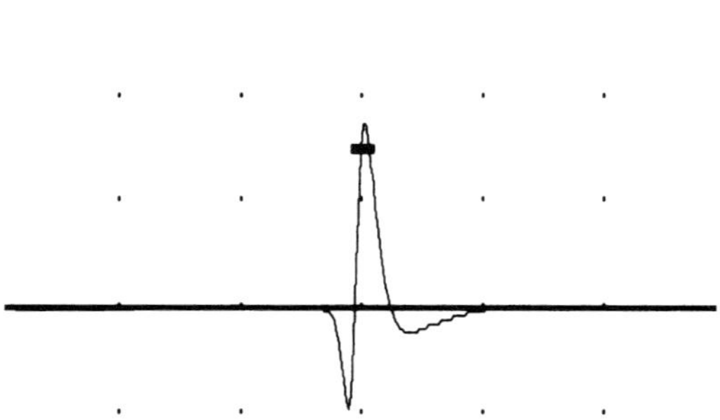

Fig. 8. Normal MUAP. This waveform was recorded by a concentric needle electrode from the biceps muscle. It was the first potential recruited during minimal voluntary contraction in a normal subject. Sweep speed is 10 msec/division, and sensitivity is 500 μV/division. This waveform amplitude is 1.4 mV, its duration is 12.5 msec, and its morphology is normal.

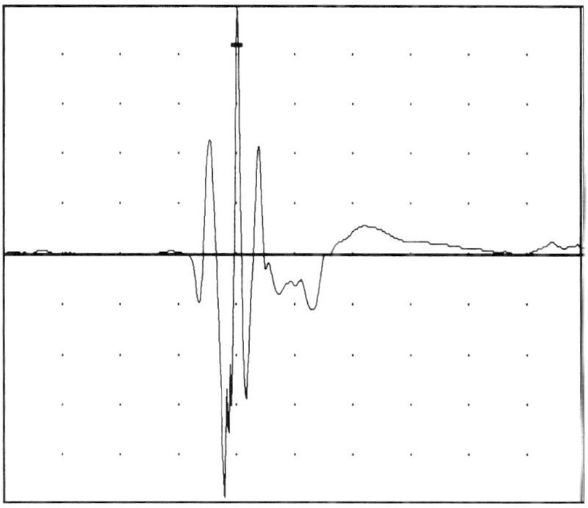

Fig. 9. Neurogenic MUAP. This waveform was recorded with a concentric needle electrode during voluntary activation of the gastrocnemius muscle in a patient with a distal, symmetric diabetic neuropathy. Sweep speed is 5 msec/division, and sensitivity is 1 mV/division. The high amplitude of 10 mV, significantly prolonged duration of 29 msec, and increased complexity (> 10 turns) reflect substantial collateral reinnervation and are markers of chronic motor axon injury and loss.

abnormal recruitment pattern. Recruitment patterns in denervating disease are marked by more rapid motor unit firing and a reduction in the number and rate at which additional motor units are added during increasingly forceful voluntary contraction. EMG of a carefully selected sample of muscles innervated by key nerves and nerve roots can delineate the degree,

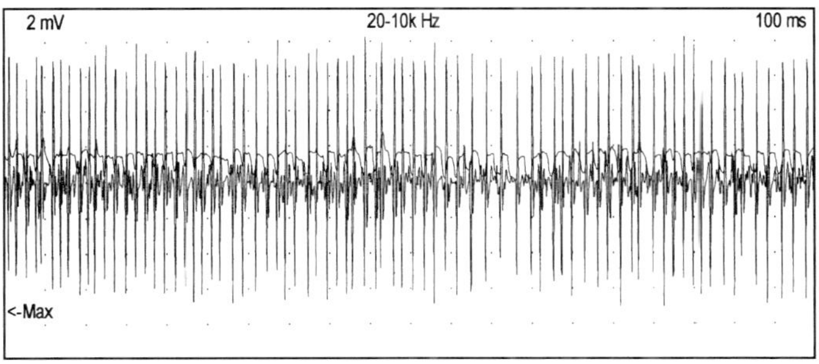

Fig. 10. Reduced interference pattern. This pattern of overlapping MUAP waveforms was recorded during needle EMG from the biceps muscle of a patient with amyotrophic lateral sclerosis during maximal voluntary contraction. The sweep speed is slow at 100 msec/division, and the sensitivity is 2 mV/division. Note the substantial gaps or "picket fence" appearance (in contrast to the normal dense band of overlapping units) caused by the loss of a significant number of motor axons. Note that the MUAP amplitude of the most prominent surviving unit is also increased in this sample (8–10 mV), consistent with concurrent collateral reinnervation by some of the surviving units.

distribution, age, and location of anterior horn cell or motor axon injury [1,8–10].

EMG and nerve conduction studies in the diagnosis of neuropathy

Axonal neuropathy

Axonal injury produces a typical pattern of abnormality on nerve conduction studies. In most instances, axonal neuropathy is a chronic process, but changes may appear on nerve conduction study as early as 3 to 5 days after the onset of acute axonopathy caused by the rapid pace of Wallerian degeneration. In the prototypic distal, symmetric sensory, or sensorimotor neuropathy (the most common types by far), there is initial loss of sensory nerve amplitude in a length-dependent fashion (ie, first in the distal lower extremities) followed by loss of motor amplitudes (in sensorimotor axonopathy), with gradual spread of these abnormalities to the shorter nerve segments in the upper extremities. This is largely because the more distal nerve segments in the legs are farther from their cell bodies (the anterior horn cells and dorsal root ganglia, in and near the spinal cord), which makes maintenance of the axon more difficult, increases its vulnerability to injury, and reduces its capacity to recover. Because myelination is relatively preserved in primary axonal injury, distal latencies, conduction velocities, and late responses are not affected. Late in the course of severe axonal disorders (usually when amplitude has markedly decreased), these parameters may become mildly abnormal because of secondary demyelination or loss of the fastest conducting fibers. Pure sensory axonopathies or dorsal root ganglionopathies affect only sensory nerve amplitudes, leaving the motor responses normal, whereas pure motor axonopathies or anterior horn cell disorders affect only motor responses. Pure motor axonopathies must be differentiated carefully from other processes causing loss of amplitudes on motor nerve conduction studies with normal sensory responses, particularly radiculopathies, anterior horn cell diseases, and distal myopathies.

EMG can provide additional information when motor involvement is suspected in a patient with neuropathy. In a distal symmetric neuropathy, changes appear first in the distal muscles and may move proximally as the neuropathy worsens and the deficits ascend. In severe, acute processes, decreased motor unit recruitment and loss of a full interference pattern on voluntary contraction are the earliest indication of axon loss. With ongoing severe denervation, increased insertional activity and spontaneous activity appear, starting approximately 3 weeks after an acute injury, and may persist as long as the disease process remains active. Neurogenic MUAPs do not appear for at least 2 to 3 months because of the time required for collateral reinnervation to become established. Using these EMG abnormalities, it is possible to estimate the time since the onset of axonal injury and its severity. The degree of axonal loss is particularly important in patients with treatable neuropathies, because an estimate of axonal integrity enables an estimate of the potential for recovery of strength. Preservation of at least a moderate degree of axonal continuity (as indicated by a mild to moderate, rather than severe, reduction in the interference pattern on full voluntary contraction during EMG) suggests a good chance for further functional recovery, because these surviving axons provide the foundation for collateral reinnervation. If the underlying disease can be controlled, collateral reinnervation is often an effective compensatory process, bringing denervated muscle fibers back into service and restoring strength. When denervating injury occurs slowly enough for collateral reinnervation to become established, nearly normal strength may be maintained even when up to half of the motor axons in a nerve have been lost [1,4,11–13].

Demyelinating neuropathy

Demyelinating neuropathy characteristically causes slowing of nerve conduction as myelin is disrupted and saltatory conduction fails, which causes prolongation of latencies, slowed nerve conduction velocities, temporal dispersion of waveforms, and prolonged or absent late responses. In contrast to axonal neuropathies, motor and sensory amplitudes are relatively preserved. Hereditary demyelinating neuropathies usually produce diffuse and symmetric abnormalities on nerve conduction studies. Most acquired demyelinating neuropathies are at least partially multifocal, however, and produce asymmetric slowing and—classically—multiple areas of conduction block caused by multifocal points of demyelination. Low amplitude waveforms also may be the result of conduction block, but this development usually can be distinguished from axonal injury by comparing the amplitudes of waveforms recorded from different segments of the same nerve. With conduction block, amplitudes from a nerve segment not affected by the block are normal, whereas amplitudes obtained from a segment containing the block are low. Rarely, a distal conduction block (eg, at the wrist) may mimic axonal injury during routine nerve conduction studies. In advanced disease with severe demyelination, secondary axonal degeneration ensues and global declines in amplitude appear.

Needle EMG abnormalities are more limited in purely demyelinating neuropathies. Most of the classic features of denervation on EMG examination are the result of axonal injury producing discontinuity of the axonal connections with the muscle fibers, which is necessary to generate abnormal insertional and spontaneous activity and trigger collateral reinnervation and motor unit remodeling. Because pure demyelination leaves the axons and their connections with the muscle fibers intact, the only abnormalities seen on EMG are changes in motor unit recruitment and loss of a complete interference pattern on full voluntary contraction. These changes occur because although the axons are physically intact, demyelination is severe enough in many of the axons to block their action potentials, functionally disabling them and preventing activation of their muscle fibers. With severe or longstanding demyelination, secondary axonal changes appear and produce the denervation changes expected with axonal neuropathy. In treatable demyelinating neuropathies, the prognosis for recovery is greatly influenced by the degree of axonal injury. Because the interference pattern may be affected by demyelination itself, axonal injury is best estimated in demyelinating processes by the degree of spontaneous activity or the number of neurogenic MUAPs observed [1,4,5,11–13].

General approach

The approach to any electrodiagnostic study begins with review of the referring information and a directed history and neurologic examination, after which a basic differential diagnosis can be established that will guide planning of the study. Although technical skill and experience are clearly important, a thorough knowledge of neuromuscular disorders and physiology is absolutely essential to the proper planning and interpretation of nerve conduction and EMG studies. Without the clinical guidance provided by a comprehensive knowledge of neuromuscular medicine, the electrical studies needed for delineation of the problem cannot be logically selected, and the generated data are irrelevant and liable to misinterpretation, despite any technical skill on the part of the examiner.

In a patient with suspected neuropathy, nerve conduction studies and EMG should define the type of nerve injury (axonal, demyelinating, or mixed), its distribution (symmetric, asymmetric, multifocal, distal, proximal, or diffuse), and severity and the degree of motor or sensory involvement. Importantly, the study also should be designed to search for other neuromuscular problems that might contribute to or account for the patient's symptoms. Common problems, such as carpal tunnel syndrome, ulnar mononeuropathy at the elbow, and lumbosacral radiculopathy, occur even more commonly in patients with neuropathy (perhaps because of the increased susceptibility of the injured nerve to additional damage from compression and other processes), but the symptoms they cause may be casually attributed to polyneuropathy by many physicians. Such potentially treatable processes may be the major source of a patient's new complaint, even if a neuropathy is also present, and these possibilities must be considered and evaluated carefully.

Nerve conduction studies for neuropathy screening typically include testing of the peroneal and tibial motor nerves and the sural (sensory) nerve in one leg and the median and ulnar motor and sensory nerves in one arm. If focal mononeuropathies are suspected (eg, peroneal mononeuropathy at the fibular head, median mononeuropathy at the wrist, ulnar mononeuropathy at the elbow) and not confirmed by routine studies, special studies may be indicated to definitively search for these focal compressive lesions. In some instances, bilateral studies are needed for side-to-side comparisons.

In patients over the age of 60, the sural and other sensory responses in the distal leg may be lost as a consequence of normal aging and may cloud a search for a mild, pure sensory distal neuropathy. Beyond this basic protocol, the next steps in any nerve conduction study depend highly on the results of these first assessments. Although this standard screen may be sufficient to make the diagnosis in many patients, others require expanded studies, with a broad range of possibilities. Uncommonly, neuromuscular junction dysfunction may be in the differential, and repetitive nerve stimulation may be indicated. Bulbar symptoms (also uncommon) may require evaluation with cranial nerve studies, such as blink reflex testing and facial nerve conduction studies [1,4,5,11–19].

Needle EMG is an important component of the diagnostic assessment of suspected neuropathy. It provides important information regarding the degree and time course of axonal injury in polyneuropathy. It also enables assessment of the proximal motor nerve segments and roots (which are not readily accessible to direct nerve conduction study), thereby providing a means of testing for plexopathy and radiculopathy. EMG also enables assessment of possible primary muscle disease, which can mimic some neuropathies or occur with them. The extent of EMG testing depends on a patient's clinical presentation and the results of the nerve conduction studies. In a clear, distal symmetric neuropathy with symptoms restricted to the lower extremities, needle EMG of one leg and lumbosacral paraspinal muscles may be adequate, but two or even three limb studies may be indicated in other cases [1,4,5,8–10].

Common sources of error during nerve conduction studies

The proper performance and interpretation of nerve conduction studies requires a thorough knowledge of the common pitfalls associated with these techniques. In many individual patients, an electrical diagnosis of peripheral neuropathy is based on a small number of abnormal values. Consequently, careful consideration of technical and physiologic factors is essential to ensure that the abnormalities found are valid and not influenced by technical error. Although some errors are discernable during a review of data after the study is concluded, many errors must be identified and corrected during the examination itself, making the presence of a trained examiner and onsite physician review essential. Faulty data may result either in the misdiagnosis of illness in a healthy patient or an erroneous or missed diagnosis in a patient with neuromuscular disease. These errors are most critical when they influence treatment decisions, prompting either the institution of potentially hazardous therapy in a normal patient or the withholding of needed therapy in a patient with disease. Erroneous electrodiagnostic conclusions may prompt costly, extensive, and sometimes invasive unwarranted diagnostic testing.

Temperature

Temperature is one of the most critical physiologic factor affecting electrodiagnostic studies. Ion channel function, acetylcholinesterase activity, and muscle contractility are a few of the temperature-dependent factors that affect nerve and muscle function [20]. Cooling of nerve profoundly affects the speed of nerve conduction, and velocity linearly increases as limb temperature rises from 29°C to 38°C (Fig. 11). Erroneously increased distal latencies and slowed conduction velocities caused by cold limbs hamper the diagnosis of peripheral neuropathy and obscure the differences between axonal and demyelinating injury; cold temperatures also reduce or mask conduction block [21]. Conventionally accepted limb temperatures range from 34°C to 36°C in the arm and from 31°C to 34°C in the leg; most published normative series use similar ranges. Despite these clear and significant effects, temperature measurement is frequently neglected during nerve conduction studies.

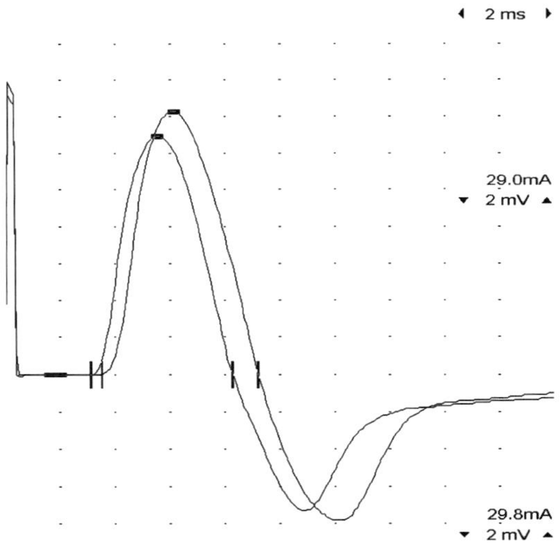

Fig. 11. Temperature effect on distal latency. These two superimposed CMAPs were recorded after stimulation of the median nerve at the wrist, with recording over the thenar eminence at exactly the same sites in a normal subject. The sweep speed is 2 msec/division, and the sensitivity is 2 mV/division. The latency change is caused by the different temperature during each recording. The later waveform (with a latency of 3.5 msec) was recorded from a normal subject at a temperature of 34.7°C, whereas the earlier waveform (with a latency of 3.1 msec) was recorded after heating of the limb with a moist hot pack for 15 minutes, which yielded a temperature of 39.0°C. This 0.4-msec change over approximately 4° is typical and emphasizes the importance of temperature control during nerve conduction studies. The slight decrease in CMAP amplitude also is the result of increased temperature but is not typically dramatic enough to impact final diagnosis.

Most contemporary EMG machines have integrated temperature probes, but reasonably accurate handheld digital devices are readily available. Surface probes measure skin but not nerve temperature, and temperatures near the nerve are generally 1° to 2°C warmer than the overlying skin in cool environments (the reverse in warm environments) [22]. Warm ambient temperature in an appropriate range helps to maintain limb temperature, whereas an excessively cool room makes adequate limb warming challenging. Warming methods include warm water immersion, thermistor-controlled infrared lamp heat, moist heat packs, hot air, and ultrasound, although no method affects each patient or limb uniformly. Warming the limb affects superficial layers more quickly than deeper layers, so brief warming may raise the skin temperature (and the reading reported by a temperature probe on the skin surface) but still not warm the more deeply situated nerve sufficiently to normalize nerve function [23]. Some researchers advocate 30 minutes of warming, but 10 to 15 minutes is more practical and probably sufficient [20,24,25]. Care must be taken not to burn patients who have heat insensitivity caused by sensory loss during heating.

Cooling increases distal latency by 0.1 to 0.3 milliseconds/°C, increases waveform duration, and decreases the severity of spontaneous activity; sensory amplitudes modestly increased in most series. Warming has the opposite effects, and it enhances the detection of conduction block and enhances the degree of decrement recorded during repetitive nerve stimulation. Some studies have calculated temperature correction factors for conduction velocity when limb temperature is abnormally cool (1.5–2.4 m/sec/°C), and some EMG/nerve conduction study devices have a fixed temperature correction option (based on one formula) that recalculates conduction velocity based on temperature probe measurements [20]. These values may be less accurate in diseased nerves, however, especially if demyelination is present, and most researchers agree that limb warming provides more accurate data than formulaic extrapolation.

Age, height, and sex

Nerve conduction velocity rapidly increases during infancy and early childhood, reaching approximately 50% of adult values at full term, 75% at 6 to 12 months of age, and 100% of adult values by 3 to 4 years. Velocity then decreases in adulthood, starting in the second and third decades, possibly because of gradual and progressive loss of the fastest conducting motor axons [26]. The rate and age at onset of this decline are debated and vary considerably between series, but the degree of slowing is relatively minor. Sensory and motor amplitudes decrease more notably with age, although few normative series include significant numbers of elderly control subjects. This effect is most evident in the distal sensory nerves of the legs, which may be unresponsive to stimulation during nerve conduction studies in normal elderly subjects. Rivner and colleagues [27] found that 11 of 46 (24%)

control subjects between the ages of 70 and 79 years and 2 of 5 subjects over the age 80 had absent sural sensory responses. Only 9 of 194 (4.6%) of sural responses in patients aged 60 to 69 were absent, however.

Height is an underappreciated factor that inversely correlates with sensory and motor nerve conduction velocity [27]. The degree of change varies considerably from subject to subject, but increased height may reduce conduction velocity more than advanced age. Velocity decreases approximately 2 to 3 m/sec for each 10 cm of height above average; amplitude is influenced much less. This slight slowing of conduction velocity in tall subjects becomes an issue when their studies are compared with normative ranges, which are based on subjects of average height. Women have slightly faster mean conduction velocity than men, but this group discrepancy does not persist after correction for height differences between the sexes [27,28].

Stimulation

Submaximal stimulation

Nerve conduction studies presume that supramaximal stimulation is delivered, which results in depolarization of all axons within the tested nerve. When stimulation of all the axons within the tested nerve is not achieved, inadequate (submaximal) stimulation occurs and artifactually low amplitude waveforms are generated during motor and sensory nerve conduction studies (Fig. 12). These artifactually low amplitudes can mimic axonal injury and partial conduction block. Conduction velocity may slow slightly if the largest—and fastest—conducting axons are not activated because conduction velocity calculations are based on the latencies of these fastest conducting fibers. Stimulating at four times the minimal threshold level needed to evoke a consistent initial response is one technique used to estimate the approximate level needed for supramaximal stimulation [29]. One common mistake is to stop progressively increasing the stimulus intensity as soon as the response amplitude crosses into the normal range, when it may be normal but still submaximal. This error especially complicates interpretation of longitudinal studies and side-to-side comparisons.

Most submaximal stimulation results from improper stimulating electrode placement (away from the intended nerve) or failure to use adequate stimulus intensity, but other factors also may play a role. Perspiration, dirt, or excess electrode paste can shunt current away from the nerve; dead skin is also a stimulation barrier. Cleaning and gently abrading the stimulus sites can minimize these factors and reduce artifact. Obesity also impedes surface nerve stimulation, most prominently sensory nerve amplitudes, which are reduced on average 20% to 25% between the highest and lowest thirds of body mass index [30]. Diseased motor axons may have reduced excitability and require high intensity and long duration stimulation (1.0 msec), especially when demyelination is present.

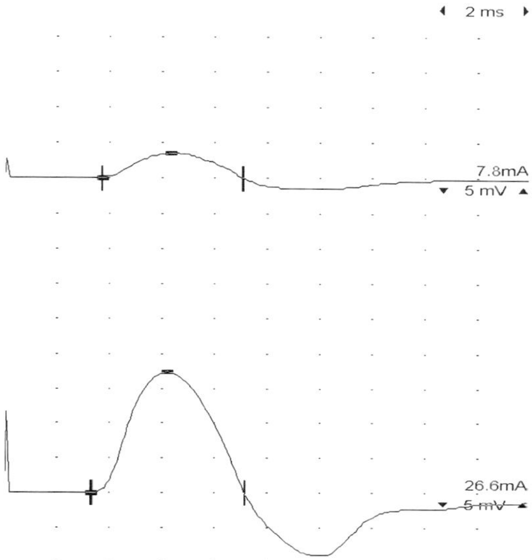

Fig. 12. Submaximal stimulation. These two CMAPs were recorded after stimulation of the median nerve at the wrist, with recording over the thenar eminence at exactly the same sites. The sweep speed is 2 msec/division, and the sensitivity is 5 mV/division for both waveforms. The stimulus intensities are also labeled to the right of each potential. The top waveform was recorded using low intensity stimulation (7.8 mA), which resulted in incomplete, submaximal stimulation of the nerve and an artifactually low CMAP amplitude of 3.5 mV. The bottom waveform was recorded with supramaximal stimulation (26.6 mA), which produced complete depolarization of all motor axons in the tested nerve and a dramatically larger amplitude of 17.5 mV. Further increases in stimulus intensity resulted in no further increases in amplitude.

At some sites, it may be challenging to fully stimulate the nerve with surface electrodes, even with maximal stimulus intensity and duration, usually because the nerves are deeply situated (eg, the brachial plexus at Erb's point, the popliteal fossa, the ulnar nerve at the cubital tunnel). Proximal conduction block across the brachial plexus can be difficult to assess in some patients because of this problem.

Excessive stimulation and stimulus spread

Exceeding supramaximal stimulus intensity does not increase waveform amplitude further but can generate erroneous data by depolarizing a larger field than desired. Such excessive stimulation increases the distance the stimulus travels from under the cathode, which results in nerve depolarization beyond the actual position of the stimulating electrode (creating a virtual cathode). As a result, the nerve segment length tested is effectively shortened and, consequently, the measured latency and calculated conduction velocity are erroneously reduced [24]. When the stimulating electrode poles (anode and cathode) are reversed, the improperly placed (more distal) anode hyperpolarizes the underlying nerve, forcing the propagating depolarization wave to pass through this hyperpolarized region and reducing stimulus effectiveness (anodal block). More critical, however, is the mistaken distance measurement point if the reversal is not identified, which adversely affects conduction velocity and distal latency.

A stimulus also can spread to an adjacent nerve when nerves are in close proximity, such as at the brachial plexus, wrist, and popliteal fossa, especially when high stimulus intensities are required. Optimal positioning of the stimulating electrodes and visualization of the muscles activated can help to confirm that the selected nerve is primarily stimulated. A change in amplitude, an initial positive deflection, or altered waveform morphology between stimulation sites alerts the examiner to this problem.

Under certain circumstances, stimulus spread can mimic conduction block when simultaneous activation of two closely situated nerves at a distal stimulation site results in artifactually high distal amplitude and a lower, but valid, amplitude results from proximal simulation where the nerves are not in close proximity. This scenario can be mistaken for focal conduction block between the proximal and distal sites. Near nerve stimulation methods can eliminate spread by delivering a supramaximal stimulus at a much lower intensity, but these techniques are more invasive and less commonly performed [29].

Recording techniques and issues

Antidromic versus orthodromic sensory recordings

Many sensory nerves can be studied using either orthodromic stimulation (distal stimulation with proximal recording, in the physiologic direction of flow for normal sensory impulses) or antidromic methods (proximal stimulation with distal recording, opposite to the physiologic direction of impulse flow). All motor studies are orthodromic (stimulation of the nerve proximally, with recording from a distal innervated muscle). Knowing which technique was used for sensory recordings is essential for valid data interpretation. Latency and velocity measures are equivalent with either method, but antidromic studies generate larger sensory amplitudes, primarily because the nerves are more superficial at distal recording sites [31]. Antidromic stimulation often activates both the motor and sensory axons in a mixed nerve, which results in concurrent muscle activation. The inadvertently triggered CMAP, which is usually much larger than the sensory response, can obscure part of the desired sensory potential and measurements of latency and amplitude can be compromised [24]. Occasionally, the motor response can obscure the sensory response entirely; however, a delayed and long duration waveform should alert the examiner to this artifact.

Distance between recording electrodes and nerve

Improper or inconsistent recording electrode placement is a common error during nerve conduction studies. Conventional electrode placement for motor nerve conduction studies involves positioning the active (G_1) electrode over the muscle belly at the motor point (the surface point closest to the neuromuscular junction) and the reference electrode (G_2) at an electrically inactive point on the muscle tendon, approximately 3 to 4 cm more distal. After motor nerve stimulation, this montage produces a diphasic waveform with a large initial negative (upward) deflection. An initial positive (downward) deflection preceding the larger negative deflection indicates incorrect G_1 electrode positioning away from the motor point or a volume conducted potential from another muscle (stimulus spread) (Fig. 13). An

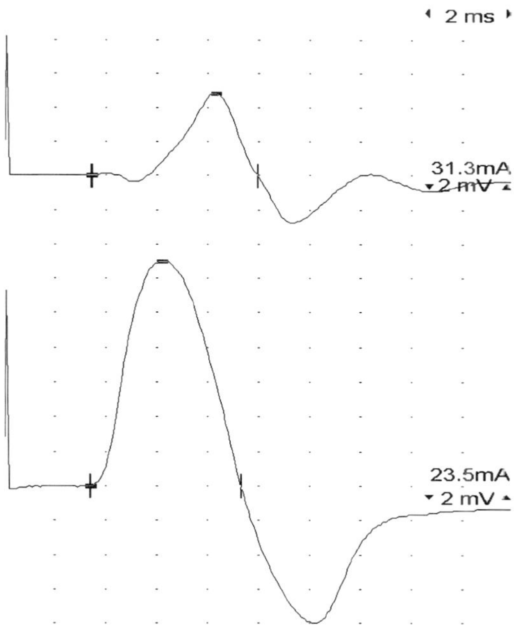

Fig. 13. Effect of recording electrode position on the CMAP. These two CMAPs were recorded after stimulation of the median nerve at the wrist. The top waveform was recorded with the active recording electrode 10 to 20 mm off the motor point of the muscle, whereas the bottom waveform was recorded with the active electrode directly over the motor point. Note the initial positive (downward) deflection immediately preceding the major negative (upward) deflection in the top waveform. This small initial positive deflection clearly indicates origination of the depolarization wave in the muscle at a distant site (the motor endplate) from the misplaced recording electrode. CMAP negative peak amplitude is also substantially reduced and latency marker placement is problematic because of the leading positive phase. Careful attention to active recording electrode placement is critical, because slight misplacement off the motor point can affect CMAP waveform parameters significantly.

inverted potential—an initial large positive wave and smaller later negative wave—occurs when the active and reference recording electrodes are reversed. For sensory studies, the recording electrode must be placed as close to the nerve as possible because sensory nerve action potential amplitude rapidly declines with increasing distance between the nerve and the recording electrode. Consequently, even gently pressing the surface electrode toward the nerve increases the SNAP amplitude by 10% to 20% [32]. Larger finger size also increases the distance between the nerve and the recording electrode. For these and other reasons, such as skin and tissue impedance, near-nerve recordings (recordings made with a needle electrode placed through the skin and next to the nerve) are typically three to seven times larger than surface recordings [24,31].

Distance between active and reference electrodes

Motor and sensory waveforms are affected by this distance, especially amplitude and waveform duration (because of differing degrees of phase cancellation and summation of the axon potentials comprising the larger SNAP waveforms) [24,33,34]. With normal human nerve conduction velocities, the optimal distance between these electrodes for proper capture of the full rising and falling phases of waveforms (recording from the nerve) is 3 to 4 cm. Most fixed bar electrodes use this distance.

Recording electrode size

Little attention is generally paid to the recording electrodes. Studies suggest that response amplitude declines slightly with larger electrodes [31,32]. Sensory amplitudes fall 10% to 15% with a 20-mm and 20% to 25% with a 40-mm recording electrode when compared with a 5-mm electrode [32]. Many modern disposable electrodes are significantly larger than the reusable electrodes used to generate most of the widely used normative data. This discrepancy is potentially relevant when amplitudes are borderline, but the issue is probably not a source of significant error and is not sufficient to discourage use of convenient, although more expensive, self-adhesive electrode sets.

Filter settings, sensitivity, and sweep speed

Most contemporary machines use standard high- and low-frequency filter settings for motor and sensory waveform recording. Changes can be made manually that can adversely affect nerve conduction studies and EMG. Filter settings affect evoked response amplitudes and latencies (eg, increasing the low-frequency [high pass] filter reduces some artifacts but also reduces response amplitudes). Examiners should be aware of the standard filter settings on their equipment and confirm that they correspond with the ranges used to record the normative data used for reference. If changes are made for any reason, the effects of these changes on the measured waveform values must be considered.

Most current machines use an internal algorithm to mark waveforms at standard sensitivity and sweep speed setting. Computerized marker placement is often incorrect, however, and each cursor must be reviewed and may require manual adjustment. Care must be taken to mark all latencies and amplitudes at a consistent sensitivity setting, because magnifying the waveform by increasing the sensitivity alters the apparent position of the latency cursors, changing latency, and conduction velocity (Fig. 14). It is tempting to record the waveform at a low sensitivity and then enlarge the waveform later by increasing the sensitivity setting to readjust the markers. The higher the sensitivity setting, the shorter the latency of a waveform appears; a gain setting of 1 mV/division is most commonly used for motor studies. Altering sweep speed causes a similar error and should be consistent

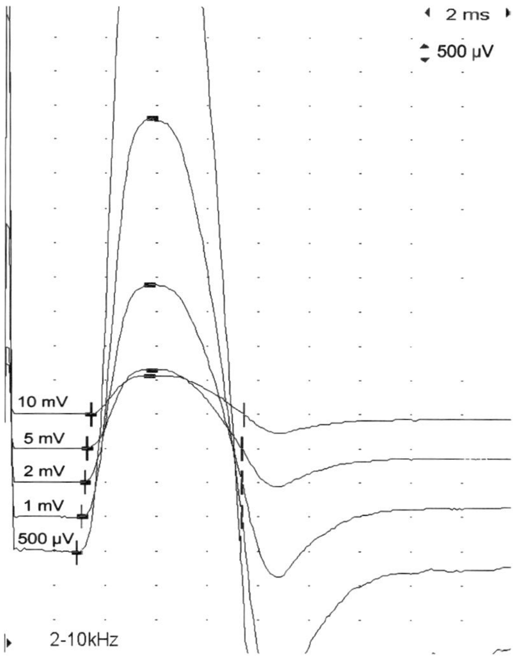

Fig. 14. Effect of sensitivity settings on measured latency. These five CMAPs were recorded after stimulation of the median nerve at the wrist, with recording over the thenar eminence at exactly the same sites. The sensitivity settings for recording of each waveform were increased from top to bottom, however (10 mV/division, then 5 mV, then 2 mV, then 1 mV, then 500 µV or 0.5 mV/division). As the sensitivity of the display is increased, the onset of the initial negative deflection becomes better defined and appears earlier, producing earlier and earlier onset latencies (3.4 msec at 10 mV, 3.3 at 5 mV, 3.2 at 2 mV, 3.1 at 1 mV, and 2.9 msec at 500 microvolts). This illustrates the importance of measuring latency at standardized and consistent sensitivities (usually 1 mV/division for motor studies) to facilitate reliable comparisons with normative data.

from study to study. A highly amplified display also can reveal a faster antidromic sensory response, not evident at conventional gain settings, that may complicate waveform marking. In instances of severe amplitude loss, higher than usual sensitivity settings may be required to measure small waveforms. In these cases a sensitivity setting as close to standard as the waveform size will allow is advised.

Effect of stimulus artifact

Excessive stimulus artifact is a common problem, especially with sensory studies. If the initial baseline is shifted and no isoelectric period occurs between the stimulus and evoked waveform, the waveform shape, measured amplitude, and onset latency are compromised; falsely increased and decreased latency and amplitude measures can result. Sensory amplitude is vital in the evaluation of peripheral neuropathy. Attention to skin preparation, appropriate and not excessive electrode gel, induced current between stimulating and recording wires, and effective grounding are primary concerns, and numerous other measures are recommended to avoid problems [24]. Shielded recording cables are used in some laboratories, and early signal digitization is accomplished by some machines to help minimize this problem.

Waveform marker placement

Conventional rules for marking nerve conduction studies waveforms differ between motor and sensory studies. The distal motor latency is marked at the onset of the initial deflection, whether positive or negative. The waveform duration is measured from its onset to the negative wave return to baseline (automated area calculations also depend on the waveform duration markers). Motor amplitudes are marked from the baseline to the primary negative waveform peak. Sensory latency is marked either at the initial positive peak of the waveform (onset latency) or the later larger negative peak (peak latency); normative latency data are published for both methods, and each laboratory typically uses one or the other for sensory latency measures. Only onset latency should be used to calculate sensory nerve conduction velocity, however. Sensory waveform duration is also measured from its onset to baseline return. Sensory amplitudes are typically measured either from the initial or terminal positive peak to the largest negative peak; the initial baseline is used if there is no initial positive peak.

Errors in marker placement, either by computer algorithm or manual settings, can alter latency (and resultant conduction velocity calculations) and duration and amplitudes, generating artifactual data, which can mimic demyelinating or axonal injury or both. Consequently, careful review of marker placement, whether automated or manual, is an essential step. If normative data from other laboratories are used for reference (rather than a locally generated normative data set), the same rules for marker placement used to acquire that normative data must be followed during testing of new patients.

Distance measurement between stimulating and recording sites

Distance measurement between stimulating and recording sites is often assumed to be simple, but measurement errors are common. Distance should be measured from the stimulating cathode center to the active recording electrode center. Slight skin movement and misreading or misplacing the measuring tape are leading causes of error. Erroneously short distances artifactually increase conduction velocity and reduce latencies, masking true abnormalities; erroneously long distances reduce velocity and increase latencies, mimicking demyelinating injury. For a 10-cm segment, a 1-cm measurement error creates approximately a 10% error in conduction velocity. This error is amplified with shorter distances and in nonlinear segments, for example, when a nerve curves around a joint. Most surface measures are slightly shorter than actual nerve length, but this difference is usually negligible unless the course is not linear [24]. Limb position is critical in some circumstances. For example, in studies of the ulnar nerve across the elbow, the nerve folds when the arm is extended and is roughly straight (but not stretched) when the elbow is slightly flexed at 70°, making standardized elbow positioning (usually 70°–130°) critical for distance measures in this segment [35,36]. A falsely slow conduction velocity across the elbow and a potential false diagnosis of ulnar mononeuropathy may result if the elbow is too straight [36]. Most nerves are measured linearly by their estimated course, regardless of whether the nerve is anatomically straight. When the course of a nerve is not linear and not affected by joint position (eg, across the spiral groove, shoulder, or pelvis), obstetric calipers provide a more accurate distance measurement.

Fixed distances are used by many laboratories for sensory studies and distal motor segments to improve consistency of latency measurements and ensure accuracy when latencies and velocities are compared with normative data. Although amplitude is typically affected less by changes in distance from study to study, sensory amplitude progressively declines with increasing distance between the stimulation and recording sites because of physiologic temporal dispersion, making standardized distances important for sensory amplitude measures as well.

Anatomic variants

Variations in peripheral nerve anatomy are prevalent but usually do not lead to misdiagnosis during routine nerve conduction studies. Two common variations can lead to errors when pronounced: the median-to-ulnar nerve anastomosis (Martin-Gruber anastomosis) and the accessory deep peroneal nerve.

The Martin-Gruber anastomosis is a bundle of ulnar nerve fibers that travel proximally with the median nerve, then cross to the ulnar nerve in the forearm and continue on to innervate selected ulnar small hand muscles. Three subtypes are described depending on the innervated muscular targets. This anastomosis occurs in 15% to 31% of the general population and is often bilateral, but the percentage of fibers involved is usually small and clinically insignificant. When enough fibers are involved, however, nerve conduction studies may be affected. The primary diagnostic clue is a difference between median or ulnar amplitude between elbow and wrist stimulation not caused by stimulating or recording errors. This difference appears as either an increase in CMAP amplitude with stimulation of the median nerve at the elbow compared with stimulation of the median nerve at the wrist or a decrease in amplitude with stimulation of the ulnar nerve at the elbow compared with stimulation of the ulnar nerve at the wrist. Normally, there is minimal change in CMAP amplitude between these sites. The anastomosis is demonstrated by performing routine median and ulnar motor studies, followed by stimulation of both nerves while recording from a single hand muscle. Ulnar mononeuropathy and conduction block are possible misdiagnoses resulting from a failure to recognize a Martin-Gruber anastomosis. A small anastomosis is frequently revealed by a superimposed median neuropathy at the wrist, which unveils the faster anomalous ulnar fibers that travel with the median nerve at the elbow but not through the carpal tunnel [37].

The accessory deep peroneal nerve is present in approximately 20% of subjects and can lead to the mistaken conclusion that reduced peroneal motor amplitude is caused by underlying peripheral neuropathy. In this variant, some axons from the superficial peroneal nerve, which normally involute during embryogenesis, instead persist to innervate a portion of the extensor digitorum brevis muscle, which is ordinarily solely innervated by the deep peroneal nerve. The extensor digitorum brevis serves as the primary recording site for routine peroneal motor nerve conduction studies. The clue to this anomaly is the presence of a smaller evoked CMAP amplitude with routine deep peroneal nerve stimulation at the ankle site (while recording over the extensor digitorum brevis) than with peroneal nerve stimulation at the knee. Because the anomalous peroneal branch is distant from the standard deep peroneal stimulation site at the ankle, the motor axons it carries are not activated with standard stimulation at the ankle and a portion of the extensor digitorum brevis remains unstimulated, generating a smaller CMAP (in contrast to stimulation at the knee, which activates the common peroneal nerve trunk above the branch point, activating all fibers and generating the full extensor digitorum brevis CMAP). If care is not taken to deliver supramaximal stimulation at the knee, artifactually low amplitudes may be seen with stimulation in both locations for different reasons, which reinforces a misdiagnosis of axonal loss. The anomalous branch is identified by stimulating behind the lateral malleolus while recording from the extensor digitorum brevis. In a subject with standard anatomy this site should contain no peroneal nerve fibers. If a response is obtained from this normally quiescent site, the presence of the branch is confirmed [38].

Late responses

F waves are low amplitude late responses best triggered by supramaximal stimulation. Waveforms potentially confused with F waves include axon reflexes, A waves, and surface recording of incompletely relaxed muscle [39–41]. Axon reflexes are uncommon, highly persistent, intermediate latency potentials triggered by submaximal stimulation, thought to be caused by ephaptic transmission of impulses between adjacent motor axons within a damaged nerve. Unlike F waves, axon reflexes are relatively fixed in shape and latency and usually occur in the setting of reinnervation. They are usually abolished by higher stimulation intensities, similar to H reflexes [39]. In contrast, A waves are common but incompletely understood phenomena found during routine F wave studies; they share some features with true F waves, but latencies are usually shorter and shape and latencies are much more constant. A waves are more prevalent in neurogenic disorders [39]. Excessive surface recorded volitional muscle activity, easily identified using the machine loudspeaker during F wave recording, also can hamper F wave identification.

The most commonly used F wave measure is minimal onset latency. An inadequate number of stimulations can affect results. Studies show that 10 stimulations produce values within 95% of true values (within 1 msec) for minimal and mean latencies (based on 100 stimulations) [40,41]. Care must be taken not to overinterpret values near the upper limit when fewer than 10 to 20 stimulations are delivered. Because minimal latency is based on the single shortest waveform, one normal axon may yield a normal overall minimal latency in an otherwise abnormal nerve. Consequently, a normal F wave study does not exclude disease. F wave persistence, the percentage of stimulations that produce a response, is 90% with 10 stimuli and 97% with 20. Persistence can be increased by slight muscular contraction, however. Peroneal nerves have lower F wave persistence than other nerves typically studied, which limits their sensitivity. Less common measures, such as amplitude comparisons and minimal to maximal latency (chronodispersion), require considerably more stimulations to produce a reliable number [41].

H reflexes from the soleus muscle stimulating the tibial nerve are sensitive indicators of large fiber polyneuropathy or S_1 root disease that correlate highly with the Achilles deep tendon reflex. Long duration, submaximal stimuli are optimal; normal responses are suppressed by excessive stimulus intensity. Also at higher intensities, possibly confounding F waves are recordable. Responses are bilaterally absent in a percentage of normal controls, more commonly in older subjects. The reflex is enhanced with activation maneuvers similar to deep tendon reflexes; latencies are affected by similar factors, such as temperature, age, nerve length, and conduction velocity. It highly correlates with the presence or absence of the deep tendon reflex on physical examination [39].

Summary

Electrodiagnostic studies are a critical tool for the identification and study of peripheral neuropathy, enabling definition of the pathophysiologic type of nerve injury, its distribution, severity, and the degree of motor or sensory nerve involvement. These data help to differentiate the varieties of neuropathy from other neuromuscular diseases. Nerve conduction studies and EMG, although widely performed, are complex techniques and are subject to a wide range of artifacts, which can result in missed or erroneous diagnoses. Important factors to consider, in addition to proper technique, include regulation of limb temperature, patient age and height, regulation of stimulus strength, recording electrode design and placement, filter settings, sensitivity and sweep speed settings, the effects of stimulus artifact, waveform marker placement, proper measurement of distance between stimulating and recording sites, and the variants of peripheral nervous system anatomy. Without proper education, training, and experience in neuromuscular disease and the techniques of electrodiagnosis and careful attention to potential sources of error, the critical information needed to properly diagnose and treat patients with neuropathy is unreliable and may lead to wasted resources and patient injury.

References

[1] Gooch C, Pullman S. Electromyography and nerve conduction studies in neuromuscular disease. In: Rowland L, editor. Merritt's textbook of neurology. 11th edition. New York: Lippincott, Williams and Wilkins; 2005. p. 89–100.
[2] Mallik A, Weir AI. Nerve conduction studies: essentials and pitfalls in practice. J Neurol Neurosurg Psychiatry 2005;76(Suppl 2):23–31.
[3] Barboi AC, Barkhaus PE. Electrodiagnostic testing in neuromuscular disorders. Neurol Clin 2004;22(3):619–41.
[4] England JD, Gronseth GS, Franklin G, et al. Distal symmetric polyneuropathy: a definition for clinical research. Report of the American Academy of Neurology, the American Association of Electrodiagnostic Medicine, and the American Academy of Physical Medicine and Rehabilitation. Neurology 2005;64(2):199–207.
[5] Cornblath DR, Sumner AJ, Daube J, et al. Conduction block in clinical practice. Muscle Nerve 1991;14(9):869–71.
[6] Kimura J. Current understanding of F-wave physiology in the clinical domain. Suppl Clin Neurophysiol 2006;59:299–303.
[7] Misiaszek J. The H-reflex as a tool in neurophysiology: its limitations and uses in understanding nervous system function. Muscle Nerve 2003;28(2):144–60.
[8] Gooch C. Clinical applications of needle electromyography. In: Basic and advanced techniques in electrodiagnostic medicine. Presented at the 15th Annual Course and Symposium, Columbia University College of Physicians and Surgeons, New York, June 8–9, 2006. p. 85–99.
[9] Daube JR. Needle examination in clinical electromyography: AAEM minimonograph #11. Muscle Nerve 1991;14(8):685–700.
[10] Buchthal F. Electromyography in the evaluation of muscle diseases. Neurol Clin 1985;3(3): 573–98.

[11] Donofrio P, Albers J. Polyneuropathy. classification by nerve conduction studies and electromyography. AAEM minimonograph #34. Muscle Nerve 1990;13(10):889–903.
[12] Gooch C, Fatimi T. Peripheral neuropathies. In: Brust J, editor. Lange's current neurologic diagnosis and treatment. New York: McGraw Hill; 2006. p. 281–319.
[13] Gooch C, Lange D, Trojaborg W. Cranial and peripheral nerve lesions. In: Rowland L, editor. Merritt's textbook of neurology. 11th edition. New York: Lippincott, Williams and Wilkins; 2005. p. 523–43.
[14] England JD, Gooch CL, Werner R. Identifying entrapment and compression neuropathies. Patient Care 1999;33:138–48.
[15] Daube JR, Gooch C, Shefner J, et al. Motor unit number estimation (MUNE) with nerve conduction studies. Suppl Clin Neurophysiol 2000;53:112–5.
[16] Bril V. Roche Neuropathy Study Group. Electrophysiologic monitoring in clinical trials. Muscle Nerve 1998;21(11):1368–73.
[17] Azrieli Y, Weimer L, Lovelace R, et al. The utility of segmental nerve conduction studies in ulnar mononeuropathy at the elbow. Muscle Nerve 2003;27(1):46–50.
[18] Weimer L, Yin J, Lovelace R, et al. Serial studies of carpal tunnel syndrome during and after pregnancy. Muscle Nerve 2002;25(6):914–7.
[19] Podwall D, Gooch C. Diabetic neuropathy: clinical features, etiology and therapy. Curr Neurol Neurosci Rep 2004;4(1):55–61.
[20] Rutkove SB. The effects of temperature in neuromuscular electrophysiology: AAEM minimonograph #14. Muscle Nerve 2001;24(7):867–82.
[21] Franssen H, Wieneke GH, Wokke JH. The influence of temperature on conduction block. Muscle Nerve 1999;22(2):166–73.
[22] De Jesus PV, Hausmanowa-Petrusewicz I, Barchi RL. The effect of cold on nerve conduction of slow and fast nerve fibers. Neurology 1973;23(11):1182–9.
[23] Halar EM, DeLisa JA. Brozovich FV. Nerve conduction velocity: relationship of skin, subcutaneous, and intramuscular temperatures. Arch Phys Med Rehabil 1980;61(5): 199–203.
[24] Oh S. Nonphysiological factors affecting nerve conduction. In: Clinical electromyography: nerve conduction studies. 3rd edition. Philadelphia: Lippincott Williams & Wilkins; 2003. p. 311–26.
[25] Franssen H, Wieneke GH. Nerve conduction and temperature: necessary warming time. Muscle Nerve 1994;17(3):336–44.
[26] Wang FC, de Pasqua V, Delwaide PJ. Age-related changes in fastest and slowest conducting axons of thenar motor units. Muscle Nerve 1999;22(8):1022–9.
[27] Rivner MH, Swift TR, Malik K. Influence of age and height on nerve conduction. Muscle Nerve 2001;24(9):1134–41.
[28] Robinson LR, Rubner DE, Wahl PW, et al. Influences of height and gender on normal nerve conduction studies. Arch Phys Med Rehabil 1993;74(11):1134–8.
[29] Krarup C. Pitfalls in electrodiagnosis. J Neurol 1999;246(12):1115–26.
[30] Buschbacher RM. Body mass index effect on common nerve conduction study measurements. Muscle Nerve 1998;21(11):1398–404.
[31] Buchthal F, Rosenfalck A. Evoked action potentials and conduction velocity in human sensory nerves. Brain Res 1966;3(1):1–122.
[32] Ven AA, Van Hees JG, Stappaerts KH. Effect of size and pressure of surface recording electrodes on amplitude of sensory nerve action potentials. Muscle Nerve 2004;30(2):234–8.
[33] Phongsamart G, Wertsch JJ, Ferdjallah M, et al. Effect of reference electrode position on the compound muscle action potential (CMAP) onset latency. Muscle Nerve 2002;25(6):816–21.
[34] Gilliatt RW, Melville ID, Velate AS, et al. Study of normal nerve action potentials using an averaging technique (barrier grid storage tube). J Neurol Neurosurg Psychiatry 1965;28: 191–200.
[35] Checkles NS, Russakov AD, Piero DL. Ulnar nerve conduction velocity: effect of elbow position on measurement. Arch Phys Med Rehabil 1971;52(8):362–5.

[36] Ulnar Neuropathy at the Elbow AANEM Task Force. Practice parameter for electrodiagnostic studies in ulnar neuropathy at the elbow: summary statement of the American Association of Electrodiagnostic Medicine, American Academy of Neurology, American Academy of Physical Medicine and Rehabilitation. Muscle Nerve 1999;22(3):408–11.
[37] Uchida Y, Sugioka Y. Electrodiagnosis of Martin-Gruber connection and its clinical importance in peripheral nerve surgery. J Hand Surg 1992;17:54–8.
[38] Sander HW, Auinto C, Chokroverty S. Accessory deep peroneal neuropathy: collision technique diagnosis. Muscle Nerve 1998;21:121–3.
[39] Bischoff C. Neurography: late responses. Muscle Nerve 2002;(Suppl 11):S59–65.
[40] Fisher MA. H reflexes and F waves: physiology and clinical indications. AAEM minimonograph #13. Muscle Nerve 1992;15(11):1223–33.
[41] Fisher MA, Hoffen B, Hultman C. Normative F wave values and the number of recorded F waves. Muscle Nerve 1994;17(10):1185–9.

ELSEVIER
SAUNDERS

Neurol Clin 25 (2007) 29–46

NEUROLOGIC
CLINICS

Antibody Testing in Peripheral Neuropathies

Steven Vernino, MD, PhD*, Gil I. Wolfe, MD

Department of Neurology, University of Texas Southwestern Medical Center, Dallas, TX, USA

Causes of peripheral neuropathy (PN) include a wide range of genetic, toxic, metabolic, and inflammatory disorders. Several PNs have an autoimmune basis, either as a consequence of systemic autoimmune disease, an autoimmune disorder specifically targeting peripheral nerve or ganglia, or a remote effect of malignancy. Several clinical presentations are distinctive for the autoimmune neuropathies. Subacute progression, asymmetric or multifocal deficits, and selective involvement of motor, sensory, or autonomic nerves are clues suggesting an autoimmune, inflammatory cause. The clinical presentation, however, may be indistinguishable from other forms of chronic length-dependent sensorimotor PN.

Antibodies against specific glycolipids or glycoproteins, such as anti-GM1 and anti–myelin-associated glycoprotein (MAG), are associated with inflammatory (often demyelinating) peripheral nerve syndromes. In some cases, these antibodies identify motor or sensory neuropathies that are responsive to immunotherapy [1–3] or those with a different prognosis [4,5]. Antineuronal nuclear and cytoplasmic antibodies (such as anti-Hu and CRMP-5) help identify patients who have paraneoplastic neuropathy resulting from remote immunologic effects of malignancy [6,7]. Various other serologic tests, although less specific, can be used to provide clues about the presence of systemic autoimmune disease that can affect the nerves. These include serologic markers for Sjögren's syndrome (SS), rheumatoid arthritis, celiac disease, and systemic vasculitides (such as Churg-Strauss syndrome) [8,9].

Because the cause of acquired neuropathies often is obscure, autoantibody testing can be of great diagnostic value in identifying autoimmune

* Corresponding author. Department of Neurology, University of Texas Southwestern Medical Center, 5323 Harry Hines Boulevard, Dallas, TX 75390-9036.

E-mail address: steven.vernino@utsouthwestern.edu (S. Vernino).

doi:10.1016/j.ncl.2006.10.002 *neurologic.theclinics.com*

neuropathy. There currently are many available antibody tests to consider when evaluating PNs. Some tests are important and specific in the appropriate clinical settings, whereas the significance of other antibodies remains unknown. As an added complication, antibody assay techniques vary among laboratories, as do the sensitivity and specificity of the serologic testing. The role of these autoantibodies in the pathogenesis of PN remains largely unproved and debated [10–12]. Nevertheless, several mechanisms recently have been elucidated by which antiganglioside antibody binding to axons or Schwann cells may exert a pathogenic effect. These include alteration of ion flux causing partial conduction block and triggering leukocyte responses resulting in cytotoxicity, cytokine production, phagocytosis, and degranulation. Furthermore, animal models that mimic sensory ataxic and motor axonal neuropathies in humans have been generated in rabbits immunized with GD1b and GM1 [13,14] Antibody results in individual patients must be correlated with clinical findings to determine the significance of the findings. Whenever possible, autoantibody tests should be selected according to the clinical presentation to enhance usefulness and cost-effectiveness.

Antibodies against glycosylated nerve components

Peripheral nerve contains many glycoprotein and glycolipid components. Gangliosides are complex acidic glycosphingolipids containing the lipid ceramide, glucose, galactose, and one or more sialic acid residues [15]. The ceramide moiety anchors the glycolipid to the nerve cell membrane. In the nomenclature, the first letter, G, stands for ganglioside, and the second letter corresponds to the number of sialic acid residues (M = 1, D = 2, T = 3, and Q = 4). The numeral represents the number of complete tetrasaccharide chains (usually 1 in humans), and the final lower-case letter (a or b) denotes the isomeric position of the sialic acid residue. At least a dozen different gangliosides are present in peripheral nerve [10]. Several glycolipids are sulfated, the most common being sulfatide (sulfated galactosylceramide). Although these gangliosides represent only a small fraction of the total glycolipid content of peripheral nerve, they typically are exposed on the surface of the nerve or myelin membrane and, therefore, are potential antigenic targets for circulating components of the immune system. Furthermore, the glycolipid structure of the nervous system is unique compared with other tissues. In theory, this could lead to an autoimmune process that is organ specific. Antibodies against glycolipids are believed an important part of the immune response against microbial carbohydrate antigens. Thus, molecular mimicry may explain the pathophysiology of postinfectious inflammatory neuropathies [16]. Lipopolysaccharide from *Campylobacter jejuni* strains that are associated closely with Guillain-Barré syndrome (GBS) or Miller Fisher syndrome (MFS) more often contain GM1 or GQ1b mimics than those bacterial strains that cause only enteritis [17]. Ganglioside and other glycolipid antibodies may be useful serologic markers of inflammatory PN (Table 1) but also may be found in a variety of other disease states and in normal healthy individuals.

Anti–myelin-associated glycoprotein antibodies

In addition to gangliosides, peripheral nerve also contains several glycoproteins, including MAG, myelin protein zero, and peripheral myelin protein 22. In 1980, Latov and colleagues [18] described a patient who had a demyelinating neuropathy and an IgM-κ gammopathy. The patient improved with immunosuppressive therapy. MAG later was identified as the target antigen for the IgM-κ monoclonal antibody. It also was determined that monoclonal proteins with and without anti-MAG activity would bind to peripheral nerve gangliosides [19]. As a result of these observations, glycoproteins and gangliosides were proposed as potential autoantigens in PN. Subsequent reports confirmed that approximately 50% of patients who have neuropathy and IgM gammopathy have IgM autoantibodies to MAG [20]. Anti-MAG autoantibodies often cross-react with other peripheral nerve glycolipids, including 3-sulfated glucuronyl paragloboside (SGPG) and sulfated glucuronyl lactosaminylparagloboside, which share an antigenic carbohydrate determinant with MAG [21].

The typical clinical presentation of the neuropathy associated with anti-MAG antibodies is a slowly progressive, distal, symmetric, predominantly sensory or sensorimotor PN [20–22]. Most patients are male. The neuropathy begins with sensory symptoms, and approximately 75% of patients

Table 1
Ganglioside autoantibodies and neuropathy syndromes

Autoantibody	Main immunoglobulin classes	Clinical syndromes
SGPG/MAG	IgM, monoclonal	Demyelinating neuropathy with IgM gammopathy [20,21]
GM1/asialo GM1	IgM > IgG	MMN [1,2,30]
	IgG or IgM	ALS/MND [30,31]
	IgG > IgM	GBS [4,5]
	IgG	AMAN
	IgG or IgM	Lower motor neuron syndromes [3]
GD1b	IgM,[a] monoclonal	Sensory PN [19,35,36]
	IgM[b]	MND [37]
	IgG > IgM[b]	GBS
GQ1b	IgG > IgM	MFS [43]
Sulfatide	IgM > IgG	Chronic sensory PN [22,47]
GALOP	IgM, monoclonal	Ataxic sensory neuropathy

Abbreviations: AMAN, acute motor axonal neuropathy; GBS, Guillain-Barre syndrome; MFS, Miller-Fisher syndrome; MND, motor neuron disease; MMN, multifocal motor neuropathy.

[a] IgM cross-reacts with other gangliosides sharing disialosyl configurations.

[b] Immunoglobulin often cross-reacts with GM1 and other gangliosides.

present with paresthesias [20]. Large-fiber sensory deficits can be severe. Gait ataxia presents a major disability in one third of patients, and hand tremor commonly is observed. Over time, the majority of patients develop motor nerve involvement with primarily distal weakness. The legs usually are affected more than the arms. Deep tendon reflexes usually are reduced or absent.

On laboratory testing, an IgM paraprotein is found in approximately 50% of cases on serum protein electrophoresis (SPEP) and immunofixation (IFE) studies, typically with a κ light chain. Nerve conduction studies demonstrate demyelination in a majority of patients [20–22]. Prolonged distal motor latencies are the most reliable finding, seen in 90% of patients. Neuropathy associated with IgM gammopathy but no anti-MAG activity may be clinically indistinguishable from the anti-MAG neuropathy [23].

A positive anti-MAG assay confirmed by Western blot is strongly suggestive of an immune-mediated PN, usually associated with an IgM paraprotein. Some patients fulfill diagnostic criteria for CIDP and should be treated appropriately. Immunotherapy regimens should be attempted in patients who have significant neurologic impairment, although the treatment response often is disappointing. The presence of an IgM paraprotein should prompt a workup for an underlying plasma cell dyscrasia.

Anti-GM1 antibodies

In 1984, Freddo and coworkers described a lower motor neuron syndrome with monoclonal IgM reactive to GM1 and gangliosides GD1b and asialo GM1 [24]. Polyclonal autoantibodies to GM1 subsequently were reported in patients who had multifocal motor neuropathy (MMN) [2]. Since then, the presence of anti-GM1 antibodies has been described in a variety of motor neuron disorders and motor-predominant neuropathies, including amyotrophic lateral sclerosis (ALS) and GBS (see Table 1).

MMN with conduction block is a potentially treatable neuropathy characterized by asymmetric, painless, slowly progressive weakness most commonly affecting the distal upper limbs [2,25]. Because of the asymmetric, distal weakness, sensory sparing, and occasional atrophy and fasciculations, MMN may resemble ALS. Upper motor neuron signs, however, are not a feature of MMN. Motor nerve conduction studies demonstrating conduction block outside of common compression sites are associated strongly with MMN and help distinguish it from MND [25,26]. There also are some patients who have clinical features of MMN without conduction block that respond to immunotherapy [27].

High-titer, anti-GM1 IgM antibodies are present in 50% to 60% of patients who have MMN [11,28]. The sensitivity of IgM anti-GM1 antibodies in MMN may be increased to 85% by complexing the GM1 antigen with secondary amino groups (co-GM1 antibody test) [29]. Because of the incomplete sensitivity, anti-GM1 antibody should not be considered a requirement for the diagnosis of MMN. Large studies of patients who had PN and MND suggest that high titers of IgM anti-GM1 antibodies are specific for immune-mediated motor-predominant neuropathies [28,30]. Lower titers of GM1 antibodies are hard to interpret, as they may be found in ALS, other PNs [1,31], or normal controls.

Anti-GM1 antibodies, predominantly of the IgG class, also are reported in a variety of acute motor neuropathies, including GBS [4,5]. Seropositivity for GM1 and related gangliosides in GBS is associated closely with evidence of *C jejuni* infection. Several GBS studies find that anti-GM1 antibodies are associated with a more severe neuropathy with widespread axonal degeneration and worse recovery [4,5], although this association is not absolute. *C jejuni* infection and anti-GM1 antibodies commonly are found in patients who have the classic, demyelinating form of GBS. Thus, the value of anti-GM1 testing in individual patients who have GBS is limited, and a positive result has no clear implication for patient management.

In addition to GM1, antibodies to a variety of other gangliosides are found in GBS, including GD1a, GD1b, and GM2. Overall, high-titer anti-ganglioside antibodies are detected in approximately 40% of GBS sera [32]. Some studies show that IgM anti-GM2 antibodies are found in approximately 50% of GBS associated with cytomegalovirus (CMV) infection, a frequency significantly higher than for other forms of GBS [33]. Another study, however, fails to find a close association between these antibodies and GBS, as anti-GM2 antibodies were found occasionally in normal subjects and also seen in acute CMV infection whether or not GBS was present [34].

Anti-GD1b and anti-GD1a antibodies

Clinical correlates for anti-GD1b antibodies are varied, including sensory and sensorimotor PN syndromes similar to those associated with antisulfatide antibodies [19,35,36], MND [37], and GBS [38]. In most settings, the antibody is of the IgM class and cross-reacts with other disialosyl-bearing gangliosides, including GD2, GD3, GT1b, and GQ1b. Although serologic testing for anti-GD1b antibodies is available through commercial laboratories, the role of this antibody in the diagnosis and treatment of neuropathy remains unclear.

Anti-GD1a antibodies are reported in several cases of axonal GBS [38]. In a recent study using a Chinese population [39], IgG anti-GD1a antibodies were detected in a high proportion (60%) of patients who had acute motor axonal neuropathy (AMAN). Only 4% of patients who had the demyelinating form of GBS harbored these antibodies. Although IgG anti-GM1 antibodies also were found frequently in the AMAN population, they were not as specific or sensitive as IgG anti-GD1a antibodies. No relationship between antiganglioside antibodies and *C jejuni* infection was found. The investigators concluded that reactivity to a GD1a-related epitope may be important in the pathogenesis of axonal GBS. The role of anti-GD1a antibodies in clinical practice, however, remains unresolved.

Anti-GQ1b antibodies

In contrast to the limited specificity of other antiganglioside antibodies, anti-GQ1b antibodies are linked closely to MFS. MFS is considered a variant of GBS characterized by the triad of ophthalmoplegia, ataxia, and areflexia. Formes frustes of MFS typically present as acute cranial motor neuropathies with ataxia [40]. GQ1b is expressed abundantly in paranodal regions of the oculomotor, trochlear, and abducens nerves [41], providing a rationale for the ophthalmoplegia common to patients who have anti-GQ1b antibodies. Several studies confirm that high titers of anti-GQ1b IgG antibodies are present in 80% to 100% of patients who have MFS [42,43]. Anti-GQ1b IgG antibodies also are reported in GBS patients who have ophthalmoplegia or ataxia [41,44] and with other neurologic disorders that bear clinical similarities to MFS, such as Bickerstaff's encephalitis [45], and acute ophthalmoparesis [46]. GQ1b epitopes are present in certain strains of *C jejuni* that are associated with antecedent infections in patients who have MFS [4,16]. As with "classic" forms of GBS, patients who have MFS respond to plasma exchange, with a corresponding reduction in anti-GQ1b antibody titers [42]. Other antiganglioside antibodies that are associated with MFS and ataxic neuropathy are anti-GT1a, anti-GD3, and anti-GD1b [40].

Antisulfatide antibodies

The discovery of cross-reactivity of anti-MAG antibodies to sulfated glycolipids encouraged researchers to investigate whether or not autoantibodies to other common sulfated glycolipids could be found in patients who have PN. Two initial studies demonstrated autoantibodies to sulfatide in approximately 25% of patients who had predominantly sensory PN that otherwise would have been classified as idiopathic [22,47]. Later studies, however, failed to show a high frequency of antisulfatide antibodies in patients who had this common clinical presentation [28,48]. The predicted frequency of IgM antisulfatide antibodies in idiopathic PN later was estimated at only 0.7% [49].

Patients who have PN and who have sulfatide antibodies tend to present with chronic, axonal, predominantly sensory PN. Sensory loss is symmetric, distal, and slowly progressive over a period of years, eventually impairing small- and large-fiber function. Pain is the predominant symptom in approximately one half of patients. Distal weakness is uncommon [50] and tends to be mild. Higher titers of antisulfatide antibodies are relatively specific for chronic, sensory-predominant PN. Monoclonal gammopathies are present in up to 50% of those cases. Low titers are found in a variety of neuropathic and non-neuropathic conditions (including idiopathic thrombocytopenic purpura, autoimmune hepatitis, and human immunodeficiency virus).

A subgroup of patients who has *g*ait disorder, *a*ntibody, *l*ate-age–*o*nset *p*olyneuropathy (GALOP) syndrome has been reported. These patients commonly have a monoclonal IgM and have antibodies to sulfatide and other antigens, including a central myelin GALOP antigen [51]. Testing for GALOP antibodies is available but the significance is not established fully.

Paraneoplastic peripheral neuropathy

Paraneoplastic neurologic disorders (PND) are immunologic disorders of the nervous system in patients who have malignancy. PND may affect any part of the nervous system. PN is encountered commonly in cancer patients, in many cases attributable to metabolic derangements or toxic effects of chemotherapeutic agents. An inflammatory/autoimmune PN can occur as a remote effect of cancer, usually preceding any systemic symptoms or diagnosis of cancer. It is believed that the most common presentation of paraneoplastic PN is a length-dependent sensorimotor axonal neuropathy indistinguishable from those of nonparaneoplastic causes. One study estimates that 4.5% of patients who have unexplained adult-onset axonal sensorimotor neuropathy have a malignancy [52]. A few clinical features may increase the suspicion of PND. The onset of paraneoplastic neuropathy tends to be more rapid with progression of symptoms, signs, and electrophysiologic changes over weeks or months. Pain is typical, and there may be unusual manifestations (such as intense itching reported in association with breast cancer) [53]. On electrophysiologic studies, there may be evidence of more widespread nerve involvement affecting nerve roots and peripheral nerves. Analysis of cerebrospinal fluid may show elevated protein or mild lymphocytic pleocytosis.

Paraneoplastic PN is associated with several cancers (small cell and non–small cell lung cancer, breast cancer, and thymoma) and with several autoantibody markers (Table 2), notably type-1 antineuronal nuclear antibodies (ANNA-1), CRMP-5, and N-type calcium channel antibodies. Antibody studies, however, can be negative in many patients who have paraneoplastic PN [52]. Typically, the neurologic syndrome precedes the diagnosis of cancer, and the detection of cancer often is delayed despite close surveillance.

Paraneoplastic sensory neuropathy

Progressive neuropathy that affects the sensory nerves exclusively is termed pure sensory neuropathy, sensory ganglionopathy, or sensory neuronopathy. Approximately 20% of cases of sensory neuronopathy are paraneoplastic; the remainder are associated with systemic autoimmune disease (notably SS) or toxin exposure or remain idiopathic. Paraneoplastic sensory neuronopathy is uncommon, affecting less than 1% of patients who have small cell lung carcinoma [54]. There is a female predominance with a median age of onset of approximately 60 years. The underlying neoplasm is small cell lung carcinoma in 80% to 90% of cases [7,55]. In nearly all patients, the neurologic syndrome and seropositivity precede diagnosis of the tumor. The pathologic correlate of paraneoplastic sensory neuronopathy is destruction of neurons and inflammation in the dorsal root ganglia.

Table 2
Neuronal paraneoplastic autoantibodies associated with peripheral neuropathy

Antibody	Usual tumor	Commonly associated syndromes
ANNA-1 (anti-Hu) [7]	SCLC	Limbic encephalitis, ataxia, sensory neuronopathy, autonomic and sensorimotor neuropathies
CRMP-5 (anti-CV2) [6]	SCLC or thymoma	Encephalomyelitis, chorea, neuropathy, optic neuritis
Amphiphysin	Lung or breast cancer	Encephalomyelitis, neuropathy, stiff-person syndrome
ANNA-2 (anti-Ri)	Lung or breast cancer	Ataxia, opsoclonus-myoclonus, neuropathy
ANNA-3	SCLC	Ataxia, limbic encephalitis and neuropathy
N-type calcium channel antibodies	Lung or breast cancer	PN and many other syndromes

Alternate nomenclature is indicated in parentheses.

Initial symptoms consist of distal pain, numbness, and paresthesias, which can be asymmetric. Clumsiness and gait unsteadiness develop as a result of marked loss of joint position sense. This sensory ataxia is distinct from ataxia because of a cerebellar disorder. Unlike cerebellar disorders, speech and eye movements are normal. Loss of balance and coordination become much worse with eyes closed, and slow wandering movements of the digits or limbs (pseudoathetosis) may be seen. Muscle stretch reflexes usually are absent. Often, paraneoplastic sensory neuropathy progresses relentlessly over weeks or months, leading to significant disability because of inability to walk or attend to basic needs. Because of marked insensitivity, patients may be unaware of serious injuries to the extremities. Nerve conduction studies show absent or low amplitude sensory responses with normal or minimally affected motor studies. The trigeminal blink reflex response usually is normal, perhaps because trigeminal sensory neurons are more centrally located than the dorsal root ganglia. Abnormalities of the trigeminal blink reflex should raise the possibility of a nonparaneoplastic inflammatory sensory neuropathy (as can be seen with SS) [55,56].

Paraneoplastic and autoimmune autonomic neuropathy

In some cases, autoimmunity can target the cells and axons of the autonomic nervous system specifically and spare the motor and sensory nerves. Autonomic dysfunction has many causes, but many cases of subacute autonomic failure have an autoimmune basis and some have an underlying malignancy. Common symptoms of autonomic neuropathy are syncope (resulting from orthostatic hypotension), heat intolerance (resulting from anhidrosis), dry mouth, severe constipation, and vomiting. The latter symptoms are the result of abnormalities of gastrointestinal motility. An autoimmune, nonparaneoplastic form of autonomic neuropathy (autoimmune autonomic neuropathy) seems to be caused by antibodies against neuronal ganglionic acetylcholine receptor (the receptor that mediates synaptic transmission in autonomic ganglia) [57].

Paraneoplastic autonomic neuropathy can present as a subacute panautonomic neuropathy (indistinguishable from nonparaneoplastic autoimmune autonomic neuropathy). Limited presentations also may occur, most notably severe gastrointestinal dysmotility without other autonomic features (paraneoplastic enteric neuropathy). As with other paraneoplastic disorders, the symptoms usually precede the diagnosis of cancer, and the tumors, when found, are limited in stage or are only locally metastatic (regional lymph nodes). Hence, because patients have no symptoms directly referable to their tumor, their autonomic symptoms cannot be attributed to direct effects of the malignancy, nonspecific consequences of chronic illness, or chemotherapy-induced neuropathy.

Paraneoplastic autonomic neuropathy commonly is associated with small cell lung cancer and anti-Hu (also known as ANNA-1) antibodies. Many patients who have paraneoplastic neuropathy have evidence of additional neurologic impairment, including limbic encephalitis, cerebellar ataxia, brainstem involvement, or myelitis [55]. Paraneoplastic gastrointestinal dysmotility is especially common and may be the presenting feature [7].

Paraneoplastic autoantibodies

The use and interpretation of antibody testing in suspected paraneoplastic neurologic disease (PND) is an area of much confusion because of the growing number of antibodies and their varied clinical associations. Antibodies that are associated with PN syndromes are presented in Table 2. The majority of paraneoplastic antibodies are directed against intracellular antigens in the nucleus or cytoplasm of neurons. In some cases, the protein antigen has been identified definitively, and testing using Western blot against recombinant protein is available. In other cases, the antibody is defined descriptively based on the pattern of immunohistochemical staining of brain sections. Many of the antibodies are shown to recognize antigens in nerve and in tumor cells. These antibodies are important as surrogate markers of a specific immune response to cancer. Each of the paraneoplastic neuronal nuclear and cytoplasmic antibodies can be associated with several different neurologic syndromes but typically are highly specific for the presence of cancer and predictive of the cancer type.

No single individual neuronal paraneoplastic antibody is a very sensitive diagnostic tool. Even when the most complete battery of paraneoplastic antibodies is obtained, many patients who have a subacute neurologic syndrome and proved cancer have no paraneoplastic antibody detected [58,59]. Thus, negative antibody tests cannot exclude a paraneoplastic cause of neuropathy, but seropositivity for a paraneoplastic antibody should mandate a thorough evaluation for occult malignancy and close oncologic follow-up if cancer is not detected on the initial search. Anti-Hu (ANNA-1) and CRMP-5 (anti-CV2) antibodies deserve special attention because of their frequent association with PN. Several other uncommon paraneoplastic antibodies, including amphyiphysin, ANNA-2 (anti-Ri) and ANNA-3 also are associated with paraneoplastic neuropathy, usually lung or breast carcinoma. Patients who have these cancers also may produce antibodies against N-type voltage-gated calcium channels. These calcium channel antibodies are different from the P/Q-type calcium channel antibodies associated with Lambert-Eaton syndrome and may be associated with several paraneoplastic syndromes, including neuropathy.

Anti-Hu (ANNA-1) antibodies

Anti-Hu antibodies (ANNA-1) bind to a family of 35–40 kd proteins expressed in the nuclei of neurons of the central nervous system, dorsal root ganglia, and myenteric plexus. These antigens also are expressed in certain tumor cells, most notably small cell lung carcinoma. Low titers of anti-Hu IgG antibodies are detected in the serum of approximately 15% of patients who have small cell lung carcinoma without a paraneoplastic syndrome [60]. Higher titers are associated with a wide variety of neurologic syndromes, ranging from limbic encephalitis to neuropathy. PN is the most common initial manifestation, occurring in 70% to 80% of patients who have anti-Hu antibody [7]. Half of these paraneoplastic neuropathies are sensory. Approximately 25% of patients who have anti-Hu have some features of gastrointestinal dysmotility.

On detection of a positive serology, patients should be screened aggressively for an underlying malignancy, beginning with chest CT if routine chest radiographs are negative. Nearly 90% of adult patients who have anti-Hu antibodies have cancer, usually small cell lung carcinoma [61]. Bronchoscopy, mediastinoscopy, or thoracotomy may identify occult tumors when radiologic studies are negative [7]. Metabolic imaging with fluorodeoxyglucose positron emission tomography scan recently has been shown to be the most sensitive test for detecting occult small cell cancer in patients who have paraneoplastic disorders [62]. There are rare reports of anti-Hu positive patients who do not develop cancer after 4 or more years. One possibility is that the vigorous immune response leads to a spontaneous cancer remission [63]. In other cases, the small cell cancer may evade detection until a patient dies of neurologic complications. If a chest malignancy is not found, the search should be widened to include other tumors, especially neuroblastoma or small cell carcinomas arising in other organs. Periodic follow-up imaging every few months is recommended if initial screening is unremarkable.

As with most paraneoplastic antibodies, a pathogenic role for anti-Hu antibodies seems unlikely as passive transfer of anti-Hu antibodies or immunization with the HuD antigen has failed to reproduce disease in animals, despite the development of high anti-Hu titers [12].

CRMP-5 (anti-CV2) antibodies

Approximately 10 years ago, in 1996, a novel paraneoplastic antibody was described, and designated anti-CV2, which recognized collapsin response-mediator proteins (CRMPs), specifically CRMP-3, and was associated with a variety of paraneoplastic syndromes [64]. More recently, another paraneoplastic antibody was characterized in more than 100 patients, which specifically recognized a 62-kd antigen that proved to be CRMP-5 [6]. CRMP-5 is a neuronal cytoplasmic protein present in adult central and peripheral neurons, and in small cell lung carcinomas. Given the similarities between CV2 and CRMP-5 antibodies, it is possible that these two paraneoplastic antibodies actually are one and the same. CRMP-5 antibodies are proving to be one of the most common markers of PND. The antibody often coexists with other paraneoplastic antibodies and is second in frequency only to anti-Hu (ANNA-1) as a marker of SCLC [6,61].

The associated neurologic syndromes are diverse (much like those associated with anti-Hu antibodies) and include PN, limbic encephalitis, ataxia, and recently recognized paraneoplastic syndromes of chorea and optic neuritis. PN, usually axonal sensorimotor type, is present in approximately one half of patients [6]. Autonomic neuropathy occurs in approximately one third. Lung carcinoma (small cell type) eventually is found in nearly 80% of seropositive patients. CRMP-5 antibodies also can be found in patients who have thymoma, with or without neurologic symptoms [6,65].

Neuropathy associated with systemic autoimmune diseases

Peripheral nerve vasculitis

In systemic vasculitis (most notably Churg-Strauss, polyarteritis nodosa, and Wegener's granulomatosis), PN occurs in 40% to 50% of patients. The neuropathy classically presents as painful mononeuritis multiplex, involvement of multiple individual nerves. Radial and peroneal nerves often are involved. A presentation with painful distal symmetric axonal neuropathy is not uncommon, however. Typically, if vasculitis affecting peripheral nerve is suspected, definitive diagnosis is obtained by biopsy of nerve (or other affected organs). Antibody tests can be useful in the initial evaluation to help raise the suspicion. These include antiproteinase 3 antibodies, antineutrophilic cytoplasmic antibodies (c-ANCA), which are found in many patients who have Wegener's granulomatosis and antimyeloperoxidase antibodies (p-ANCA), which are associated with Churg-Strauss and polyarteritis nodosa. Antinuclear antibodies (ANA) and rheumatoid factor (RF) also are associated with these vasculitides.

PN is found commonly in patients who have rheumatoid arthritis. Severe painful neuropathy or mononeuritis multiplex occurs when there is an associated vasculitis. High levels of RF and ANA may be found in patients who have vasculitic neuropathy even if joint manifestations are not evident. Patients who do not have systemic vasculitis that have had typical rheumatoid arthritis for many years often develop a mild symmetric PN.

In all cases, aggressive treatment of the underlying vasculitis with corticosteroids and other immunosuppression is the mainstay of therapy. Isolated peripheral nerve vasculitis also can occur but generally is not associated with any serologic antibody markers.

Neuropathy with Sjögren's and sicca syndromes

The exact frequency of neuropathy associated with primary SS is unknown but estimated to be approximately 10% [66]. A variety of neuropathies can be encountered, and neuropathy may be the initial presentation of the autoimmune disease. Similar patterns of neuropathy may be encountered in patients who have sicca syndrome (dry eyes and dry mouth) that do not fulfill diagnostic criteria for SS [8]. Sensory neuropathy is the most common presentation, usually a painful distal small-fiber neuropathy. Sensory ganglionopathy with sensory ataxia and trigeminal sensory loss is a distinctive but uncommon presentation. The involvement of the trigeminal sensory nerve helps distinguish this form of sensory ganglionopathy from the paraneoplastic sensory neuronopathy [56]. Autonomic features often are present in neuropathic presentations, characterized by sweating abnormalities and constipation. In a minority of cases, tonic unresponsive pupils can occur. Preliminary studies suggest that antibodies against the muscarinic acetylcholine receptor (AChR) may be associated with the autonomic neuropathy of SS [67]. Other less common neuropathic presentations include trigeminal sensory neuropathy, multiple cranial neuropathies, or vasculitis with mononeuritis multiplex. Central nervous system manifestations also can be associated with SS.

Patients who have SS predominantly are female. Diagnosis consists of symptoms and objective evidence of dry mouth and dry eyes along with confirmatory salivary gland biopsy showing inflammation or presence of antibodies. The antibodies that are associated most closely with SS are anti-Ro/SS-A and anti-La/SS-B. These antibodies are found in approximately 60% of patients who have SS. Other serologic findings include ANA and RF antibodies.

Celiac neuropathy

Celiac disease is a T-cell–mediated autoimmune disorder associated with sensitivity to ingested gluten protein in people who are genetically predisposed. Patients develop antibodies against tissue transglutaminase (TTG) and other intestinal antigens and pathologically show injury to small bowel mucosa. Typical symptoms are diarrhea, weight loss, and dermatitis herpetiformis [68]. Various studies suggest that axonal distal sensory PN is common in patients who have celiac disease [9]. It is unclear if the neuropathy results from an associated autoimmune attack against nerve or relates to nutritional deficiency resulting from impaired intestinal function. Neuropathy and other neurologic symptoms (ie, ataxia) can occur even in the absence of gastrointestinal symptoms. The neuropathy usually is a mild sensory PN. Various studies show an incidence of celiac disease that is higher than expected (2.5% or higher) in patients who have idiopathic sensory neuropathy [9]. The significance of the association between celiac disease and neuropathy, therefore still remains somewhat controversial.

For diagnostic purposes, antibody tests are useful as screening tools, but definitive diagnosis of celiac disease requires endoscopic biopsy of small bowel mucosa. The most readily available antibody tests are for antigliadin antibodies. Serum antigliadin IgA is more specific for celiac disease because gliadin IgG antibodies can be found in normal healthy controls [69]. IgA antiendomysial antibodies and TTG antibodies are more specific than gliadin antibodies. These antibodies associate with the presence of intestinal disease, however, and are less common in patients who have neurologic disease without bowel involvement. Thus, the usefulness of serologic testing for celiac disease in the evaluation of PN remains unclear. These antibody tests can be used as screening tools in patients who have idiopathic sensory or sensorimotor neuropathy (especially in patients who have gastrointestinal symptoms or the suggestive dermatitis herpetiformis rash). Positive results should prompt further evaluation with gastrointestinal endoscopic studies. Recent studies have described the frequent presence of IgG ganglioside antibodies (including anti-GM1 and anti-GD1b) in 20% to 60% of celiac patients who have neurologic symptoms [9,70,71]. The significance remains unclear because many celiac patients who do not have neurologic symptoms also may harbor ganglioside antibodies.

The current treatment for celiac disease is maintenance of a restricted gluten-free diet. Dietary modification is effective for treating the bowel manifestations, but there is no conclusive evidence that the associated PN improves.

Clinical guidelines for autoantibody testing

The initial evaluation of PN should include a thorough evaluation to define the neuropathy on clinical grounds (symmetric versus asymmetic, sensory versus motor, and so forth) and to determine (1) whether the process primarily is axonal or demyelinating and (2) whether conduction block is present. If a cause of the PN is not apparent, SPEP with IFE is important to detect the presence of a monoclonal protein. Additional specific antibody tests are warranted depending on the presenting features.

Sensorimotor or sensory polyneuropathy

In the setting of an idiopathic sensorimotor PN, autoantibody testing can be considered in certain circumstances. If there is evidence of demyelination on NCS (in particular prolonged distal latencies) anti-MAG testing may help clarify the diagnosis and help distinguish this neuropathy from CIDP. Also, because many patients who have anti-MAG antibodies have an IgM monoclonal protein, anti-MAG antibodies can be sought for any patients who have PN with IgM monoclonal proteins. Routine testing for antiganglioside or antisulfatide autoantibodies in the setting of axonal neuropathies is not established.

Testing for serologic markers of celiac disease (gliadin, endomysial, and transglutaminase antibodies) can be considered in cases of idiopathic progressive neuropathy. At present, the nature and treatment of celiac neuropathy remains unclear, so antibody testing is not a routine part of a PN evaluation. These tests might be considered when there are suggestive gastrointestinal symptoms. Further, these tests are not specific for celiac disease, so additional evaluations always are necessary to establish a diagnosis of gluten sensitivity.

In patients presenting with sensory neuronopathy (asymmetric and proximal sensory deficits), paraneoplastic antibody testing is indicated, particularly because a positive antibody result allows early diagnosis and treatment of an underlying malignancy. The role of paraneoplastic antibody testing in symmetric, slowly progressive neuropathies of unknown cause remains controversial. A rational approach is to test patients who have neuropathy and who have a significant smoking history, constitutional symptoms suggestive of cancer (such as unexplained weight loss), or additional neurologic impairment, such as cerebellar ataxia, limbic encephalitis, or gastrointestinal dysmotility. Serologic testing for SS (ANA, SS-A, and SS-B) also is appropriate in the setting of sensory predominant neuropathy, particularly if there are complaints of dry eyes and dry mouth or other rheumatologic symptoms. Sulfatide antibodies probably are not useful in routine evaluation of neuropathy, but in cases where gait ataxia is a prominent feature, testing for sulfatide and GALOP antibodies can be considered.

Painful asymmetric involvement of individual nerves (mononeuritis multiplex) is suggestive of vasculitis of nerve. In addition to nerve biopsy, antibody tests can be useful. Tests for ANCA, RF, and ANA may provide some evidence of systemic autoimmune disease.

Motor neuropathy

When evaluating a predominantly motor neuropathy, autoantibody testing can help in certain scenarios. Anti-GM1 antibodies should be considered in patients who have acquired, chronic, distal lower motor neuron syndromes whether or not there is evidence of conduction block on nerve conduction studies. When definitive upper motor neuron signs are present, anti-GM1 antibodies are not useful, because results cannot distinguish between MMN and motor neuron disease (MND). Anti-GM1 testing also can be considered in cases of GBS when electrophysiologic studies suggest significant axonal loss. Rationale for this testing mainly is to inform on prognosis because several studies demonstrate that anti-GM1 antibodies tend to predict a more severe GBS picture with worse recovery [4,5]. Anti-GM1 antibodies should not be used routinely as a diagnostic test for GBS. Anti-GD1a testing should be approached in a similar manner.

Anti-GQ1b antibodies can be used in patients who have suspected MFS or related syndromes characterized by acute ophthalmoplegia or cerebellar ataxia to distinguish these presumed immune-mediated neuropathies from other conditions, such as posterior fossa strokes and botulism. The presence of IgG anti-GQ1b antibodies suggests that treatment with plasmapheresis or intravenous gammaglobulin may be beneficial.

Autonomic neuropathy

When evaluating a predominantly autonomic neuropathy, antibody testing may help distinguish autoimmune causes from degenerative forms of autonomic failure. In recent onset autonomic failure (especially when gastrointestinal symptoms are prominent), paraneoplastic antibody testing helps identify patients who have an occult malignancy. Approximately 50% of patients who have autoimmune autonomic neuropathy have antibodies against ganglionic AChRs. Seropositivity can identify patients who may respond to plasma exchange or intravenous immunoglobulin [72].

Summary

There is a definite role for autoantibody testing in the evaluation of PN. The use and interpretation of antibody results always should depend on the clinical and electrophysiologic presentation of a patient. The presence of autoantibodies provides evidence of autoimmunity that may contribute to the pathophysiology of neuropathy. Some antibodies have clear significance in terms of guiding diagnosis (eg, paraneoplastic antibodies) or prognosis and treatment (eg, GM1 antibodies). Most of the autoantibodies, however, do not define a specific clinical syndrome and do not have a proved direct pathogenic role.

References

[1] Adams D, Kuntzer T, Burger D, et al. Predictive value of anti-GM1 ganglioside antibodies in neuromuscular diseases: a study of 180 sera. J Neuroimmunol 1991;32:223–30.

[2] Pestronk A, Cornblath DR, Ilyas AA, et al. A treatable multifocal motor neuropathy with antibodies to GM1 ganglioside. Ann Neurol 1988;24:73–8.

[3] Pestronk A, Lopate G, Kornberg AJ, et al. Distal lower motor neuron syndrome with high-titer serum IgM anti-GM1 antibodies: improvement following immunotherapy with monthly plasma exchange and intravenous cyclophosphamide. Neurology 1994;44:2027–31.

[4] Jacobs BC, van Doorn PA, Schmitz PI, et al. Campylobacter jejuni infections and anti-GM1 antibodies in Guillain-Barre syndrome. Ann Neurol 1996;40:181–7.
[5] van den Berg LH, Marrink J, de Jager AE, et al. Anti-GM1 antibodies in patients with Guillain-Barre syndrome. J Neurol Neurosurg Psychiatry 1992;55:8–11.
[6] Yu Z, Kryzer TJ, Griesmann GE, et al. CRMP-5 neuronal autoantibody: marker of lung cancer and thymoma-related autoimmunity. Ann Neurol 2001;49:146–54.
[7] Lucchinetti CF, Kimmel DW, Lennon VA. Paraneoplastic and oncologic profiles of patients seropositive for type 1 antineuronal nuclear autoantibodies. Neurology 1998;50:652–7.
[8] Grant IA, Hunder GG, Homburger HA, et al. Peripheral neuropathy associated with sicca complex. Neurology 1997;48:855–62.
[9] Chin RL, Sander HW, Brannagan TH, et al. Celiac neuropathy. Neurology 2003;60:1581–5.
[10] Asbury AK. Gangliosides and peripheral neuropathies: an overview. Prog Brain Res 1994; 101:279–87.
[11] Parry GJ. Antiganglioside antibodies do not necessarily play a role in multifocal motor neuropathy. Muscle Nerve 1994;17:97–9.
[12] Sillevis Smitt PA, Manley GT, Posner JB. Immunization with the paraneoplastic encephalomyelitis antigen HuD does not cause neurologic disease in mice. Neurology 1995;45:1873–8.
[13] Kusunoki S, Hitoshi S, Kaida K-I, et al. Monospecific anti-GD1b IgG is required to induce rabbit ataxic neuropathy. Ann Neurol 1999;45:400–3.
[14] Yuki N, Yamada M, Koga M, et al. Animal model of axonal Guillain-Barre syndrome induced by sensitization with GM1 ganglioside. Ann Neurol 2001;49:712–20.
[15] Steck AJ, Burger D, Picasso S, et al. Gangliosides and related glycoconjugates in myelin: relationship to peripheral neuropathies. Prog Brain Res 1994;101:305–12.
[16] Yuki N, Taki T, Takahashi M, et al. Molecular mimicry between GQ1b ganglioside and lipopolysaccharides of Campylobacter jejuni isolated from patients with Fisher's syndrome. Ann Neurol 1994;36:791–3.
[17] Ang CW, Laman JD, Willison HJ, et al. Structure of Campylobacter jejuni lipopolysaccharides determines antiganglioside specificity and clinical features of Guillain-Barre and Miller Fisher patients. Infect Immun 2002;70:1202–8.
[18] Latov N, Sherman WH, Nemni R, et al. Plasma-cell dyscrasia and peripheral neuropathy with a monoclonal antibody to peripheral-nerve myelin. N Engl J Med 1980;303:618–21.
[19] Ilyas AA, Quarles RH, Dalakas MC, et al. Monoclonal IgM in a patient with paraproteinemic polyneuropathy binds to gangliosides containing disialosyl groups. Ann Neurol 1985;18: 655–9.
[20] Nobile-Orazio E, Manfredini E, Carpo M, et al. Frequency and clinical correlates of antineural IgM antibodies in neuropathy associated with IgM monoclonal gammopathy. Ann Neurol 1994;36:416–24.
[21] Van den Berg L, Hays AP, Nobile-Orazio E, et al. Anti-MAG and anti-SGPG antibodies in neuropathy. Muscle Nerve 1996;19:637–43.
[22] Pestronk A, Li F, Griffin J, et al. Polyneuropathy syndromes associated with serum antibodies to sulfatide and myelin-associated glycoprotein. Neurology 1991;41:357–62.
[23] Gosselin S, Kyle RA, Dyck PJ. Neuropathy associated with monoclonal gammopathies of undetermined significance. Ann Neurol 1991;30:54–61.
[24] Freddo L, Yu RK, Latov N, et al. Gangliosides GM1 and GD1b are antigens for IgM M-protein in a patient with motor neuron disease. Neurology 1986;36:454–8.
[25] Krarup C, Stewart JD, Sumner AJ, et al. A syndrome of asymmetric limb weakness with motor conduction block. Neurology 1990;40:118–27.
[26] Chaudhry V, Corse AM, Cornblath DR, et al. Multifocal motor neuropathy: electrodiagnostic features. Muscle Nerve 1994;17:198–205.
[27] Katz JS, Wolfe GI, Bryan WW, et al. Electrophysiologic findings in multifocal motor neuropathy. Neurology 1997;48:700–7.
[28] Wolfe GI, El-Feky WH, Katz JS, et al. Antibody panels in idiopathic polyneuropathy and motor neuron disease. Muscle Nerve 1997;20:1275–83.

[29] Pestronk A, Choksi R. Multifocal motor neuropathy. Serum IgM anti-GM1 ganglioside antibodies in most patients detected using covalent linkage of GM1 to ELISA plates. Neurology 1997;49:1289–92.
[30] Taylor BV, Gross L, Windebank AJ. The sensitivity and specificity of anti-GM1 antibody testing. Neurology 1996;47:951–5.
[31] Pestronk A, Adams RN, Clawson L, et al. Serum antibodies to GM1 ganglioside in amyotrophic lateral sclerosis. Neurology 1988;38:1457–61.
[32] van Sorge NM, van der Pol WL, Jansen MD, et al. Pathogenicity of anti-ganglioside antibodies in the Guillain-Barre syndrome. Autoimmun Rev 2004;3:61–8.
[33] Khalili-Shirazi A, Gregson N, Gray I, et al. Antiganglioside antibodies in Guillain-Barre syndrome after a recent cytomegalovirus infection. J Neurol Neurosurg Psychiatry 1999; 66:376–9.
[34] Yuki N, Tagawa Y. Acute cytomegalovirus infection and IgM anti-GM2 antibody. J Neurol Sci 1998;154:14–7.
[35] Daune GC, Farrer RG. Dalakas MC, et al. Sensory neuropathy associated with monoclonal immunoglobulin M to GD1b ganglioside. Ann Neurol 1992;31:683–5.
[36] Dalakas MC, Quarles RH. Autoimmune ataxic neuropathies (sensory ganglionopathies): are glycolipids the responsible autoantigens? Ann Neurol 1996;39:419–22.
[37] Nardelli E, Steck AJ, Barkas T, et al. Motor neuron syndrome and monoclonal IgM with antibody activity against gangliosides GM1 and GD1b. Ann Neurol 1988;23:524–8.
[38] Yuki N, Yoshino H, Sato S, et al. Severe acute axonal form of Guillain-Barre syndrome associated with IgG anti-GD1a antibodies. Muscle Nerve 1992;15:899–903.
[39] Ho TW, Willison HJ, Nachamkin I, et al. Anti-GD1a antibody is associated with axonal but not demyelinating forms of Guillain-Barre syndrome. Ann Neurol 1999;45:168–73.
[40] Willison HJ. The immunobiology of Guillain-Barre syndromes. J Peripher Nerv Syst 2005; 10:94–112.
[41] Chiba A, Kusunoki S, Obata H, et al. Serum anti-GQ1b IgG antibody is associated with ophthalmoplegia in Miller Fisher syndrome and Guillain-Barre syndrome: clinical and immunohistochemical studies. Neurology 1993;43:1911–7.
[42] Yuki N, Sato S, Tsuji S, et al. Frequent presence of anti-GQ1b antibody in Fisher's syndrome. Neurology 1993;43:414–7.
[43] Willison HJ, Veitch J, Paterson G, et al. Miller Fisher syndrome is associated with serum antibodies to GQ1b ganglioside. J Neurol Neurosurg Psychiatry 1993;56:204–6.
[44] Carpo M, Pedotti R, Allaria S, et al. Clinical presentation and outcome of Guillain-Barre and related syndromes in relation to anti-ganglioside antibodies. J Neurol Sci 1999;168: 78–84.
[45] Yuki N, Sato S, Tsuji S, et al. An immunologic abnormality common to Bickerstaff's brain stem encephalitis and Fisher's syndrome. J Neurol Sci 1993;118:83–7
[46] Yuki N. Acute paresis of extraocular muscles associated with IgG anti-GQ1b antibody. Ann Neurol 1996;39:668–72.
[47] Nemni R, Fazio R, Quattrini A, et al. Antibodies to sulfatide and to chondroitin sulfate C in patients with chronic sensory neuropathy. J Neuroimmunol 1993;43:79–85.
[48] Notermans NC, Wokke JH, Franssen H, et al. Chronic idiopathic polyneuropathy presenting in middle or old age: a clinical and electrophysiological study of 75 patients. J Neurol Neurosurg Psychiatry 1993;56:1066–71.
[49] Lopate G, Parks BJ, Goldstein JM, et al. Polyneuropathies associated with high titre antisulphatide antibodies: characteristics of patients with and without serum monoclonal proteins. J Neurol Neurosurg Psychiatry 1997;62:581–5.
[50] Dabby R, Weimer LH, Hays AP, et al. Antisulfatide antibodies in neuropathy: clinical and electrophysiologic correlates. Neurology 2000;54:1448–52.
[51] Pestronk A, Choksi R, Bieser K, et al. Treatable gait disorder and polyneuropathy associated with high titer serum IgM binding to antigens that copurify with myelin-associated glycoprotein. Muscle Nerve 1994;17:1293–300.

[52] Antoine JC, Mosnier JF, Absi L, et al. Carcinoma associated paraneoplastic peripheral neuropathies in patients with and without anti-onconeural antibodies. J Neurol Neurosurg Psychiatry 1999;67:7–14.
[53] Peterson K, Forsyth PA, Posner JB. Paraneoplastic sensorimotor neuropathy associated with breast cancer. J Neurooncol 1994;21:159–70.
[54] Elrington GM, Murray NM, Spiro SG, et al. Neurological paraneoplastic syndromes in patients with small cell lung cancer. A prospective survey of 150 patients. J Neurol Neurosurg Psychiatry 1991;54:764–7.
[55] Dalmau J, Graus F, Rosenblum M, et al. Anti-Hu associated paraneoplastic encephalomyelitis/sensory neuronopathy. A clinical study of 71 patients. Medicine (Baltimore) 1992;71: 59–72.
[56] Auger RG, Windebank AJ, Lucchinetti CF, et al. Role of the blink reflex in the evaluation of sensory neuronopathy. Neurology 1999;53:407–8.
[57] Vernino S, Low PA, Fealey RD, et al. Autoantibodies to ganglionic acetylcholine receptors in autoimmune autonomic neuropathies. N Engl J Med 2000;343:847–55.
[58] Candler PM, Hart PE, Barnett M, et al. A follow up study of patients with paraneoplastic neurological disease in the United Kingdom. J Neurol Neurosurg Psychiatry 2004;75:1411–5.
[59] Lawn ND, Westmoreland BF, Kiely MJ, et al. Clinical, magnetic resonance imaging, and electroencephalographic findings in paraneoplastic limbic encephalitis. Mayo Clin Proc 2003;78:1363–8.
[60] Dalmau J, Furneaux HM, Gralla RJ, et al. Detection of the anti-Hu antibody in the serum of patients with small cell lung cancer–a quantitative western blot analysis. Ann Neurol 1990; 27:544–52.
[61] Pittock SJ, Kryzer TJ, Lennon VA. Paraneoplastic antibodies coexist and predict cancer, not neurological syndrome. Ann Neurol 2004;56:715–9.
[62] Younes-Mhenni S, Janier MF, Cinotti L, et al. FDG-PET improves tumour detection in patients with paraneoplastic neurological syndromes. Brain 2004;127(Pt 10):2331–8.
[63] Gill S, Murray N, Dalmau J, et al. Paraneoplastic sensory neuronopathy and spontaneous regression of small cell lung cancer. Can J Neurol Sci 2003;30:269–71.
[64] Honnorat J, Byk T, Kusters I, et al. Ulip/CRMP proteins are recognized by autoantibodies in paraneoplastic neurological syndromes. Eur J Neurosci 1999;11:4226–32.
[65] Vernino S, Lennon VA. Autoantibody profiles and neurological correlations of thymoma. Clin Cancer Res 2004;10:7270–5.
[66] Font J, Ramos-Casals M, de la Red G, et al. Pure sensory neuropathy in primary Sjogren's syndrome. Longterm prospective followup and review of the literature. J Rheumatol 2003; 30:1552–7.
[67] Naito Y, Matsumoto I, Wakamatsu E, et al. Muscarinic acetylcholine receptor autoantibodies in patients with Sjogren's syndrome. Ann Rheum Dis 2005;64:510–1.
[68] Farrell RJ, Kelly CP. Celiac sprue. N Engl J Med 2002;346:180–8.
[69] Hadjivassiliou M, Grunewald RA, Chattopadhyay AK, et al. Clinical, radiological, neurophysiological, and neuropathological characteristics of gluten ataxia. Lancet 1998;352:1582–5.
[70] Volta U, De Giorgio R, Granito A, et al. Anti-ganglioside antibodies in coeliac disease with neurological disorders. Dig Liver Dis 2006;38:183–7.
[71] Alaedini A, Green PH, Sander HW, et al. Ganglioside reactive antibodies in the neuropathy associated with celiac disease. J Neuroimmunol 2002;127:145–8.
[72] Schroeder C, Vernino S, Birkenfeld AL, et al. Plasma exchange for primary autoimmune autonomic failure. N Engl J Med 2005;353:1585–90.

ELSEVIER
SAUNDERS

Neurol Clin 25 (2007) 47–69

NEUROLOGIC
CLINICS

Paraproteinemic Neuropathy

Justin Y. Kwan, MD

Department of Neurology, Baylor College of Medicine, 6550 Fannin, Suite 1801, Houston, TX 77030, USA

Paraproteinemia, or monoclonal gammopathy, is the presence of excessive amounts of abnormal immunoglobulin, or monoclonal protein (M protein), in the blood produced by a single clone of plasma cells. Several distinct peripheral neuropathic syndromes are associated with monoclonal gammopathies of non-neoplastic or neoplastic origin. It is important to identify the presence of M proteins in patients who have peripheral neuropathy, because the detection of paraproteins may lead to the discovery of underlying systemic disorders, such as primary amyloidosis, multiple myeloma, osteosclerotic myeloma, Waldenström's macroglobulinemia, cryoglobulinemia, lymphoma, Castleman's disease, or chronic leukemias.

An intact M protein consists of two identical class and subclass of heavy polypeptide chains and two light chains of the same type. The different types of immunoglobulins are designated by the class of heavy chains: IgA, IgD, IgE, IgG, or IgM. The light chains are either kappa (κ) or lambda (λ). Monoclonal or polyclonal plasma cell proliferation can occur. A monoclonal gammopathy may be malignant or potentially malignant, whereas increased polyclonal immunoglobulins composed of different heavy chains and light chains result from inflammatory or reactive conditions.

The presence of an M protein is detected by screening patients' serum with agarose gel electrophoresis [1]. If a monoclonal spike is detected on the serum protein electrophoresis (SPEP), immunofixation electrophoresis is the preferred method to confirm the presence of the M protein and to determine the heavy chain class and light chain type. Immunofixation is recommended if a monoclonal gammopathy is suspected, even if the SPEP is normal. It is more sensitive than SPEP [1]. Urine electrophoresis and immunofixation also should be examined for the presence of light chain if plasma cell malignancy or light chain amyloidosis is suspected.

E-mail address: jkwan@bcm.tmc.edu

0733-8619/07/$ - see front matter
doi:10.1016/j.ncl.2006.12.002 *neurologic.theclinics.com*

There is a high prevalence of paraproteinemia in the elderly population. M protein without evidence of multiple myeloma or related conditions is present in 1% of people over the age of 25 [2]. Other studies report prevalence of 3% in persons older than 70 [3] and 10% of people older than 80 [4]. There also are racial differences, with a higher prevalence of monoclonal gammopathy noted among African Americans in a community-based sample [5].

One of the earliest observations that peripheral neuropathy is associated with monoclonal gammopathy was made by Chazot and colleagues [6] and, subsequently, Read and coworkers [7], who described three additional cases. Epidemiologic studies provided further evidence supporting the causal link between the presence of M protein and the development of peripheral neuropathy. The prevalence of paraproteins in patients who have idiopathic peripheral neuropathy is 10%. In contrast, only 2.5% of patients who have neuropathy of known cause have a monoclonal gammopathy [8]. Neuropathy also seems more common in patients who have a monoclonal gammopathy compared with the general population [9,10].

Monoclonal gammopathy of undetermined significance

Monoclonal gammopathy of undetermined significance (MGUS) is defined by the following: a M protein concentration of less than 3 g/dL; less than 10% plasma cells in the bone marrow; little or no M protein in the urine; absence of lytic bone lesions; and no related anemia, hypercalcemia, or renal insufficiency [11]. Approximately two thirds of patients who have a paraproteinemia have MGUS [12]. MGUS once was considered a benign process; however, epidemiologic studies show that 26% of patients who have MGUS eventually develop multiple myeloma, Waldenström's macroglobulinemia, primary amyloidosis, or lymphoproliferative disease [11]. The previous finding has been confirmed by a long-term study of the prognosis in MGUS that showed a risk for progression to a hematologic malignancy of 1% per year and a cumulative probability for progression of 10% at 10 years, 21% at 20 years, and 26% at 25 years [13]. Furthermore, patients remain at risk for malignant transformation even after 25 years or more of stable MGUS [13]. It is suggested that the risk for developing hematologic malignancies in patients who have polyneuropathy and MGUS may be different from those patients who do not have a neuropathy. In a 5-year prospective study, 9% of patients who had polyneuropathy associated with MGUS developed a lymphoproliferative malignancy during follow-up [14]; however, only 3 of 50 patients developed a hematologic malignancy in a retrospective study of patients who had peripheral neuropathy associated with MGUS [15]. More recently, a higher frequency of malignant transformation of 25% has been noted in patients who have polyneuropathy and MGUS. Unexplained weight loss, progression of polyneuropathy, and M protein concentration of more than 1 g/L are independent predictors of an underlying cancer [16]. Early detection of a hematologic malignancy is important so that potential treatments can be initiated. Careful investigation must be undertaken in patients who have risk factors for malignant transformation, such as significant concentration of M protein level at the time of the diagnosis of MGUS [13], increased M protein level during follow-up [17], presence of Bence Jones proteinuria, bone marrow plasmacytosis greater than 10%, age over 70 [18], polyclonal immunoglobulin reduction, and high erythrocyte sedimentation rate [19].

Neuropathy associated with monoclonal gammopathy of undetermined significance

Most patients who have peripheral neuropathy and paraproteinemia have MGUS-associated neuropathy [8]. Neuropathy associated with MGUS is a heterogeneous entity with several different clinical presentations, including symmetric polyneuropathy, mononeuritis multiplex, mononeuropathy, and cranial nerve palsies [20]. MGUS-associated neuropathy can be classified into two groups, depending on the class of M protein that is present, IgM or non-IgM associated. Within the IgM-associated group, further subdivisions can be made based on the presence or absence of antibodies targeting specific neural antigens.

Clinical features

MGUS-associated neuropathies typically affect men over age 50. Symptoms are insidious in onset in the distal legs and predominantly are sensory, consisting of numbness, paresthesia, pain, or unsteady gait. Gradually, over months to years, there is progression of sensory deficits, and weakness and atrophy of distal leg muscles develop [21–23]. Rare cases of pure lower motor neuron syndrome are reported [24]. Neurologic examination reveals distal symmetric sensorimotor polyneuropathy or polyradiculoneuropathy, hypoactive or absent reflexes predominantly in the lower extremities, and mild to moderate distal leg weakness. All sensory modalities usually are affected, but vibration sense may be affected to a greater degree than proprioception, pinprick, and light touch [21,23]. Action and postural tremor in the upper limbs may be prominent [22,25]. Electrophysiologic testing can show features of demyelination, axonal degeneration, or both [26]. Cerebrospinal fluid analysis in most patients shows elevated protein without pleocytosis (Table 1) [21,22].

Association of monoclonal gammopathy of undetermined significance and peripheral neuropathy

The high prevalence of M proteins in persons older than 25 [2] may indicate that in some cases MGUS and neuropathy coexist by chance. Several epidemiologic and laboratory studies suggest, however, a pathogenic role of MGUS in the development of neuropathy. A disproportionate increase

Table 1
Clinical and laboratory features of paraproteinemic neuropathy

	Peripheral neuropathy	Neurologic deficits	Systemic involvement	Electrophysiology	Monoclonal heavy chain	Monoclonal light chain
MGUS	5%	Sensory > motor	—	Demyelinating	IgM, IgG, IgA	κ > λ
Multiple myeloma	3%–13%	Sensorimotor	Multisystemic	Demyelinating or axonal	IgG, IgA	κ > λ
Waldenström's macroglobuinemia	7%–46%	Sensorimotor	Multisystemic	Demyelinating or axonal	IgM	κ > λ
POEMS syndrome	100%	Sensorimotor	Multisystemic	Demyelinating	IgG, IgA, IgM	λ > κ
Primary amyloidosis	15%–20%	Sensorimotor and autonomic	Multisystemic	Axonal or demyelinating	IgG, IgA, IgM	λ > κ

in the number of cases of peripheral neuropathy is noted in patients who have monoclonal gammopathy without evidence of multiple myeloma and Waldenström's macroglobulinemia [10,27]. In addition, the most common heavy chain class in a group of patients who had MGUS was IgG (74%), followed by IgM and IgA (15% and 12%, respectively). In contrast, the frequency of heavy chain class in patients who had MGUS and neuropathy was 48% IgM, 37% IgG, and 15% IgA [21]. Up to two thirds of patients who have a peripheral neuropathy and MGUS have an IgM monoclonal gammopathy [28]. Consistent overrepresentation of IgM in patients who have MGUS and neuropathy indicates more than a mere coincidental association [14,22,23,29]. Immunohistochemistry studies also show direct binding of IgM and light chain to the peripheral myelin in patients who have monoclonal gammopathy and neuropathy; the IgM and light chain correspond to the M protein type, implicating a causative role [30–32]. In addition, higher titers of IgM antibodies to one or more neural antigens are present and at high frequency in patients who have neuropathy and IgM monoclonal gammopathy compared with patients who have monoclonal gammopathy without neuropathy [33]. Furthermore, more than 70% of the IgM antibodies from patients who have IgM monoclonal gammopathy and neuropathy bind to one of the components of the peripheral nerve [28].

Neuropathy with myelin-associated glycoprotein reactive antibody

In approximately 50% of patients who have a benign IgM paraproteinemia and a peripheral neuropathy, the M protein reacts against myelin-associated glycoprotein (MAG) [34,35]. Patients who have IgM MGUS and high titers of anti-MAG antibody (greater than 1:6400) who have no symptom of neuropathy or have a subclinical neuropathy have an increased frequency of developing clinically symptomatic neuropathy. Subclinical neuropathy is also more common in patients who have a high anti-MAG antibody titer [36]. These findings support the role of anti-MAG antibody in the pathogenesis of neuropathy.

MAG is a 110-kd glycoprotein located in the central and peripheral nerve myelin sheaths [37]. It accounts for less than 1% of total myelin protein [38]. Unlike the P0, the major glycoprotein in peripheral myelin, and peripheral myelin protein-22 (PMP-22), it is present only in noncompacted myelin. MAG is concentrated in the periaxonal Schwann's cell membrane and paranodal loops of myelin. It has five extracellular immunoglobulin-like domains, which have eight sites for N-linked glycosylation. The carbohydrate epitopes on MAG are shared by the immune and nervous systems and reacts with HNK-adhesion molecule. MAG also shares epitopes with P0, PMP-22, other adhesion molecules in the immunoglobulin superfamily, and glycosphingolipids, such as SGPG [39]. MAG seems to play a role in glia axon interaction and may act as a ligand for a receptor that regulates axon properties [38].

The symptoms in anti-MAG reactive polyneuropathy are insidious in onset and characteristically begin in the distal lower extremity with paresthesia that slowly extends proximally. Romberg's sign and impairment of light touch, vibration and joint position sense are present. There usually is minimal autonomic involvement or loss of pain and temperature. Distal muscle weakness and atrophy may occur as the disease progresses. Motor symptoms frequently are overshadowed by the prominent sensory disturbances, although rare cases with more pronounced motor dysfunction are reported. Gait ataxia and action or positional tremors frequently are present [20,40,41]. This disorder most commonly afflicts men in their 60s or 70s and worsens slowly over 1 or 2 decades [28]. The majority of patients have a favorable long-term prognosis. After an average of 11 years of follow-up, 44% of the patients are disabled by severe hand tremors, gait ataxia, tremor and gait disorder, and fatigue [42].

Anti-MAG antibodies usually are detected in the setting of MGUS; however, some patients may lack a monoclonal spike on routine SPEP or the monoclonal gammopathy may be discovered later [43]. The light chain component usually is κ [44]. The antibody is directed against the carbohydrate epitopes on MAG and can cross react with other components of the myelin that share the same carbohydrate antigenic determinant [45,46]. MAG reactive antibodies also are present in a minority of patients who have Waldenström's macroglobulinemia, lymphoma, or chronic lymphocytic leukemia [34]. The titer of anti-MAG antibodies does not correlate with disease severity [33].

There is slowing of conduction velocity and prolongation of the distal latencies and F-wave latencies on the electrophysiologic studies, consistent with a demyelinating neuropathy [40,47]. Accentuation of slowing of conduction distally with disproportionately prolonged distal latencies is described as the hallmark of demyelinating paraproteinemic neuropathy [48]. Despite the absence of cranial nerve involvement clinically, there can be an increase in blink reflex R1 response latency and prolongation of P100 latency on visual evoked potential [40].

Nerve biopsy shows segmental demyelination more frequently, although features of axonal degeneration and demyelination can be present [33,40]. Direct immunofluorescent studies show deposition and binding of IgM M protein to the periphery of the myelin sheath. IgM is localized to areas of myelin splitting, which represent regions of noncompaction of myelin [33,49]. Colocalization of complement with IgM antibodies to the myelin sheath is noted, suggesting a pathogenic role of complement in mediating demyelination [20,50]. Ultrastructural studies show widening of myelin lamellae (WML), which at times is restricted to the periphery. This abnormality may be the result of insinuation by anti-MAG antibodies between the densely packed layers of myelin lamellae [39]. "Irregular" uncompacted myelin lamellae (UML) may be a more specific finding of monoclonal gammopathy with anti-MAG reactivity and is suggested to differ from the "regular" and "complex" forms that can be associated with other acquired and hereditary neuropathies [51]. The finding of WML is suggested as a characteristic pathologic marker of neuropathy associated with anti-MAG antibodies [40].

Non–myelin-associated glycoprotein–associated IgM monoclonal gammopathy of undetermined significance neuropathy

Neuropathy associated with IgM MGUS but unreactive to anti-MAG antibodies represents a more diverse group of disorders. There is no predominant clinical pattern of either greater sensory or motor involvement. Pathologic studies show demyelination or axonal degeneration, and these patients do not have IgM myelin deposits or WML. The monoclonal IgM reacts to several different peripheral nerve antigens [28,33]. Furthermore, the neuropathy may be asymmetric, involve the cranial nerves, and have a more rapid progression. Peripheral neuropathy often is not the initial symptom leading to the discovery of the monoclonal gammopathy [28,52].

Chronic inflammatory demyelinating polyradiculoneuropathy and monoclonal gammopathy of undetermined significance

Chronic inflammatory demyelinating polyradiculoneuropathy (CIDP) is a chronic progressive or relapsing-remitting acquired neuropathy. It is characterized by a symmetric sensorimotor neuropathy, with predominant motor symptoms, and demyelinating changes on electrophysiologic testing and nerve biopsy. CIDP seldom is confused with MGUS-associated neuropathy. Although up to 25% of patients diagnosed with CIDP have a monoclonal gammopathy, the implication of this finding remains unclear [53]. The M protein detected can react with several myelin antigens, including MAG and SGPG [54]. Several differences between patients who have CIDP with and without MGUS are reported. Patients who have both CIDP and MGUS are older; the course of disease is slowly progressive without relapsing and remitting episodes; fewer motor deficits and greater sensory impairment are present, and the neuropathy is symmetric and more often affects the distal legs [53,55,56]. Another study reports less severe weakness, greater vibration loss in the distal upper limb, gait ataxia, and involuntary upper limb tremors [57]. Findings on electrodiagnostic testing are similar in the two groups [22,57]. All patients respond to treatment, although patients who have CIDP without MGUS may have a better response and the response rate is greatest with plasma exchange [53,57].

Antisulfatide-associated neuropathy

Sulfatide is a major glycosphingolipid concentrated in central and peripheral nerve myelin. Antisulfatide antibodies are present in several different neurologic and systemic conditions, raising the question of the diagnostic relevance of these antibodies [58–60]. Several types of polyneuropathies are associated with elevated titers of IgM sulfatide antibodies, including sensory and sensorimotor, both demyelinating and axonal neuropathies [33,61,62]. Antisulfatide associated neuropathy pleomorphic entity may be classified into two groups based on the presence or absence of paraproteinemia. Antisulfatide neuropathy not associated with a monoclonal gammopathy predominantly is an axonal painful sensory neuropathy without significant motor deficits. In contrast, neuropathy associated with an M protein manifests clinically as weakness without pain or dysesthesia and electrophysiologically as a demyelinating neuropathy [63]. In 25 patients who had highly elevated sulfatide antibody, 92% had either a sensory or sensorimotor neuropathy, and 80% of the neuropathy was predominantly axonal [64]. Pathologic studies show complement and IgM deposits on myelin sheath and antisulfatide antibodies binding to the surface of dorsal root ganglia neurons or myelin sheath, suggesting a pathogenic role for these antibodies [65–67].

Non-IgM monoclonal gammopathy of undetermined significance neuropathy

Unlike neuropathies associated with IgM monoclonal gammopathy, in particular anti-MAG antibodies, polyneuropathy with IgG or IgA M proteins represents a heterogeneous group. Several types of neuropathies are reported, including those that are predominantly sensory, sensorimotor, and predominantly motor [14,22,26]. Axonal degeneration, primary demyelination, and mixed axonal/demyelinating changes are noted on electrophysiologic and histologic studies [68]. A few studies have attempted to correlate the clinical features and electrophysiologic findings with the type of paraprotein present. When compared with IgG/IgA MGUS neuropathies, patients who have IgM MGUS neuropathies have increased frequency of sensory loss and gait ataxia and more severe abnormalities on nerve conduction studies [21,23]. Another prospective study of patients who have polyneuropathy associated with MGUS shows greater clinical progression and more pronounced abnormalities on nerve conductions studies in patients who have IgM MGUS [14]. These differences between IgG/IgA and IgM MGUS neuropathies, however, are not confirmed in another case series [29].

The pathogenic role of IgG and IgA paraproteins in neuropathy is uncertain. Typical ultrastructural and immunohistochemical changes seen in IgM MGUS neuropathy, such as WML or immunoglobulin deposition on myelin seen in IgM MGUS neuropathy, rarely are present in IgG/IgA neuropathies [22]. There seems to be an overlap between CIDP and IgG/IgA MGUS neuropathy. In some patients who have IgG/IgA MGUS neuropathy, the clinical findings, alterations on electrodiagnostic studies, morphologic abnormalities, and response to treatment are nearly identical to patients who have CIDP [69–71]. This raises the possibility that the IgG and IgA monoclonal gammopathies may be the consequence of neuronal injury rather than the perpetrator.

Pathophysiology

Polyneuropathy associated with MGUS is believed an autoimmune disorder mediated by pathologenic activity of the M protein. Studies on the deposition of complement and IgM of the same light chain type as the M protein on the peripheral myelin sheath have provided the foundation for the possible pathogenic role of these antibodies in mediating neuronal damage. The unique ultrastructural changes and the selective presence of IgM paraprotein within the split myelin sheath further support a link between the neuropathic process and paraproteins in IgM MGUS neuropathy [32,49]. Subsequent studies have identified specific antigens on the peripheral myelin to which the paraproteins from patients who have MGUS-related neuropathy bind, such as MAG, SGPG, and sulfatide [45,72,73]. Passive transfer of disease to animals by injecting serum from a patient who has MGUS-related neuropathy is strong evidence for an antibody-mediated process. Mice injected with purified IgG from patients who have monoclonal gammopathy and multiple myeloma develop a demyelinating polyneuropathy [74]. Serum from patients who have neuropathy and anti-MAG antibody injected into feline sciatic nerve produce widespread demyelination and splitting in the myelin sheath, suggesting the myelinolysis potential of paraproteins [75]. Peritoneal injection into chicken with human IgM anti-MAG antibody shows demyelination in areas where the myelin debris reacted strongly with human IgM, WML, and concentrated IgM deposits in the node of Ranvier and Schmidt-Lanterman incisure [76]. Although the animals are asymptomatic, the pathologic lesions are nearly identical to those seen in humans who have the disease. Rats injected with serum from patients who have MGUS show sensory nerve dysfunction by electrophysiologic testing and degenerative changes in the myelinated nerve fibers [77].

Treatment

Demonstration of a possible pathogenic role of immunoglobulins reactive to myelin components in some patients who have demyelinating neuropathy and monoclonal gammopathies have led to the use of immunomodulatory agents in the treatment of these conditions. Unfortunately, only a few randomized controlled treatment trials have been performed, and most studies involve only a small number of participants. In addition, the long-term benefits of these therapeutic agents and the impact on the natural history of this slowly progressive disease remain uncertain. A double-blind randomized trial of plasma exchange and sham exchanges in 39 patients who had neuropathy and MGUS of IgG, IgA, or IgM subtypes shows improvement in the weakness score of the neuropathy disability scale, average neuropathy disability score, and compound muscle action potential (CMAP) of motor nerve. Patients who had IgG and IgA MGUS had a better response [78]. An uncontrolled study comparing IgM and IgG MGUS polyneuropathy shows a response rate of 27% and 33%, respectively, to plasma exchange with no significant difference between these two groups [29]. A comparative trial of chlorambucil with and without plasma exchanged shows an improvement of the clinical neuropathy disability score (CNDS) with treatment, but the combination of the two therapies is not more effective than chlorambucil alone [79]. A doubleblind, randomized, controlled study of high-dose intravenous immunoglobulin (IVIg) in 11 patients who had IgM MGUS–related neuropathy, most of whom had antibodies reactive to MAG, shows only a modest benefit in motor function in two patients and sensation in one patient [80]. A subsequent randomized, double-blind, placebo-controlled study of IVIg in 22 patients who had demyelinating neuropathy associated with IgM MGUS (11 of the 19 patients who were tested had MAG reactivity) shows a statistically significant decrease in the Inflammatory Neuropathy Cause and Treatment disability score and several other secondary outcome measures in the IVIg-treated group [81].

Corticosteroid when given alone does not seem effective; however, when given in conjunction with other immunosuppressants, there seems to be a 50% response rate [42]. A multicenter, randomized, comparative study of IVIg and interferon-α of 20 patients who had IgM MGUS–related polyneuropathy with anti-MAG antibody activity shows a greater than 20% improvement of the CNDS in 8 of the 10 patients treated with interferon-α compared with 1 of 10 patients treated with IVIg [82]. This finding was not confirmed in a later randomized, placebo-controlled, double-blind multicenter trial [83]. Several other cytotoxic agents have been used alone or in combination with other therapies, including cyclophosphamide [84,85], fludarabine [86,87], and cladribine [88]. High-dose chemotherapy followed by autologous bone marrow transplantation was beneficial to the neuropathy in a patient who had Waldenström's macroglobulinemia and anti-MAG antibody [89]. More recently, rituximab, a monoclonal antibody that binds to the CD20 antigen on B lymphocytes, has been shown to benefit patients who had MGUS-related neuropathy [90,91]; however, an absence of response also is reported [92,93].

Multiple myeloma

Multiple myeloma is a plasma cell dyscrasia characterized by monoclonal proliferation of plasma cells producing a specific immunoglobulin. It comprises 10% of all hematologic malignancies and has an annual incidence of approximately 4 per 100,000 per year [94]. The age of onset ranges from 40 to 80 and peaks in the seventh decade [95]. Patients typically have symptoms of fatigue, weakness, bone pain, and recurrent infections [95]. It may be difficult to differentiate multiple myeloma from other plasma cell dyscrasias; however, several factors may suggest this diagnosis. Serum M protein greater than 3 g/dL, Bence Jones proteinuria, presence of more than 10% plasma cells in the bone marrow, osteolyic lesions, increased plasma cell labeling index, anemia, hypercalcemia, and renal insufficiency all strongly indicate the diagnosis of multiple myeloma [12].

The most common neurologic manifestation of multiple myeloma is nerve root pain resulting from the direct compression of the nerve root by plasmacytomas, foraminal stenosis secondary to pathologic fracture, and collapse of the vertebrae. Leptomeningeal disease is less common [96]. Spinal cord compression is present in 5% of patients, causing back pain, lower extremity motor deficits, and bowel or bladder incontinence [96]. The prevalence of peripheral neuropathy in multiple myeloma is considered low, with only 3% of patients found to have polyneuropathy in a large case series [97]; however, a subsequent prospective study notes a higher incidence of 13% [98], and a subclinical neuropathy was detected in 40% to 60% of patients based on electrodiagnostic or histopathologic studies [99].

Neuropathy associated with multiple myeloma without amyloidosis is a heterogeneous entity. The clinical features of myeloma neuropathy are reported to be similar to that of carcinomatous neuropathy, which can present as a mild sensorimotor, a pure sensory, or a subacute or relapsing-remitting polyneuropathy [100]. Demyelination and axonal degeneration can be seen on nerve biopsy [100,101]. The exact cause of neuropathy associated with multiple myeloma is controversial. Several mechanisms are proposed for the pathogenesis of the neuropathy, including production of humoral substance by the tumor [100], pathogenic effect of the light chain [102], or humoral immune-mediated response [103]. Two cases of multifocal neuropathy resulting from infiltration of the peripheral nerves by malignant plasma cells are described [104]. Treatment of myeloma does not improve the neuropathy, and polyneuropathy also may be caused by medications that are part of the therapeutic regimen for multiple myeloma, such as thalidomide or bortezomib [94].

Waldenström's macroglobulinemia

Waldenström's macroglobulinemia is an uncommon plasma cell dyscrasia characterized by infiltration of lymphocytes and plasma cells in the bone marrow and IgM monoclonal gammopathy. The presence of IgM M protein in isolation is insufficient for the diagnosis and the serum concentration of the monoclonal IgM can vary in macroglobulinemia [105]. Some patients are diagnosed incidentally after the detection of M protein on routine laboratory studies but otherwise are asymptomatic. Most patients have systemic symptoms, such as fever, weight loss, and bleeding; they also may have symptoms resulting from direct tumor infiltration, hyperviscosity syndrome, cold agglutinin disease, and amyloidosis [106].

Peripheral neuropathy is a commonly reported complication of Waldenström's macroglobulinemia with symptoms and findings similar to that of neuropathy associated with other IgM monoclonal gammopathies. The incidence varies from 7% to 46% [107,108]. It is a slowly progressive distal symmetric sensorimotor polyneuropathy. Paresthesia in the distal leg is a frequent early symptom, and sensory abnormalities dominate the clinical picture with mild motor weakness appearing later. Tremor in the arms can be prominent [108]. Electrophysiologic studies show findings of demyelination, although cases of distal axonal neuropathy and neuropathy with axonal and demyelinating features also are reported. Anti-MAG antibodies are present in 50% of patients who have neuropathy [108]. Prolongation of P100 latency on visual evoked response may be present in patients who have neuropathy and IgM M protein that reacts with MAG, suggesting a subclinical central involvement [109]. Morphologic studies of the sural nerve show reduction in the number of myelinated nerve fibers and findings of demyelination and remyelination on teased nerve fiber preparation [108]. In addition, small collections of atypical lymphocytes may be present in the perineurium or endoneurium [110]. Immunofluorescence studies show binding of monoclonal IgM to the myelin sheaths or the endoneurium [108,110–112], and ultrastructural studies show WML [110,113].

Asymptomatic individuals who have Waldenström's macroglobulinemia are not treated [105]. Once symptoms begin, however, alkylating agents or nucleoside analogs, such as chlorambucil and fludarabine, are common first-line therapeutic agents [114]. A combination of plasmapheresis and chlorambucil may be effective in treatment of peripheral neuropathy [115]. Other treatment options for systemic symptoms include combination chemotherapy, splenectomy, and high-dose therapy followed by autologous stem cell transplantation. Newer agents, such as rituximab, interferon-α, thalidomide, and bortezomib, seem beneficial in the treatment of macroglobulinemia [105].

Polyneuropathy, organomegaly, endocrinopathy, M protein, and skin changes syndrome (osteosclerotic myeloma)

Polyneuropathy, organomegaly, endocrinopathy, M protein, and skin changes (POEMS) syndrome—also known as Crow-Fukase syndrome; plasma cell dyscrasia, endocrinopathy, and polyneuropathy (PEP) syndrome; or Takatsuki syndrome—is a rare cause of demyelinating and axonal polyneuropathy [116–118]. The acronym, POEMS, coined by Bardwick and colleagues [119] in 1980, encompasses some of the salient features of this disorder. In addition to these dominant clinical findings, other associated features include sclerotic bone lesions, Castleman's disease, papilledema, thrombocytosis, peripheral edema, ascites, effusions, polycythemia, fatigue, and clubbing. It is not necessary for all of these findings to be present to make the diagnosis. It is suggested that at a minimum, patients should have the two major criteria, which are peripheral neuropathy and a monoclonal plasma cell proliferative disorder, and at least one of the other clinical features [120,121]. The peak incidence of POEMS syndrome is in the fifth decade of life. New symptoms can develop over time, during relapses in patients who previously responded to treatment, and even 10 years after the initial presentation. The monoclonal light chain is all λ restricted in a series of 99 patients [120].

The most prominent clinical manifestation of POEMS syndrome is the progressive symmetric sensorimotor polyneuropathy. All patients have peripheral neuropathy and typically it is the presenting symptom [120]. The initial symptoms, consisting of tingling, paresthesia, and coldness, begin in the feet and seldom are painful. Distal motor weakness follows the sensory symptoms, and both gradually spread proximally. Patients may have severe proximal leg muscle weakness, causing difficulty in rising from a chair or climbing the stairs and distal upper extremity involvement resulting in a weak grip [122]. Motor weakness often overshadows the sensory deficits [120].

Electrophysiologic studies show slowing of the nerve conduction velocity, predominantly in the intermediate nerve segment, and more severe reduction in the CMAP and sensory nerve action potential in the lower than upper limbs [123,124]. Prolongation of the distal latencies can be present but is less prominent than in patients who have CIDP. Conduction block also is less common than CIDP [123]. Electromyography demonstrates distal fibrillation potentials and enlarged, polyphasic voluntary motor unit action potentials with decreased recruitment. Cerebrospinal fluid analysis shows elevated protein levels [122]. Histologic examination of nerve biopsies reveals reduction in the density of myelinated nerve fibers, mild endoneurial and subperineurial edema, and few scattered endoneurial mononuclear cells. There is evidence of axonal degeneration and primary demyelination, as evidenced by the presence of clusters of regenerating meylinated fibers and segmental demyelination and Wallerian degeneration on teased nerve fiber preparations [125,126]. Electron microscopy demonstrates deposition of immunoglobulin that corresponds to the class of the M protein in the endoneurium and in the myelin sheath [125]. UML is suggested to distinguish POEMS syndrome from CIDP and other demyelinating peripheral nerve disorders [126].

The cause of POEMS syndrome is unknown but increased levels of cytokines, specifically vascular endothelial growth factor (VEGF), have been implicated in the pathogenesis [127,128]. VEGF is a multifunctional cytokine that can induce angiogenesis and microvascular permeability by acting on the endothelial cells. It normally is expressed by osteoblasts and also is an important regulator of osteoblastic differentiation [121]. The level of serum VEGF decreases with treatment and this correlates with improvement in symptoms of POEMS and further supports the pathogenic role of this cytokine [129]. VEGF can account for several of the clinical features in POEMS syndrome, including organomegaly, edema, and skin lesions; however, its role in neuropathy is less certain. There is increased expression of VEGF in the vasa nervorum of POEMS syndrome nerve and in nonmyelin-forming Schwann's cells. An inverse relationship between VEGF and erythropoietin has been noted, suggesting involvement of VEGF and erythropoietin in the pathogenesis of the neuropathy [130].

There is no standard treatment for POEMS syndrome. Substantial improvement of neuropathy can result from irradiation of an isolated plasmacytoma or multiple lesions in a limited area. Multiple widespread lesions require systemic chemotherapy (alkylating agents and corticosteroids) and peripheral blood stem cell transplantation should be considered [131]. Intravenous gamma globulin and plasmapheresis are not helpful. Patients who have POEMS syndrome have a relatively favorable prognosis. The median survival is up to 13.8 years in patients who do not receive peripheral blood stem cell transplant. The prognosis is independent of the number of clinical features at the time of diagnosis [120].

Primary (light chain) amyloidosis

Amyloidosis is not a single pathologic entity but describes several disorders characterized by extracellular deposition of misfolded proteins that aggregate as insoluble fibrils in various soft tissues. Amyloid binds to Congo red and displays apple green birefringence when viewed under polarized light [132]. The current classification of amyloidosis is based on the identity of the protein that forms the deposit [133]. Amyloidosis can be familial (ATTR), primary (AL), or secondary (AA). AA occurs as a complication of long-standing inflammation [134]. AL is the most common form in western countries and is associated with the presence of monoclonal light chain or heavy chain (AH) in the serum or urine [135]. Unlike multiple myeloma in which the most common light chain is κ, λ light chains predominate in AL amyloidosis with the ratio of κ to λ light chain of 1:3 [132]. λ VI Subclass is especially common [136]. It is presumed that the unique structure of immunoglobulin light chain in AL results in the greater propensity to form beta pleated sheet. Mice injected with immunoglobulin light chain extracted from patients who have AL have amyloid deposits, whereas injecting Bence Jones protein from patients who have multiple myeloma without amyloidosis does not show amyloid deposits [137]. Multiple myeloma is uncommon in AL and progression to multiple myeloma from amyloidosis is rare [138].

AL amyloidosis is a multisystem disorder that can involve almost any organ. The clinical manifestation depends on the organ or organs most involved. The most common presentations are nephrotic syndrome with or without renal insufficiency, restrictive cardiomyopathy, hepatomegaly, and idiopathic peripheral neuropathy. Certain constellations of physical findings may be diagnostic of amyloidosis, including macroglossia, hepatomegaly, and purpura [135]. Rarely, there can be dramatic spontaneous acral ulcerations. Peripheral neuropathy is the initial feature in up to 17% of patients who have AL amyloidosis with symptoms consisting of numbness, burning, and lancinating pain in the distal legs [139]. Pain and temperature sensory loss are more affected than discriminative perception, although dissociated sensory loss is absent in half of cases. Weakness appears after sensory loss, and sensory and motor deficits gradually extend proximally and involve the upper limbs [140,141]. Carpal tunnel syndrome is present in half of the patients [135]. Unusual presentations are reported, including cranial neuropathy, motor neuron disease, multiple mononeuropathies, and demyelinating polyneuropathy [142–144]. Symptoms of dysautonomia can be prominent, including postural hypotension, diarrhea or constipation, bladder dysfunction, and impotence [145].

Nerve conduction studies are consistent with an axonal polyneuropathy, with the sensory nerve affected more severely than the motor nerves. Needle electromyography shows fibrillation potential and neurogenic changes [140]. Noninvasive autonomic function testing demonstrates abnormalities in variation of heart rate with deep breathing, cardiovascular response to the Valsalva maneuver and orthostatic hypotension. Definite diagnosis requires histopathologic detection of amyloid deposition by biopsy of the sural nerve, abdominal fat pad, rectal mucosa, skin, salivary glands, and bone marrow [141]. The absence of amyloid deposits on the sural nerve does

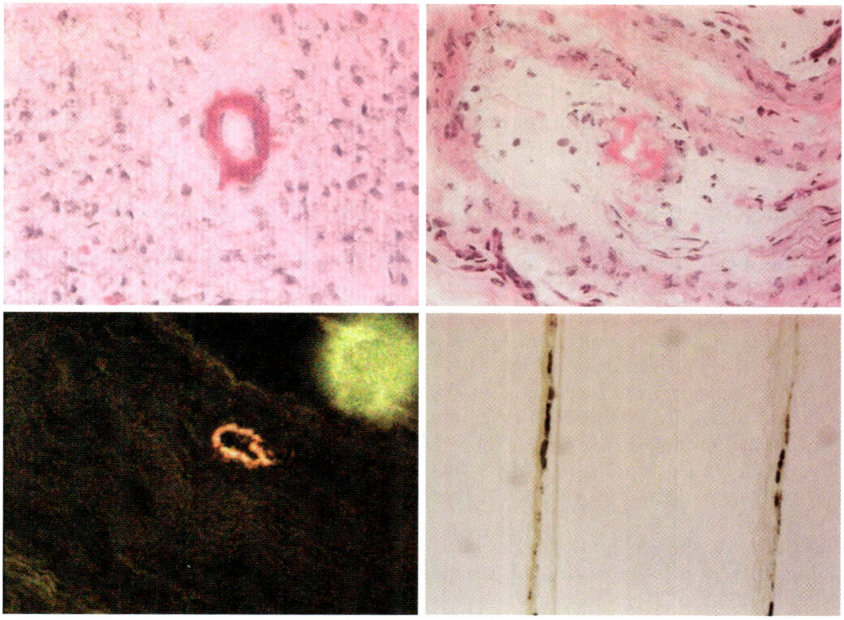

Fig. 1. Top left (crystal violet): crystal violet positive endoneurial amyloid deposit. Top right (hematoxylin-eosin): amorphous endoneurial eosinophilic amyloid deposit. Bottom left (Congo red): congophilic endoneurial amyloid deposit. Bottom right (teased nerve preparation): axonal degeneration.

not exclude the diagnosis of amyloidosis, and multiple biopsies of other tissues or superficial nerves may be needed to confirm the diagnosis (Fig. 1).

The median duration of survival ranges from 2 to 3.8 years [146]. Progressive cardiomyopathy and sudden death resulting from cardiac arrhythmia are the most common causes of death. Symptomatic congestive heart failure is a negative predictor of survival [147]. Exertional syncope is a predictor of sudden death [148]. Current treatment options include alkylating agents and other chemotherapeutic agents, corticosteroid, cardiac transplantation, and stem cell transplantation. Melphalan and prednisone combinations are shown to prolong survival when compared with colchicine in two randomized studies and they are the first-line therapy [138,149,150]. Iododeoxydoxorubicin is shown to cause amyloid resorption and represents a novel treatment option [151]. The therapeutic regimen must be tailored to the extent of systemic disease and the ability of patients to tolerate the treatment.

Summary

Neuropathy associated with M protein represents several distinct syndromes. The presence of a monoclonal gammopathy in patients who have peripheral neuropathy mandates further investigation and surveillance of other organ involvement to detect the presence of a systemic disorder. Although definitive treatment for some of these entities remains limited at this time, an improved understanding of the mechanism of disease will lead to more effective therapeutic regimens.

References

[1] Keren DF. Procedures for the evaluation of monoclonal immunoglobulins. Arch Pathol Lab Med 1999;123:126–32.

[2] Axelsson U, Holmberg A. Frequency of pathological proteins (M-components) in 6,995 sera from an adult population. Acta Med Scand 1966;179:235–47.

[3] Kyle RA, Finkelstein S, Elveback LR, et al. Incidence of monoclonal proteins in a Minnesota community with a cluster of multiple myeloma. Blood 1972;40:719–24.

[4] Crawford J, Eye MK, Cohen HJ. Evaluation of monoclonal gammopathies in the 'well' elderly. Am J Med 1987;82:39–45.

[5] Cohen HJ, Crawford J, Rao MK, et al. Racial differences in the prevalence of monoclonal gammopathy in a community-based sample of the elderly. Am J Med 1998;104: 439–44.

[6] Chazot G, Berger B, Carrier H, et al. Manifestations neurologiques des gammapathies monoclonales [Neurological manifestations of the monoclonal gammopathies]. Rev Neurol 1976;132:195–212 [in French].

[7] Read DJ, Vanhegan RI, Matthews WB. Peripheral neuropathy and benign IgG paraproteinaemia. J Neurol Neurosurg Psychiatry 1978;41:215–9.

[8] Kelly JJ, Kyle RA, O'Brien PC, et al. Prevalence of monoclonal protein in peripheral neuropathy. Neurology 1981;31:1480–3.

[9] Nobile-Orazio E, Marmiroli P, Baldini L, et al. Peripheral neuropathy in macroglobulinemia: incidence and antigen-specificity of M proteins. Neurology 1987;37:1506–14.
[10] Osby E, Noring L, Hast R, et al. Benign monoclonal gammopathy and peripheral neuropathy. Br J Haematol 1982;51:531–9.
[11] Kyle RA. Monoclonal gammopathy of undetermined significance. Natural history in 241 cases. Am J Med 1978;64:814–26.
[12] Kyle RA, Therneau TM, Rajkumar SV, et al. Long-term follow-up of IgM monoclonal gammopathy of undetermined significance. Blood 2003;102:3759–64.
[13] Kyle RA, Therneau TM, Rajkumar SV, et al. A long-term study of prognosis in monoclonal gammopathy of undetermined significance. N Engl J Med 2002;346:546–9.
[14] Notermans NC, Wokke JH, Lokhorst HM, et al. Polyneuropathy associated with monoclonal gammopathy of undetermined significance. A prospective study of the prognostic value of clinical and laboratory abnormalities. Brain 1994;117:1385–93.
[15] Ponsford S, Willison H, Veitch J, et al. Long-term clinical and neurophysiological follow-up of patients with peripheral neuropathy associated with benign monoclonal gammopathy. Muscle Nerve 2000;23:164–74.
[16] Eurelings M, Notermans NC, Van de Donk NW, et al. Risk factors for hematological malignancy in polyneuropathy associated with monoclonal gammopathy. Muscle Nerve 2001; 24:1312–8.
[17] Vuckovic J, Ilic A, Knezevic N, et al. Prognosis in monoclonal gammopathy of undetermined significance. Br J Haematol 1997;97:649–51.
[18] Baldini L, Guffanti A, Cesana BM, et al. Role of different hematologic variables in defining the risk of malignant transformation in monoclonal gammopathy. Blood 1996; 87:912–8.
[19] Cesana C, Klersy C, Barbarano L, et al. Prognostic factors for malignant transformation in monoclonal gammopathy of undetermined significance and smoldering multiple myeloma. J Clin Oncol 2002;20:1625–34.
[20] Nobile-Orazio E. IgM paraproteinaemic neuropathies. Curr Opin Neurol 2004;17:599–605.
[21] Gosselin S, Kyle RA, Dyck PJ. Neuropathy associated with monoclonal gammopathies of undetermined significance. Ann Neurol 1991;30:54–61.
[22] Yeung KB, Thomas PK, King RHM, et al. The clinical spectrum of peripheral neuropathies associated with benign monoclonal IgM, IgG and IgA paraproteinemia: comparative clinical, immunological and nerve biopsy findings. J Neurol 1991;238:383–91.
[23] Suarez GA, Kelly JJ Jr. Polyneuropathy associated with monoclonal gammopathy of undetermined significance: further evidence that IgM MGUS neuropathies are different than IgG-MGUS. Neurology 1993;43:1304–8.
[24] Younger DS, Rowland LP, Latov N, et al. Motor neuron disease and amylotrophic lateral sclerosis: relation of high CSF protein content to paraproteinemia and clinical syndromes. Neurology 1990;40:595–9.
[25] Bain PG, Britton TC, Jenkin IH, et al. Tremor associated with benign IgM paraproteinaemic neuropathy. Brain 1996;119:789–99.
[26] Nobile-Orazio E, Barbieri S, Baldini L, et al. Peripheral neuropathy in monoclonal gammopathy of undetermined significance: prevalence and immunopathogenetic studies. Acta Neurol Scand 1992;85:383–90.
[27] Kahn SN, Riches PG, Kohn J. Paraproteinaemia in neurological disease: incidence, associations, and classification of monoclonal immunoglobulins. J Clin Pathol 1980;33: 617–21.
[28] Steck AJ, Murray N, Dellagi K, et al. Peripheral neuropathy associated with monoclonal IgM autoantibody. Ann Neurol 1987;22:764–7.
[29] Simovic D, Gorson KC, Ropper AH. Comparison of IgM-MGUS and IgG-MGUS polyneuropathy. Acta Neurol Scand 1998;97:194–200.
[30] Latov N, Braun PE, Gross RB, et al. Plasma cell dyscrasia and peripheral neuropathy. Proc Natl Acad Sci U S A 1981;78:7139–42.

[31] Smith IS, Kahn SN, Lacey BW, et al. Chronic demyelinating neuropathy associated with benign IgM paraproteinaemia. Brain 1983;106:169–95.
[32] Takatsu M, Hays AP, Latov N, et al. Immunofluorescence study of patients with neuropathy and IgM M proteins. Ann Neurol 1985;18:173–81.
[33] Nobile-Orazio E, Manfredini E, Carpo M, et al. Frequency and clinical correlates of antineural IgM antibodies in neuropathy associated with IgM monoclonal gammopathy. Ann Neurol 1994;36:416–24.
[34] Latov N, Hays AP, Sherman WH. Peripheral neuropathy and anti-MAG antibodies. Crit Rev Neurobiol 1988;3:301–2.
[35] Hafler DA, Johnson D, Kelly JJ, et al. Monoclonal gammopathy and neuropathy: myelin-associated glycoprotein reactivity and clinical characteristics. Neurology 1986;36: 777–84.
[36] Meucci N, Baldini L, Cappellari A, et al. Anti-myelin-associated glycoprotein antibodies predict the development of neuropathy in asymptomatic patients with IgM monoclonal gammopathy. Ann Neurol 1999;46:119–22.
[37] Kyle RA, Dyck PJ. Neuropathy associated with the monoclonal gammopathies. In: Dyck PJ, Thomas PK, editors. Peripheral neuropathy, vol. 2. 4th ed. Philadelphia: Elsevier Saunders; 2005. p. 2255–76.
[38] Quarles RH. Myelin sheaths: glycoproteins involved in their formation, maintenance and degeneration. Cell Mol Life Sci 2002;59:1851–71.
[39] Ropper AH, Gorson KC. Neuropathies associated with paraproteinemia. N Engl J Med 1998;338:1601–7.
[40] Ellie E, Vital A, Steck A, et al. Neuropathy associated with "benign" anti-myelin-associated glycoprotein IgM gammopathy: clinical, immunological, neurophysiological pathological findings and response to treatment in 33 cases. J Neurol 1996;243:34–43.
[41] Kelly JJ Jr. Dysproteinemic neuropathies. In: Kitirji B, Kaminski HJ, Preston DC, et al, editors. Neuromuscular disorders in clinical practice. 1st edition. Boston: Butterworth Heinemann; 2002. p. 589–97.
[42] Nobile-Orazio E, Meucci N, Baldini L, et al. Long-term prognosis of neuropathy associated with anti-MAG IgM M-proteins and its relationship to immune therapies. Brain 2000;123: 710–7.
[43] Nobile-Orazio E, Latov N, Hays AP, et al. Neuropathy and anti-MAG antibodies without detectable serum M-protein. Neurology 1984;34:218–21.
[44] Hafler DA, Johnson D, Kelly JJ, et al. Monoclonal gammopathy and neuropathy: myelin-associated glycoprotein reactivity and clinical characteristics. Neurology 1986;36: 75–8.
[45] Ilyas AA, Quarles RH, MacIntosh TD, et al. IgM in a human neuropathy related to paraproteinemia binds to a carbohydrate determinant in the myelin-associated glycoprotein and to a ganglioside. Proc Nat Acad Sci U S A 1984;81:1255–9.
[46] Nobile-Orazio E, Hays AP, Latov N, et al. Specificity of mouse and human monoclonal antibodies to myelin-associated glycoprotein. Neurology 1984;34:1336–42.
[47] Kelly JJ Jr. The electrodiagnostic findings in polyneuropathies associated with IgM monoclonal gammopathies. Muscle Nerve 1990;13:1113–7.
[48] Smith IS. The natural history of chronic demyelinating neuropathy associated with benign IgM paraproteinaemia. A clinica neurophysiological study. Brain 1994;117:949–57.
[49] Mendell JR, Sahenk Z, Whitaker JN, et al. Polyneuropathy and IgM monoclonal gammopathy: studies on the pathogenetic role of anti-myelin-associated glycoprotein antibody. Ann Neurol 1985;17:243–54.
[50] Monaco S, Bonetti B, Ferrari S, et al. Complement-mediated demyelination in patients with IgM monoclonal gammopathy and polyneuropathy. N Engl J Med 1990;332: 649–52.
[51] Vital C, Vital A, Bouillot S, et al. Uncompacted myelin lamellae in peripheral nerve biopsy. Ultrastruct Pathol 2003;27:1–5.

[52] Chassande B, Leger J, Younes-Chennoufi AB, et al. Peripheral neuropathy associated with IgM monoclonal gammopathy: correlations between M-protein antibody activity and clinical/electrophysiological features in 40 cases. Muscle Nerve 1998;21:55–62.
[53] Simmons Z, Albers JW, Bromberg MB, et al. Presentation and initial clinical course in patients with chronic inflammatory demyelinating polyradiculoneuropathy: comparison of patients without and with monoclonal gammopathy. Neurology 1993;43:2202–9.
[54] Tagawa Y, Yuki N, Hirata K. Anti-SGPG antibody in CIDP: nosological position of IgM anti-MAG/SGPG antibody-associated neuropathy. Muscle Nerve 2000;129:678–80.
[55] Simmons Z, Albers JW, Bromberg MB, et al. Long-term follow-up of patients with chronic inflammatory demyelinating polyradiculoneuropathy, without and with monoclonal gammopathy. Brain 1995;12:565–84.
[56] Notermans NC, Franssen H, Eurelings M, et al. Diagnostic criteria for demyelinating polyneuropathy associated with monoclonal gammopathy. Muscle Nerve 2000;23:73–9.
[57] Gorson KC, Allam G, Simovic D, et al. Improvement following interferon-alpha 2A in chronic inflammatory demyelinating polyneuropathy. Neurology 1997;48:777–80.
[58] Ryberg B. Multiple specificities of antibrain antibodies in multiple sclerosis and chronic myelopathy. J Neurol Sci 1978;38:357–82.
[59] van Vliet HH, Kappers-Klunne MC, van der Hel JW, et al. Antibodies against glycosphingolipids in sera of patients with idiopathic thrombocytopenic purpura. Br J Haematol 1987; 67:103–8.
[60] Toda G, Ikeda Y, Kashiwagi M, et al. Hepatocyte plasma membrane glycosphingolipid reactive with sera from patients with autoimmune chronic active hepatitis: its identification as sulfatide. Hepatology 1990;12:664–70.
[61] Pestronk A, Li F, Griffin J, et al. Polyneuropathy syndromes associated with serum antibodies to sulfatide and myelin-associated glycoprotein. Neurology 1991;41:357–62.
[62] van den Berg LH, Lankamp CL, de Jager AE, et al. Anti-sulphatide antibodies in peripheral neuropathy. J Neurol Neurosurg Psychiatry 1993;56:1164–8.
[63] Lopate G, Parks BJ, Goldstein JM, et al. Polyneuropathies associated with high titre anti-sulphatide antibodies: characteristics of patients with and without serum monoclonal proteins. J Neurol Neurosurg Psychiatry 1997;62:581–5.
[64] Dabby R, Weimer LH, Hays AP, et al. Antisulfatide antibodies in neuropathy: clinical and electrophysiologic correlates. Neurology 2000;54:1448–52.
[65] Ferrari S, Morbin M, Nobile-Orazio E, et al. Antisulfatide polyneuropathy: antibody-mediated complement attack on peripheral myelin. Acta Neuropathol (Berl) 1998;96: 603–9.
[66] Quattrini A, Corbo M, Dhaliwal SK, et al. Anti-sulfatide antibodies in neurological disease: binding to rat dorsal root ganglia neurons. J Neurol Sci 1992;112:152–9.
[67] Lopate G, Pestronk A, Kornberg AJ, et al. IgM anti-sulfatide autoantibodies: patterns of binding to cerebellum, dorsal root ganglion and peripheral nerve. J Neurol Sci 1997;151: 189–93.
[68] Simmons Z, Bromberg MB, Feldman EL, et al. Polyneuropathy associated with IgA monoclonal gammopathy of undetermined significance. Muscle Nerve 1993;16:77–83.
[69] Di Troia A, Carpo M, Meucci N, et al. Clinical features and anti-neural reactivity in neuropathy associated with IgG monoclonal gammopathy of undetermined significance. J Neurol Sci 1999;164:64–71.
[70] Vital A, Lagueny A, Julien J, et al. Chronic inflammatory demyelinating polyneuropathy associated with dysglobulinemia: a peripheral nerve biopsy study in 18 cases. Acta Neruopathol 2000;100:63–8.
[71] Magy L, Chassande B, Maisonobe T, et al. Polyneuropathy associated with IgG/IgA monoclonal gammopathy: a clinical and electrophysiological study of 15 cases. Eur J Neurol 2003;10:677–85.
[72] Freddo L, Ariga T, Saito M, et al. The neuropathy of plasma cell dyscrasia: binding of IgM M-proteins to peripheral nerve glycolipids. Neurology 1985;35:1420–4.

[73] Maeda Y, Brosnan CF, Miyatani N, et al. Preliminary studies on sensitization of Lewis rats with sulfated glucuronyl paragloboside. Brain Res 1991;541:257–64.
[74] Besinger UA, Toyka KV, Anzil AP, et al. Myeloma neuropathy: passive transfer from man to mouse. Science 1981;213:1027–30.
[75] Hays AP, Latov N, Takatsu M, et al. Experimental demyelination of nerve induced by serum of patients with neuropathy and an anti-MAG IgM M-protein. Neurology 1987;37: 242–56.
[76] Tatum AH. Experimental paraprotein neuropathy, demyelination by passive transfer of human IgM anti-myelin-associated glycoprotein. Ann Neurol 1993;33:502–6.
[77] Lawlor MW, Richards MP, Fisher MA, et al. Sensory nerve conduction deficit in experimental monoclonal gammopathy of undetermined significance (MGUS) neuropathy. Muscle Nerve 2001;24:806–16.
[78] Dyck PJ, Low PA, Windebank AJ, et al. Plasma exchange in polyneuropathy associated with monoclonal gammopathy of undetermined significance. N Engl J Med 1991;325: 1482–6.
[79] Oksenhendler E, Chevret S, Leger JM, et al. Plasma exchange and chlorambucil in polyneuropathy associated with monoclonal IgM gammopathy. IgM-associated Polyneuropathy Study Group. J Neurol Neurosurg Psychiatry 1995;59:243–7.
[80] Dalakas MC, Quarles RH, Ferrer RG, et al. A controlled study of intravenous immunoglobulin in demyelinating neuropathy with IgM gammopathy. Ann Neurol 1996;40: 792–5.
[81] Comi G, Roveri L, Swan A, et al. Inflammatory Neuropathy Cause and Treatment Group. A randomised controlled trial of intravenous immunoglobulin in IgM paraprotein associated demyelinating neuropathy. J Neurol 2002;249:1370–7.
[82] Mariette X, Chastang C, Clavelou P, et al. A randomised clinical trial comparing interferon-alpha and intravenous immunoglobulin in polyneuropathy associated with monoclonal IgM. The IgM-associated Polyneuropathy Study Group. J Neurol Neurosurg Psychiatry 1997;63:28–34.
[83] Mariette X, Jean-Claude B, Chevret S, et al. A randomised double blind trial versus placebo does not confirm the benefit of alpha-interferon in polyneuropathy associated with monoclonal IgM. J Neurol Neurosurg Psychiatry 2000;69:279–80.
[84] Notermans NC, Lokhorst HM, Franssen H, et al. Intermittent cyclophosphamide and prednisone treatment of polyneuropathy associated with monoclonal gammopathy of undetermined significance. Neurology 1996;47:1227–33.
[85] Blume G, Pestronk A, Goodnough LT. Anti-MAG antibody-associated polyneuropathies: improvement following immunotherapy with monthly plasma exchange and IV cyclophosphamide. Neurology 1995;45:1577–80.
[86] Sherman WH, Latov N, Lange DE, et al. Fludarabine for IgM antibody-mediated neuropathies [abstract]. Ann Neurol 1994;36:336–7.
[87] Wilson HC, Lunn MP, Schey S, et al. Successful treatment of IgM paraproteinaemic neuropathy with fludarabine. J Neurol Neurosurg Psychiatry 1999;66:575–80.
[88] Ghosh A, Littlewood T, Donaghy M. Cladribine in the treatment of IgM paraproteinemic polyneuropathy. Neurology 2002;59:1290–1.
[89] Rudnicki SA, Harik SI, Dhodapkar M, et al. Nervous system dysfunction in Waldenstrom's macroglobulinemia: response to treatment. Neurology 1998;51:1210–3.
[90] Levine TD, Pestronk A. IgM antibody-related polyneuropathies: B-cell depletion chemotherapy using Rituximab. Neurology 1999;52:1701–4.
[91] Renaud S, Fuhr P, Gregor M, et al. High-dose rituximab and anti-MAG-associated polyneuropathy. Neuology 2006;66:742–4.
[92] Rojas-Garcia R, Gallardo E, de Andres I, et al. Chronic neuropathy with IgM anti-ganglioside antibodies: lack of long term response to rituximab. Neurology 2003;61:1814–6.
[93] Broglio L, Lauria G. Worsening after rituximab treatment in anti-MAG neuropathy. Muscle Nerve 2005;32:378–9.

[94] Rajkumar SV, Kyle RA. Multiple myeloma: diagnosis and treatment. Mayo Clin Proc 2005;80:1371–82.
[95] Kyle RA, Gertz MA, Witzig TE, et al. Review of 1027 patients with newly diagnosed multiple myeloma. Mayo Clin Proc 2003;78:21–33.
[96] Dispenzieri A, Kyle RA. Neurological aspects of multiple myeloma and related disorders. Best Prac Res Clin Haematol 2005;18:673–88.
[97] Silverstein A, Doniger DE. Neurologic complications of myelomatosis. Arch Neurol 1963; 9:534–44.
[98] Walsh JC. The neuropathy of multiple myeloma. An electrophysiological and histological study. Arch Neurol 1971;25:404–14.
[99] Hesselvik M. Neuropathological studies on myelomatosis. Acta Neurol Scand 1969;45: 95–108.
[100] Kelly JJ, Kyle RA, Miles JM, et al. The spectrum of peripheral neuropathy in myeloma. Neurology 1981;31:24–31.
[101] Ohi T, Kyle RA, Dyck PJ. Axonal attenuation and secondary segmental demyelination in myeloma neuropathies. Ann Neurol 1985;17:255–61.
[102] Dayan AD, Stokes MI. Peripheral neuropathy and experimental myeloma in the mouse. Nat New Biol 1972;236:117–8.
[103] Eng AS. Pathogenesis of myeloma neuropathy through sharing epitopes with myelin basic protein. Lancet 1983;2:801.
[104] Denier C, Lozeron P, Adams D, et al. Multifocal neuropathy due to plasma cell infiltration of peripheral nerves in multiple myeloma. Neurology 2006;66:917–8.
[105] Dimopoulos MA, Kyle RA, Anagnostopoulos A, et al. Diagnosis and management of Waldenstrom's macroglobulinemia. J Clin Oncol 2005;23:1564–77.
[106] Dimopoulos MA, Panayiotidis P, Moulopoulos LA, et al. Waldenstrom's macroglobulinemia: clinical features, complications, and management. J Clin Oncol 2000;18: 214–26.
[107] Logothetis J, Silverstein P, Coe J. Neurologic aspects of Waldenstrom's macroglobulinemia; report of a case. Arch Neurol 1960;3:564–73.
[108] Nobile-Orazio E, Marmiroli P, Baldini L, et al. Peripheral neuropathy in macroglobulinemia: incidence and antigen-specificity of M proteins. Neurology 1987;37:1506–14.
[109] Barbieri S, Nobile-Orazio E, Baldini L, et al. Visual evoked potentials in patients with neuropathy and macroglobulinemia. Ann Neurol 1987;22:663–6.
[110] Vital C, Vallat JM, Deminiere C, et al. Peripheral nerve damage during multiple myeloma and Waldenstrom's macroglobulinemia: an ultrastructural and immunopathologic study. Cancer 1982;50:1491–7.
[111] Propp RP, Means E, Deibel R, et al. Waldenstrom's macroglobulinemia and neuropathy. Deposition of M-component on myelin sheaths. Neurology 1979;25:980–8.
[112] Vital C, Deminiere C, Bourgouin B, et al. Waldenstrom's macroglobulinemia and peripheral neuropathy: deposition of M-component and kappa light chain in the endoneurium. Neurology 1985;35:603–6.
[113] Vital C, Vital A, Deminiere C, et al. Myelin modifications in 8 cases of peripheral neuropathy with Waldenstrom's macroglobulinemia and anti-MAG activity. Ultrastruct Pathol 1997;21:509–16.
[114] Chen CI. Treatment for Waldenstrom's macroglobulinemia. Ann Oncol 2004;15:550–8.
[115] Dalakas MC, Flaum MA, Rick M, et al. Treatment of polyneuropathy in Waldenstrom's macroglobulinemia: role of paraproteinemia and immunologic studies. Neurology 1983;33: 1406–10.
[116] Crow R. Peripheral neuritis in myelomatosis. BMJ 1956;2:802–4.
[117] Nakanishi T, Sobue I, Toyokura Y, et al. The Crow-Fukase syndrome: a study of 102 cases in Japan. Neurology 1984;34:712–20.
[118] Driedger H, Pruzanski W. Plasma cell neoplasia with peripheral polyneuropathy: a study of five cases and a review of the literature. Medicine 1980;59:301–10.

[119] Bardwick PA, Zvaifler NJ, Gill GN, et al. Plasma cell dyscrasia with polyneuropathy, organomegaly, endocrinopathy, M protein and skin changes: the POEMS syndrome; report on two cases and a review of the literature. Medicine 1980;59:311–22.
[120] Dispenzieri A, Kyle RA, Lacy MQ, et al. POEMS syndrome: definitions and long-term outcome. Blood 2003;101:2496–506.
[121] Dispenzieri A. POEMS syndrome. Hematology Am Soc Hematol Educ Program 2005;360–7.
[122] Kelly JJ, Kyle RA, Miles JM, et al. Osteosclerotic myeloma and peripheral neuropathy. Neurology 1983;33:202–10.
[123] Sung JY, Kuwabara S, Ogawara K, et al. Patterns of nerve conduction abnormalities in POEMS syndrome. Muscle Nerve 2002;26:189–93.
[124] Min J, Hong Y, Lee K. Electrophysiological features of patients with POEMS syndrome. Clin Neurophysiol 2005;116:965–8.
[125] Adams D, Said G. Ultrastructural characterization of the M protein in nerve biopsy of patients with POEMS syndrome. J Neurol Neurosurg Psychiatry 1998;64:809–12.
[126] Vital C, Vital A, Ferrer X, et al. Crow-Fukase (POEMS) syndrome: a study of peripheral nerve biopsy in five new cases. J Peripher Nerv Syst 2003;8:136–44.
[127] Watanabe O, Maruyama I, Arimura K, et al. Overproduction of vascular endothelial growth factor/vascular permeability factor is causative in Crow-Fukase (POEMS) syndrome. Muscle Nerve 1998;2:1390–7.
[128] Hashiguchi T, Arimura K, Matsumuro K, et al. Highly concentrated vascular endothelial growth factor in platelets in Crow-Fukase syndrome. Muscle Nerve 2000;23:1051–6.
[129] Kuwabara S, Misawa S, Kanai K. Autologous peripheral blood stem cell transplantation for POEMS syndrome. Neurology 2006;66:105–7.
[130] Scarlato M, Previtali SC, Carpo M, et al. Polyneuropathy in POEMS syndrome: role of angiogenic factors in the pathogenesis. Brain 2005;128:1911–20.
[131] Dispenzieri A, Gertz M. Treatment of POEMS syndrome. Curr Treat Options Oncol 2004; 5:249–57.
[132] Falk RH, Comenzo RL, Skinner M. The systemic amyloidosis. N Engl J Med 1997;337: 898–909.
[133] Nomenclature Sub-Committee WHO-IUIS. Nomenclature of amyloid and amyloidosis. Bull World Health Organ 1993;71:105–12.
[134] Gertz MA. Secondary amyloidosis (AA). J Intern Med 1992;232:517–8.
[135] Gertz MA, Lacy MQ, Dispenzieri A. Amyloidosis. Hematol Oncol Clin North Am 1999;13: 1211–33.
[136] Solomon A, Frangione B, Franklin EC. Bence Jones proteins and light chains of immunoglobulins. Preferential association of the V lambda VI subgroup of human light chains with amyloidosis AL (lambda). J Clin Invest 1982;70:453–60.
[137] Solomon A, Weiss DT, Pepys MB. Induction in mice of human light-chain-associated amyloidosis. Am J Pathol 1992;140:629–37.
[138] Gertz MA, Rajkumar SV. Primary systemic amyloidosis. Curr Treat Options Oncol 2002;3: 261–71.
[139] Kyle RA, Gertz MA. Primary systemic amyloidosis: clinical and laboratory features in 474 cases. Semin Hematol 1995;32:43–59.
[140] Kelly JJ, Kyle RA, O'Brien PC, et al. The natural history of peripheral neuropathy in primary systemic amyloidosis. Ann Neurol 1979;6:1–7.
[141] Adams D. Hereditary and acquired amyloid neuropathies. J Neurol 2001;248:647–57.
[142] Traynor AE, Gertz MA, Kyle RA. Cranial neuropathy associated with primary amyloidosis. Ann Neurol 1991;29:451–4.
[143] Abarbanci JM, Frisher S, Osimani A. Primary amyloidosis with peripheral neuropathy and signs of motor neuron disease. Neurology 1986;36:1125–7.
[144] Vucic S, Chong PS, Cros D. Atypical presentations of primary amyloid neuropathy. Muscle Nerve 2003;28:696–702.

[145] Obici L, Perfetti V, Palladini G, et al. Clinical aspects of systemic amyloid diseases. Biochim Biophys Acta 2005;1753:11–22.
[146] Palladini G, Kyle RA, Larson DR, et al. Multicentre versus single centre approach to rare diseases: the model of systemic light chain amyloidosis. Amyloid 2005;12:120–6.
[147] Kyle RA, Greipp PR, O'Fallon WM. Primary systemic amyloidosis: multivariate analysis to prognostic factors in 168 cases. Blood 1986;68:220–4.
[148] Charnathi B, Dubrey SW, Cha K. Features and prognosis of exertional syncope in light-chain associated AL cardiac amyloidosis. Am J Cardiol 1997;80:1242–5.
[149] Kyle RA, Gertz MA, Greipp PR. A trial of three regimens for primary amyloidosis: colchicine alone, melphalan and prednisone, and melphalan, prednisone, and colchicine. N Engl J Med 1997;336:1202–7.
[150] Skinner M, Anderson J, Simms R, et al. Treatment of 100 patients with primary amyloidosis: a randomized trial of melphalan, prednisone and colchicine versus colchicine only. Am J Med 1996;100:290–8.
[151] Gianni L, Bellotti V, Gianni AM, et al. New drug therapy of amyloidosis: resorption of AL-type deposits with 4'-iodo-4'deoxydoxorubicin. Blood 1995;86:855–61.

ELSEVIER
SAUNDERS

Neurol Clin 25 (2007) 71–87

NEUROLOGIC
CLINICS

Chronic Inflammatory Demyelinating Polyneuropathy

Richard A. Lewis, MD

Wayne State School of Medicine, 8-D University Health Center, 4201 St. Antoine, Detroit, MI 48201, USA

In 1958, as part of a review of 32 patients who had recurrent polyneuropathies, James Austin presented a patient who, over a 5-year period, repeatedly responded to steroids during relapses of the illness. He made the observation that this disorder most likely was related to segmental demyelination and it is clear that he was describing the disorder now recognized as chronic inflammatory demyelinating polyneuropathy (CIDP) [1]. In 1975, the clinical, electrodiagnostic, and pathologic features of 53 patients seen at the Mayo Clinic defined the disorder. That description did not include "demyelinating" in the title but subsequent reports have made it clear that demyelination is a cardinal feature of the disorder [2]. Over the past 30 years, different variants have been described and associated systemic disorders identified. Despite this, there continues to be discussion as to how best to define CIDP and classify the various disorders that are chronic, acquired, immune mediated, and demyelinating. Understanding the different disorders and their similarities, differences, and characteristic features allows clinicians to make appropriate treatment decisions. Box 1 considers CIDP as a symmetric disorder with proximal and distal weakness. The disorders, which have some characteristics that are unique but otherwise have clinical, electrophysiologic, laboratory, and therapeutic aspects similar to CIDP, are considered variants. Some disorders, however, originally considered as variants, now are shown to have characteristic features that make them distinct from CIDP. In particular, these disorders have distinctive clinical, eletrophysiologic or laboratory features and respond differently to therapies. As such, it is imperative to recognize the differences between these disorders.

The reason to consider multifocal motor neuropathy (MMN), the neuropathies associated with IgM paraproteins (IgM neuropathies), and the neuropathy involved in POEMS (polyneuropathy, organomegaly,

E-mail address: rlewis@med.wayne.edu

doi:10.1016/j.ncl.2006.11.003

Box 1. Chronic acquired demyelinating polyneuropathies

I. CIDP and variants
   A. Symmetric proximal and distal motor predominant CIDP
   B. Lewis-Sumner syndrome (LSS) (or multifocal acquired demyelinating sensory and motor neuropathy)
   C. Demyelinating neuropathy with IgG or IgA paraprotein
   D. Sensory predominant demyelinating neuropathy
   E. CIDP neuropathy with central nervous system (CNS) demyelination
   F. Demyelinating neuropathy associated with systemic disorders
      1. Hepatitis B or C
      2. HIV
      3. Lymphoma
      4. Diabetes mellitus
      5. Systemic lupus erythematosus or other collagen vascular disorders
      6. Thyrotoxicosis
      7. Organ or bone marrow transplants
      8. Nephrotic syndrome
      9. Inflammatory bowel disease
   G. CIDP in patients who have inherited neuropathy

II. Distinct from CIDP
   A. Multifocal motor neuropathy (MMN)
   B. IgM paraprotein–related neuropathies
      1. Distal demyelinating neuropathy
         a. With anti–myelin-associated glycoprotein (MAG) antibodies
         b. Without anti-MAG antibodies
      2. Chronic ataxic neuropathy ophthalmoplegia M-protein agglutination disialosyl antibodies (CANOMAD)
      3. Polyneuropathy, organomegaly, endocrinopathy, monoclonal gammopathy, and skin changes syndrome (POEMS)

endocrinopathy, M-protein, and skin changes) as distinct is because they all have features that are unique or not found in CIDP. MMN does not respond to corticosteroids in the same manner as CIDP. POEMS also does not respond to CIDP treatments and the relationship with osteosclerotic myeloma, or Castleman's syndrome, points to the unique pathophysiology of this disorder. The IgM neuropathy associated with antibodies directed against myelin-associated-glycoprotein (anti-MAG) typically is a distal sensory predominant disorder with the distinctive electrodiagnostic featue of distal accentuated slowing and does not usually respond to CIDP treatments. This and the other IgM-related neuropathies, therefore, are clearly distinct from CIDP. The relationship of IgA and IgG paraproteins to demyelinating neuropathies is less clear, however. Patients who have demyelinating neuropathies and IgG or IgA paraproteins have features identical to those of patients who have CIDP. Thus patients with CIDP and IgG or IgA paraproteins are considered as CIDP variants.

Epidemiology

The prevalence of CIDP is difficult to ascertain but estimates range from 0.8 to 1.9 per 100,000 [3,4]. The disorder can affect all ages but is more common in older males. The disease is believed more likely to be progressive in the older age group and relapsing-remitting in younger patients. No specific predisposing factors have been identified. There are conflicting studies on HLA-type associations but no clear genetic predisposition is identified.

The temporal continuum of Guillain-Barré syndrome and chronic inflammatory demyelinating polyneuropathy

The distinction between the demyelinating form of Guillain-Barré syndrome (GBS), acute inflammatory demyelinating polyneuropathy (AIDP), and CIDP is a somewhat arbitrary one based on the time of progression. Acute inflammatory demyelinating polyneuropathy is a monophasic subacute illness that reaches its nadir within 3 to 4 weeks. CIDP is defined as a disorder that continues to progress or has relapses for more than 8 weeks. Patients who have presentations in-between these two time periods are designated as having subacute inflammatory demyelinating polyneuropathy [5,6]. This delineation is complicated in practice, because depending on when physicians see patients, therapeutic interventions likely are initiated before patients reach a specific time point that distinguishes between these entities. Some patients who have CIDP have a subacute, GBS-like onset and the only way to recognize that patients have CIDP is when relapses or progression occurs over the ensuing few months.

The onset of GBS usually is identified easily whereas this is less clear with CIDP. Antecedent events are recognized more clearly in GBS than in CIDP, with more than 70% of patients who have GBS having an identifiable infectious illness, vaccination, or surgery preceding, by 3 to 4 weeks, the onset of symptoms. Most studies, however, find an antecedent event in less than 30% of patients who have CIDP. There are other differences between GBS and

CIDP. The IgG antibodies are found primarily in the axonal form of GBS, acute motor axonal neuropathy, which has some parallels with MMN. Table 1 shows some of the similarities and differences between GBS and CIDP.

Clinical manifestations

The initial description of CIDP in 1975 [2] pointed out the major cardinal features of the disorder. Since then, the following aspects have been emphasized:

1. Progression over at least 2 months
2. Predominant motor symptoms
3. Symmetric involvement of arms and legs
4. Proximal muscles involved along with distal muscles
5. Deep tendon reflexes reduction or absence
6. Cerebrospinal fluid (CSF) protein elevation without pleocytosis
7. Nerve conduction evidence of a primary demyelinating neuropathy

CIDP can be distinguished from chronic length-dependent peripheral neuropathies by the more global muscle weakness of upper and lower extremities (proximally and distally), the general reduction or absence of deep tendon reflexes, and the more aggressive course of the disease. These features point to the multifocal or generalized nature of the disease even at early stages of the illness. Typical cases of CIDP are fairly symmetric, and motor involvement is greater than sensory. Cranial nerve involvement and bulbar involvement occur in 10% to 20% and painful dysesthesias

Table 1
Parallels and differences between Guillain-Barré syndrome and chronic inflammatory demyelinating polyneuropathy GBS and CIDP

Parallels	
Acute	Chronic
AIDP: no antibody	CIDP: no antibody
AMAN: IgG anti-GM1	MMN: IgM anti-GM1
Fisher syndrome: IgG anti-GQ1B	CANOMAD: IgM anti-GQ1B and GT1A
Differences	
Acute	Chronic
Antecedent event in 70%	No antecedent event
Monophasic	Requires continued Rx
Steroids ineffective	Steroids effective in CIDP
IgG antibodies	IgM antibodies
Both axonal and demyelinating forms	Axonal forms not as well described

Abbreviations: AIDP, acute inflammatory demyelinating polyneuropathy; AMAN, acute motor axonal neuropathy; CANOMAD, chronic ataxic neuropathy ophthalmoplegia M-protein agglutination disialosyl antibodies; CIDP, chronic inflammatory demyelinating polyneuropathy; GBS, Guillain Barre syndrome; MMN, multifocal motor neuropathy.

are described in a similar minority of patients. The course is slowly progressive in the majority but a relapsing-remitting course is noted in at least one third, more commonly in younger patients. This latter issue is more difficult to characterize now that treatments are initiated early in the disease, making it difficult to tell whether or not remissions are treatment related rather than the natural course of the disease. The sensory involvement usually is greater for vibration and position sense than for pain and temperature, reflecting the involvement of larger myelinated fibers. As opposed to the motor involvement, the sensory involvement tends to follow a distal to proximal gradient, although finger involvement frequently is as early as toe/foot involvement. Constipation and urinary retention can occur but usually is not an early symptom. Back pain may be present and, rarely, if there is marked nerve root hypertrophy, symptoms of lumbar spinal stenosis and cauda equina syndrome can occur, which may be considered for surgical intervention.

Clinical variants

Lewis-Sumner syndrome

The LSS variant is distinguished by its striking multifocal picture. Originally described in 1982 as a true mononeuropathy multiplex with sensory or motor symptoms in individual nerve distributions [7], the disorder became confused with MMN. There now are several series with more than 100 patients described [8–12] and it has become clear that there are important differences between LSS and MMN (Table 2). The increased incidence of MMN in men is not noted as consistently as in LSS. Pain, paresthesias, and Tinel's signs are seen only in patients who have sensory symptoms. Sural nerve biopsies of patients who have LSS reveal significantly more abnormalities consistent with a demyelinating neuropathy than do biopsies of patients who have MMN. High titers of GM1 antibodies are not reported in LSS, although Oh and colleagues [10] note one patient out of 16 who had mildly elevated titers. CSF protein, although not very elevated, tends to be higher than in patients who have MMN, suggesting

Table 2
Multifocal motor neuropathy versus Lewis-Sumner syndrome

Factors	Multifocal motor neuropathy	Lewis-Sumner syndrome
Gender	Male > female (.2:1)	Male = female
Sensory symptoms	No	Yes
Pain and Tinel's	No	Yes
Sensory conduction	Normal	Abnormal
Anti-GM1 Abs	High titers in 35%–80%	Normal in all patients
CSF protein	Minimal increase	Mild to moderate increase
Nerve biopsy	Normal	90% with demyelination
Prednisone	Poor response	Good response
Plasmapheresis	No response	Some respond

that nerve roots may be more involved in LSS. A significant number of patients who have LSS respond to corticosteroids; 50% (3 of 6) in Saperstein and coworkers' series [8] and 79% (11 of 14) in Oh and colleagues' series [10]. This is in distinct contrast to patients who have MMN, in whom corticosteroids have been remarkably ineffective and possibly deleterious [13]. Most patients who had MMN, who were reported to respond to corticosteroids, at closer view had sensory signs or symptoms that more likely indicated LSS [14,15].

The findings on motor conduction studies in LSS are indistinguishable from those found in MMN. Sensory abnormalities usually are seen, however, particularly if proximal stimulation is used. Whether or not the distal sensory response is abnormal depends on whether or not the conduction block lesion is distal or whether or not secondary wallerian degeneration has occurred. Most patients tend to show some distal sensory amplitude reduction, however. In contradistinction to MMN, in which many reports show normal sensory conduction through areas of motor block, there now is at least one case of LSS demonstrating sensory conduction block that improved with treatment [16].

The pathology of LSS has become more clear. Sural nerve biopsies of patients who have LSS show demyelination in a remarkably high number of patients. An autopsy study of two patients who had LSS showed multifocal inflammatory demyelinating changes as seen in CIDP [17].

Although there are compelling reasons to differentiate LSS from MMN, there seems to be a "gray zone" in which occasional patients cannot be labeled easily as MMN or LSS. There are anecdotal reports of patients who present with a pure motor syndrome but then develop sensory symptoms years later. It also is apparent that some patients have a few sensory symptoms or minor changes on sensory conduction studies and it becomes difficult to decide whether or not these changes are significant enough to warrant a diagnosis of LSS. LSS responds to treatments virtually identically to patients who have typical CIDP and except for the persistent multifocal pattern, there are no other features to distinguish LSS from CIDP. It, therefore, is reasonable to consider LSS as a CIDP variant.

Sensory variants

The sensory predominant form of CIDP may have only clinical sensory symptoms and signs with balance problems, pain, paresthesias, and dysesthesias. As many as 15% of patients who have CIDP may have sensory signs and ataxia as the predominant or only feature [18]. Despite the lack of weakness, the nerve conduction studies demonstrate significant motor conduction slowing and other demyelinating features [18–20]. Some patients may present with sensory symptoms, then develop weakness, and then behave as with the motor predominant form. Some patients only have sensory symptoms, however, despite the motor conduction abnormalities.

The distal acquired demyelinating sensory (DADS) neuropathy frequently is associated with an IgM paraprotein and usually has a more slowly progressive course [21,22]. There are patients, however, who have DADS without a paraprotein. Although half of the patients who have DADS and IgM paraprotein have anti-MAG antibodies, it is not clear that the presence of anti-MAG antibodies distinguishes these patients clinically. With or without anti-MAG antibodies, patients who have IgM neuropathy tend to be resistant to standard CIDP immunosuppressant/immunomodulatory therapies. DADS with an IgM paraprotein with or without anti-MAG antibodies is usually considered distinct from CIDP. The response to treatment of patients who have DADS without IgM parparotein, however, may be more favorable and is considered a variant of CIDP.

CIDP and central nervous system (CNS) disease

The disorders with associated CNS involvement may have optic nerve disorders, hyperreflexia, Babinski's signs, and MRI abnormalities of CNS demyelination but whether or not there is a true association or just coincidental problems remains unclear [23].

Immunopathogenesis

Although the cause of CIDP and its variants is unknown, there is strong evidence to support the concept that the disorders are immunologically based. The cellular and humoral components of the immune system seem to be involved. T-cell activation and crossing of the blood-nerve barrier by activated T cells have been demonstrated along with expression of cytokines, tumor necrosis factor, and interferon and interleukins. As for humoral immunity, immunoglobulin and complement deposition on myelinated nerve fibers have been seen and passive transfer experiments using serum or purified IgG from patients who have CIDP have induced conduction block and demyelination when injected into rats. Despite awareness of the role of gangliosides as target antigens in GBS, anti-MAG, and other neuropathies, however, specific antigens are not identified clearly in CIDP. As such, the immunologic causes of CIDP remain unclear and the disorder likely has multiple triggers [24–26].

Electrodiagnostic features

The cardinal pathophysiologic feature of CIDP is demyelination, which must be determined by electrodiagnostic findings (Box 2) [27] or by nerve biopsy. Nerve conduction studies, therefore, are a critical component of the evaluation. Demyelination causes conduction slowing and conduction block, which can be detected in different segments using different techniques.

Box 2. Electrodiagnostic findings suggestive of demyelination

1. Conduction block
2. Conduction velocity slowing greater than can be explained by axonal loss
   A. Prolonged distal motor latencies
   B. Slow conduction velocity
   C. Prolonged F-wave latency
   D. Prolonged H-reflex latency
3. Temporal dispersion of the duration of the compound motor action potential (CMAP) on proximal stimulation compared with distal stimulation
4. Prolongation of the duration of the distal CMAP

Electromyographers must be able to determine if the latencies and velocities observed are too slow to be accounted for by axonal loss alone. The diameters of motor nerve fibers are between 6 and 14 microns, with longer fibers tapering such that the diameters of the peroneal and tibial nerve fibers in the lower leg are thinner than the median and ulnar nerve fibers at the wrist. The corresponding conduction velocities for motor fibers, dependent on the diameter of the fibers, range from 30 to 70 m/sec in the arms and 25 to 60 m/sec in the leg. When velocities are less than 30 m/sec in the arm (or 25 m/sec in the lower leg), then no normal motor fiber could be involved and a demyelinating lesion is apparent. The problem arises when the velocities are between 30 and 40 m/sec. To determine whether or not that degree of slowing is secondary to demyelination or axonal loss requires a careful comparison of velocity and amplitude. The lower the amplitude, the more likely axonal loss is playing a significant role. With higher amplitudes, axonal loss is less likely to be involved. Electromyographers must be careful, however, because in chronic neuropathies, amplitudes can be normal despite severe axonal loss as a result of collateral sprouting and large motor units. Although needle EMG can help sort this out, it can be difficult to determine whether or not the conduction studies point clearly to demyelination. In addition, the determination of conduction block is problematic. How much amplitude reduction on proximal stimulation should be used as the criteria for block varies depending on the distance between stimuli. There also are several potential technical pitfalls that can confuse electromyographers. In CIDP, it is less crucial than in other disorders to differentiate block from amplitude reduction as a result of temporal dispersion, because both suggest segmental demyelination. Although it is customary to equate conduction block with demyelination, in actuality block is determined by changes at the nodes of Ranvier and paranode and is not exclusively the result of demeyelinating lesions.

Because of all these issues, there has been a great deal of interest in developing criteria to assist clinicians in determining whether or not a neuropathy is demyelinating. There are more than 10 published criteria designed to explicitly define the parameters of conduction changes that reflect a demyelinating neuropathy, not only for CIDP but also for GBS, MMN, and other demyelinating neuropathies. They differ in the degree of slowing, the number of abnormalities required, and the definition of conduction block to determine definite, probable, and possible demyelination. A comparison study of 10 criteria in patients who had GBS, CIDP, ALS, and or diabetic neuropathy revealed sensitivities ranging from 39% to 89% for CIDP. One set identified a patient who had ALS and demyelinating features, and eight of the criteria overlapped with diabetic neuropathy. The three most sensitive criteria to CIDP each overlapped with diabetic neuropathy in more than 50%, which is not surprising because diabetic neuropathies frequently have slowing greater than can be accounted for by axonal loss. Based on these findings, the investigators devised another set of criteria but could come up with only 75% sensitivity while avoiding overlaps with diabetic neuropathy [28]. Despite the inability to obtain ideal sensitivity and specificity, these criteria can be helpful to clinicians and are important for clinical trials when uniformity of diagnosis is critical. Expert electromyographers sometimes can recognize subtle changes in conduction that are beyond the scope of most of these criteria. Prolongation of the distal CMAP duration recently has been shown to be helpful in determining demyelinating disorders and is included in more recent diagnostic criteria [27]. A retrospective analysis of six published criteria with and without prolongation of the duration of the distal CMAP concludes that the addition improved sensitivity and that extensive studies of the upper extremities or all four limbs is important to improve diagnostic yield [29]. This point cannot be overemphasized. To determine whether or not a conduction study points to a demyelinating neuropathy, electromyographers must be confident that the findings are not the result of axonal loss, compression, or technical issues. Enough segments need to be studied to overcome some of these issues. They should be suspect if only one or two segmental changes are found and four limbs should be studied if need be.

Pathologic findings

Sural nerve biopsy has been used to determine demyelination and was a mandatory component of some of the earlier criteria for diagnosing CIDP. It has been shown occasionally to find other abnormalities that occasionally may mimic CIDP (amyloidosis, sarcoidosis, and vasculitis). Because CIDP is a multifocal disorder, and motor nerve fibers tend to be more affected than sensory nerves (the usual nerves used for biopsy), the biopsy sample may not demonstrate the demyelination. In addition, although there is an inflammatory component to CIDP, this may not be prominent and may not be apparent on biopsy. The necessity of nerve biopsy in the diagnosis of CIDP remains controversial. The more recent diagnostic criteria no longer require biopsy for diagnosis, but others argue the importance of biopsy in finding unsuspected disorders or in finding demyelination when electrophysiologic criteria are not met [30,31,68].

The characteristic pathologic features of CIDP are segmental demyelination and remyelination and onion bulb formation [32], usually with some degree of axonal degeneration. Although axonal loss is considered a secondary, bystander product of the inflammatory demyelinating process, the exact mechanism of axonal degeneration is not determined completely. There are varying degrees of interstitial edema and endoneurial inflammatory cell infiltrates, including lymphocytes and macrophages. The macrophages are believed to initiate the demyelination by unraveling and degrading the myelin [33]. Unfortunately, this is not found commonly on most biopsy specimens.

Diagnosing chronic inflammatory demyelinating polyneuropathy

The work-up of any neuropathy includes the electrodiagnostic study to determine if there is demyelination and laboratory studies to look for disorders that either are associated with neuropathy or cause the disorder. If CIDP is suspected, then laboratory studies that are important in helping define or exclude the disorder include serum glucose, glycated hemoglobin, thyroid function studies, hepatitis profiles, HIV testing, and serum immunofixation electropheresis. A lumbar puncture is helpful in that the classic albuminocytologic dissociation is present in more than 90% [33]. A cellular CSF ($>10/\mu L$) suggests that other disorders may be present except when patients are HIV positive, in which case more cells may be seen in the CSF. Nerve biopsy no longer is considered a necessary and required procedure, but is used when the other studies fail to establish the diagnosis clearly. It is recognized that certain genetic disorders of peripheral nerve myelin have characteristics that can mimic the clinical or electrodiagnostic features of CIDP or its variants. A careful family history and appropriate genetic testing should be considered. In particular, Charcot-Marie-Tooth (CMT)-1A, adult-onset CMT-1B, CMT-1X, and hereditary neuropathy with liability to pressure palsies on occasion may be confused with CIDP. In children and patients who have hypertrophic neuropathy, other genetic disorders, including recessive disorders, should be considered.

Diagnostic criteria of chronic inflammatory demyelinating polyneuropathy

During the past 20 years, there have been at least eight different published criteria for CIDP [21,34–38] and there still is no consensus as to the optimal approach to the diagnosis. They all give clinical, laboratory, and electrodiagnostic criteria and most describe definite, probable, and possible categories. The differences between them are related to definitions of the clinical picture, the requirements for nerve biopsy, electrodiagnostic criteria for demyelination, and the number of features required to make the diagnosis. The American Academy of Neurology criteria, designed for research purposes, are considered specific but not sensitive enough for clinical use. Others are sensitive but less specific and may overdiagnose the disorder. The most recent European Federation of Neurological Societies/Peripheral Nerve Society (EFNS/PNS) guideline attempts to provide criteria and recommended practice guidelines based on the currently available literature plus expert consensus [38]. This carefully considered report defines CIDP as typical or atypical, with or without concomitant diseases. MRI with gadolinium of the cauda equina, brachial and lumbar plexus, and other nerve regions to look for enlarged or enhancing nerves may assist in diagnosis, and response to immunotherapy is considered supportive evidence. The diagnostic categories are determined by clinical, electrodiagnostic, and supportive criteria. For definite CIDP, there must be a typical or atypical clinical picture, with clear-cut demyelinating electrodiagnostic changes in two nerves or probable demyelinating features in two nerves plus at least one supportive feature (CSF, biopsy, MRI, or treatment response). CIDP with concomitant disease is relegated to a possible category. Without explanation, these guidelines consider IgM paraprotein–related neuropathies with anti-MAG antibodies as distinct from CIDP but IgM disorders without anti-MAG as a CIDP variant.

The large number of criteria for the electrophysiologic identification of demyelination and conduction block and for the clinical diagnosis of CIDP, with continuing attempts to develop more specific and yet sensitive criteria, point to the difficulties in trying to develop strict criteria for problems that have multiple variations. The EFNS/PNS guidelines have much to recommend them and are an excellent point of reference. Clinicians must assess all patients carefully and individually and convince themselves that patients have a clinical picture that is consistent with the diagnosis and that the electrophysiology or other studies (CSF, nerve biopsy, or MRI) have features suggesting a demyelinating neuropathy. In those instances in which the diagnosis remains unclear, a treatment trial may be indicated and the response to therapy may add clarity to the situation. Although a conclusion may be that response to immunotherapy suggests an inflammatory or immunologic disease, it does not point to a specific disorder.

Treatment

Although there are many treatments available for CIDP, there still is a need for new therapies that are more specific, less toxic, and more beneficial than those currently available. Intravenous immunogolobulin (IVIg) and plasmapheresis (PE) are shown to be effective in double-blind trials and, along with corticosteroids, are the mainstays of treatment. Several immunosuppressive agents are reported to be beneficial (Box 3) but none has been studied rigorously in randomized controlled trials with enough power to provide convincing evidence of efficacy [39]. Many of these remain promising, however.

The use of high-dose cyclophosphamide without stem cell rescue is shown in small series as effective in patients unresponsive to other treatments [40]. The potential benefits must be weighed against potentially life-threatening complications. More experience is needed before strongly recommending this approach.

Azathioprine was tested in 14 patients and not found to have added benefit to prednisone [59].

Although interferon-α and etanercept are considered potential treatments for CIDP, they also are reported potentially to cause the disorder [51–53,55,56]. This points to the potential concerns as treatments are targeted to different cytokines, and neurotrophic factors may have beneficial and injurious immunologic effects.

The strongest evidence of efficacy is for IVIg; four double-blind trials show evidence of benefit in more than 100 patients [60–63]. The benefit of IVIg is not found to be greater than that of PE [64] or prednisone [36]. The problems with IVIg are that the treatment does not, by itself, usually lead to remission and it requires repeated expensive treatments every 2 to 6 weeks. In a 20-year review of 95 patients treated with IVIg, van Doorn and colleagues [65] found that more than 75% improved with IVIg. Of these, however, 85% required repeated treatment but some were able to discontinue treatment at a mean of 3.5 years (median 2 years). Severity at onset and residual deficit were negative predictors of discontinuation. Therefore,

Box 3. Immunosuppressants considered for chronic inflammatory demyelinating polyneuropathy

1. Cyclophosphamide [40,41]
2. Cyclosporine [42–46]
3. Mycophenolate mofetil [47,48]
4. Interferon-β [49,50]
5. Interferon-α [51–53]
6. Methotrexate [54]
7. Etanercept [55,56]
8. Rituximab (anti-CD 20) [14,57]
9. FK-506 [15,58]
10. Azathioprine

although IVIg can control the disorder, unless other treatments are added, many patients may require infusions for many years.

PE also is shown to be efficacious in double-blind trials [66,67] and is equally effective as IVIg [64]. Like IVIg, it is unlikely, by itself, to lead to remission and has the added concerns of venous access, somewhat more complications, and lack of availability in many locales.

Corticosteroids have been reported to be beneficial for more than 20 years, but no large double-blind study has been performed. One randomized controlled study of 14 patients placed on high-dose prednisone (120 mg/day) compared with 14 patients treated with placebo showed clinically meaningful improvement over 12 weeks. Despite the lack of large trials, there have been years of clinical use of oral prednisone and the overwhelming consensus is that corticosteroids, despite the significant side effects, are effective in CIDP. It is more likely than either IVIg or PE to produce a clinical remission. Dosing of corticosteroids, however, is not agreed upon, with different suggested regimens, including daily and alternate-day oral prednisone and monthly or weekly pulse methylprednisolone.

Corticosteroids are compared with IVIg in a double-blind, crossover study of 32 patients and no significant difference is identified with the two treatment modalities [37].

Therapeutic regimens

There are some patients who have CIDP who, at certain times have mild disease with minimal impact on function and quality of life. Treatment might not be initiated in these cases. Most patients are impaired significantly, however, by the disorder and some treatment should be considered. If severe and fulminant, then treatment with an agent with rapid improvement should be considered. This has the advantage potentially of helping patients quickly, reducing the chance for axonal degeneration, and allowing clinicians to determine effectiveness in a short period of time. Either IVIg or PE could be used. Although studies tend to favor IVIg because of fewer side effects, this is somewhat dependent on the center providing the treatment. The major problems with pheresis are related to the use of indwelling catheters. If these can be avoided, then pheresis may, in some instances, be a better choice. If the disorder is more insidious and the goal is to put patients in remission, then corticosteroids might be initiated without IVIg. If IVIg is used, then the optimal regimen is 2 gms/kg divided into 2 to 5 doses. The trial conducted by Mendell and colleagues [63] added a second treatment, 1 gm/kg at 3 weeks, and treatment response was evident within 6 weeks. If patients have a response but then relapse after a few weeks, repeated treatments are considered. A small portion of patients (<20%) may respond to one treatment and not require further therapy. The other patients who respond require treatment at intervals, usually ranging from 2 to 6 weeks. The timing and dosing is titrated to avoid relapses. If patients continue to require high doses of IVIg for many months, then the addition of corticosteroids or other immunosuppressants might be considered. Failure to respond to IVIg triggers intervention with PE or immunosuppression.

If treatments other than corticosteroids, IVIg, or PE are considered, the choice of immunosuppressant depends on several factors and must be individualized. These factors include the severity of the disease, which may indicate more aggressive but more risky treatments; the age and gender of patients, which might limit the use of agents that lead to infertility; and coincident medical problems, which may be complicated by certain treatments. Although most patients respond to one or a combination of treatments, there is a significant minority that continue to progress despite all attempts. This seems to be the appropriate time to consider the high-dose cyclophosphamide regimen [40].

References

[1] Austin JH. Recurrent polyneuropathies and their corticosteroid treatment: with five-year observations of a placebo-controlled case treated with corticotrophin, cortisone and prednisone. Brain 1958;81:157.

[2] Dyck PJ, Lais AC, Ohta M, et al. Chronic inflammatory demyelinating polyradiculoneuropathy. Mayo Clin Proc 1975;50:621.

[3] Lunn MP, Manji H, Choudhary PP, et al. Chronic inflammatory demyelinating polyradiculoneuropathy: a prevalence study in south east England. J Neurol Neurosurg Psychiatry 1999;66:677.

[4] McLeod JG, Pollard JD, Macaskill P, et al. Prevalence of chronic inflammatory demyelinating polyneuropathy in New South Wales, Australia. Ann Neurol 1999;46:910.

[5] Hughes R, Sanders E, Hall S, et al. Subacute idiopathic demyelinating polyradiculoneuropathy. Arch Neurol 1992;49:612.

[6] Oh SJ, Kutkawa K, de Almeida DF, et al. Subacute inflammatory demyelinating polyneuropathy. Neurology 2003;61:1507.

[7] Lewis R, Sumner A, Brown MJ, et al. Chronic multifocal demyelinative neuropathy: a unique disorder with persistent conduction block. Neurology 1982;32:958–62.

[8] Saperstein DS, Amato AA, Wolfe GI, et al. Multifocal acquired demyelinating sensory and motor neuropathy: the Lewis-Sumner Syndrome. Muscle Nerve 1999;22:560–6.

[9] Van den Berg-Vos RM, Van den berg LH, Franssen H, et al. Multifocal inflammatory demyelinating neuropathy: a distinct clinical entity? Neurology 2000;54:26–32.

[10] Oh SJ, Claussen GC, Kim DS. Motor and sensory demyelinating mononeuropathy multiplex (multifocal motor and sensory demyelinating neuropathy): a separate entity or a variant of chronic inflammatory demyelinating polyneuropathy. J Periph Nervous System 1997;2:362–9.

[11] Verschueren A, Azulay JP, Attarian S, et al. Lewis-Sumner syndrome and multifocal motor neuropathy. Muscle Nerve 2005;31:88–94.

[12] Viala K, Renie L, Maisonobe T, et al. Follow-up study and response to treatment in 23 patients with Lewis-Sumner syndrome. Brain 2004;127:2010–7.

[13] Donaghy M, Mills KR, Boniface SJ, et al. Pure motor demyelinating neuropathy: deterioration after steroid treatment and improvement with intravenous immunoglobulin. J Neurol Neurosurg Psych 1994;57:778–83.

[14] Briani C, Zara G, Zambello R, et al. Rituximab-responsive CIDP. Eur J Neurol 2004;11:788.

[15] Ahlmen J, Andersen O, Hallgren G, et al. Positive effects of tacrolimus in a case of CIDP. Transplant Proc 1998;30:4194.
[16] Nikhar NJ, Lewis RA. Multifocal sensorimotor demyelinating neuropathy with persistent conduction block is distinct from multifocal motor neuropathy. Neurology 1998; 50(Suppl):A206.
[17] Oh SJ, LaGanke C, Powers R, et al. Multifocal motor sensory demyelinating neuropathy: inflammatory demyelinating polyradiculoneuropathy. Neurology 2005;65:1639–42.
[18] Rotta FT, Sussman AT, Bradley WG, et al. The spectrum of chronic inflammatory demyelinating polyneuropathy. J Neurol Sci 2000;173:129–39.
[19] Oh SJ, Joy JJ, Kuruoglu R. "Chronic sensory demyelinating neuropathy": chronic inflammatory demyelinating polyneruopathy presenting as a pure sensory neuropathy. J Neurol Neurosurg Psychiatry 1992;55:677.
[20] Sinnreich M, Klein CJ, Daube JR, et al. Chronic immune sensory polyradiculopathy: a possibly treatable sensory ataxia. Neurology 2004;63:1662–9.
[21] Saperstein DS, Katz JS, Amato AA, et al. The clinical spectrum of chronic acquired demyelinating polyneuropathy. Muscle Nerve 2001;24:311.
[22] Katz JS, Saperstein DS, Gronseth G, et al. Distal acquired demyelinating symmetric neuropathy. Neurology 2000;54:615.
[23] Feasby TE, Hahn AF, Koopman WJ, et al. Central lesions in chronic inflammatory demyelinating polyneuropathy: an MRI study. Neurology 1990;40:476.
[24] Kieseier BC, Dalakas MC, Hartung H-P. Inflammatory mechanisms in chronic inflammatory demyelinating neuropathy. Neurology 2002;59(Suppl 6):S7–12.
[25] Rezania K, Gundogdu B, Soliven B. Pathogenesis of chronic inflammatory demyelinating polyradiculoneuropathy. Front Biosci 2004;9:939–45.
[26] Quattrini A, Previtali SC, Keiseier BC, et al. Autoimmunity in the peripheral nervous system. Crit Rev Neurobiol 2003;151:1–39.
[27] Thaisetthawatkul P, Logigian EL, Herrman DN. Dispersion of distal compound muscle action potential as a diagnostic criterion for chronic inflammatory demyelianting polyneuropathy. Neurology 2002;59:1526–32.
[28] van den Bergh PYK, Piéret F. Electrodiagnostic criteria for acute and chronic inflammatory demyelinating polyradiculoneuropathy. Muscle Nerve 2004;29:565–74.
[29] Rajabally YA, Jacob S, Hbahbih M. Optimizing the use of electrophysiology in the diagnosis of chronic inflammatory demyelinating polyneuropathy: a study of 20 cases. J Periph Nervous System 2005;10:282–92.
[30] Bosboom WM, van den Berg LH, Franssen H. Diagnostic value of sural nerve demyelination in chronic inflammatory demyelinating polyneuropathy. Brain 2001;124:2427.
[31] Molenaar DS, Vermeulen M, de Haan RJ. Diagnostic value of sural nerve biopsy in chronic inflammatory demyelinating polyneuropathy. J Neurol Neurosurg Psychiatry 1998; 64:84.
[32] Dyck PJ, Engelstad J, Dyck PJ. Pattern of onion bulbdistribution predicts acquired versus inherited hypertrophic neuropathy. Ann Neurol 1999;46:482.
[33] Prineas JW. Demyelination and remyelination in recurrent idiopathic polyneuropathy: an electron microscope study. Acta Neuropathol (Berl) 1971;18:34.
[34] Barohn RJ, Kissel JT, Warmolts JR, et al. Chronic inflammatory demyelianting polyradiculoneuropathy: clinical characteristics, course, and recommendations for diagnostic criteria. Arch Neurol 1989;46:878.
[35] Ad hoc subcommittee of the American Academy of Neurology AIDS task force. Research criteria for the diagnosis of chronic inflammatory demyelinating polyradiculoneuropathy. Neurology 1991;41:617–8.
[36] Hughes R, Bensa S, Willison H, et al. Randomized controlled trial of intravenous immunoglobulin versus oral prednisolone in chronic inflammatory demyelinating polyradiculoneuropathy. Ann Neurol 2001;50:195–201.

[37] Saperstein DS, Katz JS, Amato AA, et al. Clinical spectrum of chronic acquired demyelinating polyneuropathy. Muscle Nerve 2001;24:311–24.
[38] Joint task force of the EFNS and PNS. European Federation of Neurological Societies/Peripheral Nerve Society guideline on management of chronic inflammatory demyelinating polyradiculoneuropathy. J Periph Nerv Syst 2005;10:220–8.
[39] Hughes RA, Swan AV, van Doorn PA. Cytotoxic drugs and interferons for chronic inflammatory demyelinating polyradiculoneuropathy. Cochrane Database Syst Rev 2004: CD003280.
[40] Gladstone DE, Prestrud AA, Brannagan TH. High-dose cyclophosphamide results in long-term disease remission with restoration of a normal quality of life in patients with severe refractory chronic inflammatory demyelinating polyneuropathy. J Peripher Nerv Syst 2005;10:11–6.
[41] Good JL, Chehrenama M, Mayer RF, et al. Pulse cyclophosphamide therapy in chronic inflammatory demyelinating polyneuropathy. Neurology 1998;51:1735–8.
[42] Odaka M, Tatsumoto M, Susuki K, et al. Intractable chronic inflammatory demyelinating polyneuropathy treated successfully with ciclosporin. J Neurol Neurosurg Psychiatry 2005; 76:1115–20.
[43] Visudtibhan A, Chiemchanya S, Visudhiphan P. Cyclosporine in chronic inflammatory demyelinating polyradiculoneuropathy. Pediatr Neurol 2005;33:368–72.
[44] Matsuda M, Hoshi K, Gono T, et al. Cyclosporin A in treatment of refractory patients with chronic inflammatory demyelinating polyradiculoneuropathy. J Neurol Sci 2004;224:29–35.
[45] Barnett MH, Pollard JD, Davies L, et al. Cyclosporin A in resistant chronic inflammatory demyelinating polyradiculoneuropathy. Muscle Nerve 1998;21:454–60.
[46] Mahattanakul W, Crawford TO, Griffin JW, et al. Treatment of chronic inflammatory demyelinating polyneuropathy with cyclosporin-A. J Neurol Neurosurg Psychiatry 1996;60: 185–7.
[47] Radziwill AJ, Schweikert K, Kuntzer T, et al. Mycophenolate mofetil for chronic inflammatory demyelinating polyradiculoneuropathy: aAn open-label study. Eur Neurol 2006;56: 37–8.
[48] Gorson KC, Amato AA, Ropper AH. Efficacy of mycophenolate mofetil in patients with chronic immune demyelinating polyneuropathy. Neurology 2004;63:715–7.
[49] Cocco E, Mamusa E, Carboni N, et al. Treatment of refractory chronic inflammatory demyelinating polyneuropathy with interferon beta 1B. J Neurol 2005;252:1420–2.
[50] Vallat JM, Hahn AF, Leger JM, et al. Interferon beta-1a as an investigational treatment for CIDP. Neurology 2003;60(8, Suppl 3):S23–8.
[51] Pavesi G, Cattaneo L, Marbini A, et al. Long-term efficacy of interferon-alpha in chronic inflammatory demyelinating polyneuropathy. J Neurol 2002;249:777–9.
[52] Meriggioli MN, Rowin J. Chronic inflammatory demyelinating polyneuropathy after treatment with interferon-alpha. Muscle Nerve 2000;23:433–5.
[53] Lisak RP. Type I interferons and chronic inflammatory demyelinating polyneuropathy: treatment or cause? Muscle Nerve 2000;23:307–9.
[54] Fialho D, Chan YC, Allen DC, et al. Treatment of chronic inflammatory demyelinating polyradiculoneuropathy with methotrexate. J Neurol Neurosurg Psychiatry 2006;77:544–7.
[55] Chin RL, Sherman WH, Sander HW, et al. Etanercept (Enbrel) therapy for chronic inflammatory demyelinating polyneuropathy. J Neurol Sci 2003;210:19–21.
[56] Richez C, Blanco P, Lagueny A, et al. Neuropathy resembling CIDP in patients receiving tumor necrosis factor-alpha blockers. Neurology 2005;64:1468–70.
[57] Gorson KC, Natarajan N, Ropper AH, et al. Rituximab treatment in patients with IVIg-dependent immune polyneuropathy: a prospective pilot trial. Muscle Nerve 2006;35:66–9.
[58] Wilson JR, Conwit RA, Eidelman BH, et al. Sensorimotor neuropathy resembling CIDP in patients receiving FK506. Muscle Nerve 1994;17:528–32.
[59] Dyck PJ, O'Brien P, Swanson C, et al. Combined azathioprine and prednisone in chronic inflammatory polyneuropathy. Neurology 1985;35:1173–6.

[60] van Doorn PA, Brand A, Strngers PF, et al. High-dose intravenous immunoglobulin treatment in chronic inflammatory demyelinating polyneuropathy: a double-blind, placebo-controlled, crossover study. Neurology 1990;40:209–12.

[61] Vermeulen M, van Doorn PA, Brand A, et al. Intravenous immunoglobulin treatment in patients with chronic inflammatory demyelinating polyneruopathy: a double blind, placebo controlled study. J Neurol Neurosurg Psychiatry 1993;56:36–9.

[62] Hahn AF, Bolton CF, Zochodne D, et al. Intravenous immunoglobulin treatment (IVIg) in chronic inflammatory demelingating polyneuropathy (CIDP): a double-blind placebo-controlled cross-over study. Brain 1996;119:1067–78.

[63] Mendell JR, Barohn RJ, Freimer ML, et al. Randomized controlled trial of IVIg in untreated chronic inflammatory demyelinating polyradiculoneuropathy. Neurology 2001;56:445–9.

[64] Dyck PJ, Litchy WJ, Kratz KM, et al. A plasma exchange versus immune globulin infusion trial in chronic inflammatory demyelinating polyradiculoneuropathy. Ann Neurol 1994;36: 838–45.

[65] van Doorn PA, Dippel DWJ, van Burken MMG, et al. Long term IV immunoglobulin treatment in CIDP. J Periph Nerv Syst 2003;8(Suppl 1):70.

[66] Dyck PJ, Daube J, O'Brien, et al. Plasma exchange in chronic inflammatory demyelinating polyradiculoneuropathy. N Engl J Med 1986;314:461–5.

[67] Hahn AF, Bolton CF, Pillay N, et al. Plasma exchange therapy in chronic inflammatory demyelinating polyneuropathy (CIDP): a double-blind, sham-controlled cross-over study. Brain 1996;119:1055–66.

[68] Vallat JM, Tabaraud F, Magy L, et al. Diagnostic value of nerve biopsy for atypical chronic inflammatory demyelinating polyneuropathy: evaluation of eight cases. Muscle Nerve 2003; 27:478–85.

ELSEVIER
SAUNDERS

Neurol Clin 25 (2007) 89–113

NEUROLOGIC
CLINICS

Vasculitic Neuropathies

Ted M. Burns, MD[a], Gregory A. Schaublin, MD[a], P. James B. Dyck, MD[b,*]

[a]*Department of Neurology, University of Virginia, Charlottesville, VA 22908, USA*
[b]*Peripheral Neuropathy Research Laboratory, Mayo Clinic College of Medicine, 200 First Street SW, Rochester, MN 55905, USA*

The various forms of vasculitis comprise a heterogenous group of disorders that can affect different organ systems and different blood vessel calibers. Many forms of vasculitis share the common feature of frequently affecting the peripheral nervous system. Several schemes aimed at classifying the vasculitides are offered. The purpose of this review is to bring neurologists up to date on the current classification and treatment of the most common forms of vasculitic neuropathy.

Classification

The classification of the vasculitides has become increasingly sophisticated over the past half-century [1–4]. The classification, however, remains complex and still is unsettled. For neurologists, it is helpful to conceptualize the classification in terms of (1) clinical characteristics (eg, systemic or nonsystemic, chronic or acute, or monophasic) and (2) histopathologic features (nerve large arteriole vasculitis or nerve microvasculitis). This construct has limits, however, because any binary classification scheme of vasculitis necessitates dividing what likely is actually a continuum. For example, it is proposed that some cases of nonsystemic vasculitic neuropathy (NSVN) actually are a relatively localized form of (systemic) microscopic polyangiitis (MPA) [5]. With regard to classification based on vessel size, the marked overlap in vessel size involvement among the various vasculitides also must be considered. Nonetheless, the authors believe classification based on clinical and histopathologic features has merit because it allows for a characterization of an individual's vasculitic neuropathy that provides

* Corresponding author.
E-mail address: dyck.pjames@mayo.edu (P.J.B. Dyck).

doi:10.1016/j.ncl.2006.11.002

information about prognosis and provides a blueprint for treatment and other management.

From a clinical standpoint, vasculitis of nerve needs to be thought of as systemic or nonsystemic. The systemic vasculitides commonly are divided into primary systemic vasculitis, of which there is no known cause, and secondary systemic vasculitis, in which a virus, drug, or connective tissue disease is responsible for vessel wall inflammation [6–8]. Vasculitides are classified further by the kind and size of blood vessels involved, organ involvement, disease associations, underlying mechanisms, and, sometimes, autoantibody profiles [9]. The primary systemic vasculitides most likely to cause vasculitic neuropathy include polyarteritis nodosa (PAN), Wegener's granulomatosis, Churg-Strauss syndrome, and MPA [1,2,7,10]. Of these, MPA is perhaps the one that causes vasculitic neuropathy most commonly [10]. Secondary causes of systemic vasculitis involving peripheral nerves include connective tissue diseases, such as rheumatoid arthritis (RA), systemic lupus erythematosis, and Sjögren's syndrome. For example, RA, which affects 1% to 2% of the population, may evolve into rheumatoid vasculitis in 2% to 15% of patients who have RA, and half of these patients develop neuropathy on a vasculitic basis [11–14]. Mixed type II cryoglobulinemic vasculitis associated with hepatitis C infection is another secondary form of vasculitis. Other viruses associated with vasculitis are HIV and cytomegalovirus. Sarcoidosis affecting nerve also may cause an angiitis [15,16]. Vasculitis that seems confined to the nerve and muscle classically is termed NSVN [5,17–19]. An important distinction between systemic vasculitic neuropathy (SVN) and NSVN is that NSVN usually is not fatal, whereas untreated SVN often is fatal. Early on, it may be difficult to distinguish NSVN from SVN; approximately 10% of cases of initially what seems to be NSVN ultimately become systemic vasculitis [19,20]. For this reason, the evaluation in the early phase for what seems to be NSVN should be no different than that for SVN. Some investigators suggest, however, that NSVN simply is part of a continuum in the spectrum of systemic vasculitis. In favor of this view is the demonstration of clinicopathologic and pathologic similarities between NSVN and MPA. Alternatively, NSVN and MPA differ in age of onset, severity, and presence of antineutrophil cytoplasmic antibody (ANCA) with perinuclear immunofluorescence pattern directed against myeloperoxidase (MPO) (p-ANCA), which is absent in NSVN [5].

From the perspective of peripheral nerve histopathology, the authors favor a separation of necrotizing vasculitis of nerve into two groups, nerve large arteriole vasculitis (Fig. 1) and nerve microvasculitis (Fig. 2) [4]. The separation is based on differences in the size and kind of vessels involved, disease associations, and, perhaps, course, outlook, and treatment considerations. Again, classification based on vessel size must acknowledge the overlap of vessel involvement [9]. Large arteriole vasculitis of nerve has involvement of small arteries, large arterioles, and a varying degree of smaller vessels [4]. In large arteriole SVN, pathologic changes typically are found in epineural and perineural vessels 75 to 200 microns in diameter

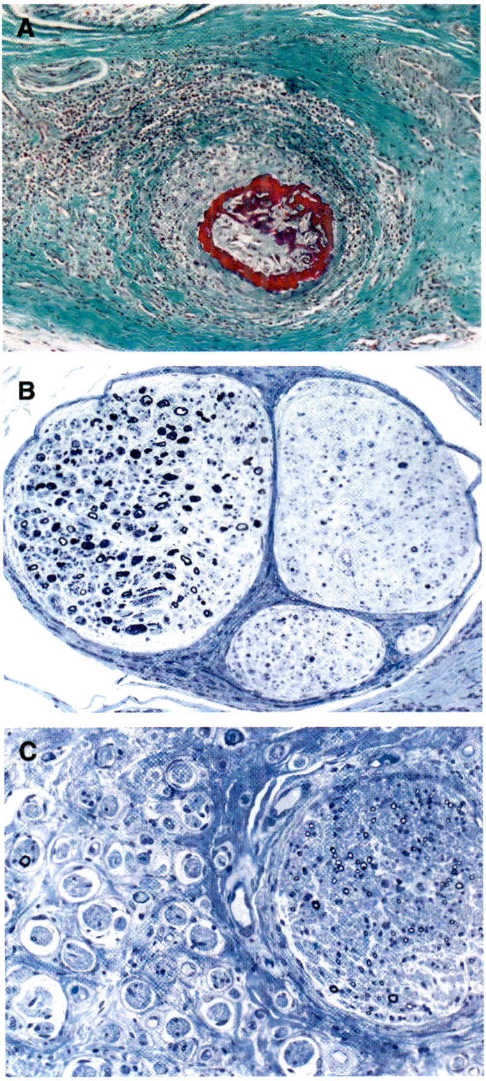

Fig. 1. Nerves from patients who have large nerve vessel necrotizing vasculitis demonstrating changes typically seen in chronic ischemic damage. (*A*) A cross-section of sural nerve in paraffin showing an arteriole with an inflammatory mononuclear cell infiltrate and fibrinoid necrosis of a sector of the wall (red) (trichrome stain). (*B*) Transverse semithin epoxy sections stained with methylene blue demonstrating multifocal fiber loss. The fascicle on the left shows relative preservation of myelinated fibers, whereas the fascicles on the right are devoid of myelinated fibers. (*C*) Transverse semithin epoxy section showing the injury neuroma and microfascicular (*left*). Note the parent fascicle on the right. These ischemic changes (multifocal fibers loss at injury neuroma) are found frequently in nerves of patients who have either large nerve vessel (arteriole) or small nerve vessel (microvessel) vasculitis.

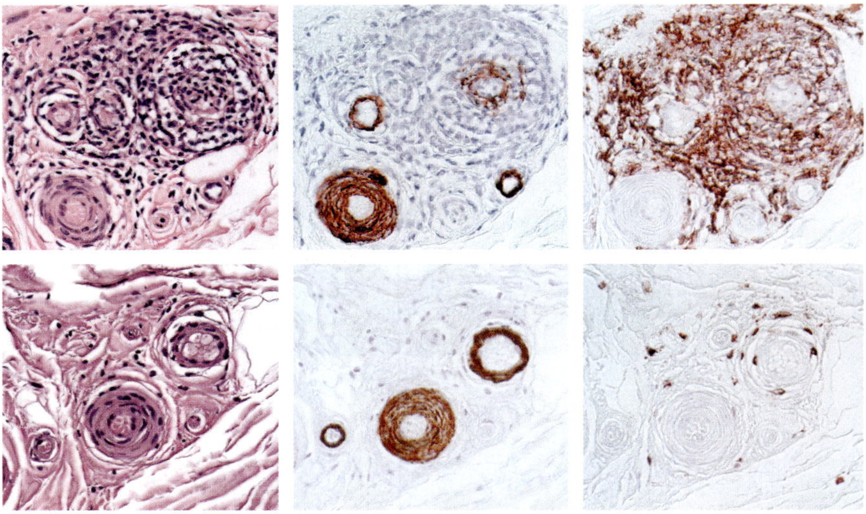

Fig. 2. Serial skip paraffin sections of a microvessel at (*upper row*) and below (*lower row*) regions of microvasculitis in the sural nerve of a patient who has LRPN. The sections in the left column are stained with hematoxylin and eosin; the sections in the middle column are reacted with antihuman smooth muscle actin; and the sections in the right column are reacted with CD45 (lymphocytes). The smooth muscle of the tunica media in the regions of the microvasculitis (*upper row, middle panel*) are separated by mononuclear cells, fragmented, and decreased in amount. The changes are those of a focal microvasculitis. These changes are seen in the diabetic and the nondiabetic conditions.

[17,21]. Almost all nerve vessels are small vessels, so nerve large arteriole vasculitis still is a "small vessel" vasculitis, but the nerve vessels involved—although small—are larger than those in nerve microvasculitis. Nerve large arteriole vasculitis usually is associated with RA, PAN, Churg-Strauss syndrome, or Wegener's granulomatosis. Nerve microvasculitis is less well defined but involves a different spectrum of vessels—the smallest arterioles (<40 μm), microvessels, venules, and not the large arterioles [4]. Nerve microvasculitis occurs in NSVN, MPA, immune sensorimotor polyneuropathies sometimes associated with sicca, classic Sjögren's syndrome, paraneoplastic neuropathies, and virus-associated neuropathies (some cases of HIV, cytomegalic, hepatitis C, and perhaps others).

The authors also believe that many autoimmune, monophasic, or relapsing plexopathies—or, more accurately, radiculoplexus neuropathies (RPNs)—also should be classified as nerve microvasculitis. These include diabetic lumbosacral RPN (DLRPN) (also known by diabetic amyotrophy, proximal diabetic neuropathy, and other names), nondiabetic LRPN, and immune and inherited brachial plexus neuropathies (BPNs) (also called neuralgic amyotrophy and hereditary neuralgic amyotrophy). Histopathologic study of LRPN has demonstrated features suggesting nerve microvasculitis (see Fig. 2). The pathology of BPN (eg, cervical RPN) has not been studied as extensively as LRPN but nerve microvasculitis is demonstrated in some cases [22–24]. With respect to clinical classification, RPN is interesting because it does not fall clearly on one side of the systemic versus nonsystemic scheme. RPN probably has more features in common with NSVN: vessel involvement seems to be confined primarily to nerves and does not evolve to involve other organs (nonetheless, the unexplained weight loss of RPN indicates at least some effects outside of the peripheral nervous system); vessels involved in NSVN and RPN are similar in size; and NSVN and RPN are not fatal disorders. But it must be recognized that RPN differs from NSVN in the distribution of nerve involvement and by being monophasic. This unique temporal profile places the focus of RPN (and BPN) treatment on acute intervention rather than on relapse prevention. Thus, treatment of RPN (and BPN) differs from treatment of more typical NSVN or SVN. Nonetheless, the authors believe that the RPNs probably are stereotypical, monophasic forms of NSVN.

Clinical and diagnostic features of vasculitic neuropathy

The typical clinical features of vasculitic neuropathy are acute to subacute onset of painful sensory or sensorimotor deficits [8,25]. The most common presentations are of multiple mononeuropathies or an asymmetric polyneuropathy [12,17,21,26–33]. Commonly, the progression of mononeuropathies is so rapid that on presentation the deficits seem confluent. For this reason, it is imperative that patients are queried in detail about the clinical course of the initial and all subsequent deficits. Although any nerve may be affected, most patients who have SVN or NSVN experience their initial symptoms in the lower extremities, typically the peroneal or tibial divisions of the sciatic nerve (the distribution of nerve involvement is different for RPN and BPN). A distal, symmetric polyneuropathy is less common, but vasculitic neuropathy infrequently may present in this manner [10,27,30,31]. Accompanying constitutional symptoms may include myalgias, arthralgias, weight loss, respiratory symptoms, hematuria, abdominal pain, rash, or night sweats. These systemic symptoms infrequently may be minimal or absent early [12,17,21,26–33].

Electrodiagnostic studies help reveal characteristic vasculitic neuropathy findings, including acute-to-subacute axonal loss of sensory and motor nerve fibers, often in a patchy, multifocal distribution. In contrast, studies that show only conduction slowing or block at common entrapment sites (such as median neuropathy at the wrist or peroneal neuropathy across the fibular head) should lead clinicians to consider other causes that increase the likelihood for compression neuropathies, such as some forms of diabetic neuropathies (carpal tunnel syndrome and ulnar neuropathy at the elbow), nonvasculitic RA, or hereditary neuropathy with liability to pressure palsies [18].

Laboratory evaluation of suspected cases of vasculitic neuropathy should include a complete blood count (CBC), metabolic panel (electrolytes, blood urea nitrogen, creatinine, and glucose), erythrocyte sedimentation rate (ESR), C-reactive protein, antinuclear antibody, rheumatoid factor, ANCA with cytoplasmic immunofluorescence pattern directed against the neutrophil serine protease proteinase 3 (PR3/c-ANCA) and MPO/p-ANCA, hepatitis B and C panel, and cryoglobulins [34]. Serum complement determinations are appropriate in suspected mixed cryoglobulinemia or systemic lupus syndromes. In many cases, it also is appropriate to check extractable nuclear antigen, serum angiotensin-converting enzyme level, serum protein electrophoresis, and HIV. Cerebrospinal fluid analysis usually is not helpful, except to aid in the investigation of mimickers, including infectious (eg, Lyme disease) or other inflammatory causes (eg, carcinomatous root involvement). In SVN, serologic testing is abnormal and helps define the cause or syndrome further (Table 1). In NSVN, the ESR or C-reactive protein may be elevated slightly, but other markers of inflammation or systemic disease usually are normal.

Because of the need for long-term treatment with potentially toxic medications, the diagnosis of vasculitis usually requires histologic confirmation. This is so especially for Churg-Strauss syndrome, Wegener's granulomatosis, and MPA. Alternatively, because PAN affects larger vessels, diagnostic confirmation sometimes can be achieved by angiography. In general, the sensitivity of a nerve or nerve and muscle biopsy is believed to be approximately 60% for vasculitis if inflammation and vessel wall destruction are mandatory criteria [30,35]. Sensitivity of nerve biopsy increases but specificity decreases if other features, such as ischemic injury (multifocal nerve fiber loss) with inflammation but without vessel wall destruction [30,32,35], are considered sufficient for diagnosis. Some investigators recommend biopsy of nerve and muscle, for example the superficial peroneal nerve and ipsilateral peroneus brevis muscle [30,35]. The sensitivity of a nerve biopsy depends on several factors, including patient selection, which nerve is biopsied, timing in relation to symptoms, and the histologic criteria required for diagnosis.

In large arteriole SVN, pathologic changes typically are found in epineural and perineural vessels 75 to 200 microns in diameter [17,21]. The vessels involved in microvasculitis usually are smaller arterioles without an internal elastic lamina (ie, <40 μm), microvessels, and venules [4]. Whereas in nerve large arteriole vasculitis, fibrinoid necrosis of the tunica media often is prominent and characteristic, obvious fibrinoid necrosis usually is not found in nerve microvasculitis. In microvasculitis, there is inflammation of the vessel wall with separation, fragmentation, and necrosis of the thin tunica media (see Fig. 2). In both groups of necrotizing vasculitis, evidence of ischemic injury or repair (multifocal fiber loss, injury neuroma, neovascularization, and perineurial thickening) often is found [36–39]. Inflammatory cells separate muscle layers. With increased severity there is separation of the muscle leaflets, which become fragmented and separated from the microvessel. Obvious occlusion of vessels usually is not encountered but recent or previous bleeding (hemosiderin in macrophages) is typical. Hemosiderin typically is found adjacent to affected microvessels. Typical of vessel inflammation is angioneogenesis—closely spaced, thin-walled microvessels in regions of previously ischemic areas. The authors have found all stages of perineurial injury associated with microvasculitis—from acute fibrinoid degeneration to thickening and scarring and regrowth of microfasciculi through the perineurium into the epineurium (injury neuroma). Although segmental demyelination may be found in acute ischemic injury, it usually is at borders of ischemic injury and may relate to axonal atrophy (distal to sites of axonal stasis) or to sites of axonal enlargement. Immune complex deposition in vessel walls is seen commonly in SVN and NSVN.

Clinical features of the primary systemic vasculitides

Microscopic polyangiitis

MPA is perhaps the form of systemic vasculitis associated most commonly with vasculitic neuropathy [10]. In MPA, arterioles, capillaries, and venules are affected. Many of these patients present with systemic, renal, or cutaneous manifestations of vasculitis (see Table 1). More than half of patients who have MPA develop neuropathy.

Polyarteritis nodosa

PAN is a primary vasculitis affecting vessels larger than those affected by the other vasculitides that affect nerves, namely the medium and small muscular arteries (typically not arterioles, capillaries, and venules) [40,41]. PAN is distinct from and less common than the ANCA-related systemic vasculitides. In one analysis of systemic vasculitis, only 2% of the patients could be classified as true PAN [42]. Vasculitic neuropathy occurs in up to 75% of patients who have PAN [28]. Other clinical features of PAN are listed in Table 1. PAN commonly is associated with hepatitis B (one third to one half of patients) and may behave more aggressively in cases where it is associated with hepatitis B [28,43].

Churg-Strauss syndrome

Churg-Strauss syndrome affects small- to medium-sized vessels (arterioles, venules, capillaries, and small arteries). The presentation usually is of asthma, pulmonary infiltrates, fever, and eosinophilia (see Table 1). Neuropathy is common, occurring in 65% to 80% of patients [27,32,42,44]. Of the ANCA-related syndromes, Churg-Strauss syndrome is most likely to present as a vasculitic neuropathy, occurring in more than 20% of cases [42].

Table 1
A partial list of clinical characteristics and treatments for six common forms of systemic vasculitis affecting small or medium-sized vessels of nerve

Characteristic	Wegener's Granulomatosis	Churg-Strauss syndrome	Polyarteritis nodosa	Microscopic polyangiitis	Rheumatoid vasculitis	Mixed cryoglobulinemia
Peripheral nerve disease	40%–50%	65%–80%	35%–75%	60%–70%	50% (of cases of rheumatoid vasculitis—a secondary vasculitis that occurs in 5%–15% of cases of RA)	20%–90%
Upper airway disease	95%	50%–60%	No	No		No
Pulmonary disease, radiographic nodule/infiltrates	70%–85%	40%–70%	No	15%–70%	5%–30%	No
Glomerulonephritis	70%–80%	10%–40%	No	75%–90%	10%–25%	33%–55%
Gastrointestinal	<5%	30%–50%	15%–55%	30%	10%–30%	<20%
Arthralgia/arthritis	60%–70%	40%–50%	50%–75%	40%–60%	90%–100%	20%–90%
Cardiac	10%–25%	10%–40%	5%–30%	10%–15%	10%–30%	No
Skin	40%–50%	50%–55%	25%–60%	50%–65%	30%–90%	60%–100% (eg, palpable purpura)
Central nervous system	5%–10%	5%–30%	3%–30%	10%–15%	5%–15%	No
c-ANCA (PR3)	75%–90%	3%–35%	Rare	10%–50%		No
p-ANCA (MPO)	5%–20%	2%–50%	Rare	50%–80%		No

Vessel size involved	Small to medium vessels (eg, capillaries, venules, arterioles, arteries)	Small to medium vessels	Medium to small arteries (not arterioles, capillaries or venules)	Small vessels (eg, capillaries, arterioles, venules)	Medium to small arteries (histologically indistinguishable from polyarteritis nodosa)	Small (eg, capillaries, arterioles, venules)
Other features		Asthma, fever, hypereosinophilia	Fever, hypertension	Fever	Elevated serum rheumatoid factor and ESR, extraarticular disease (eg, nodules) fever, weight loss, scleritis	Hepatitis C infection, mixed cryoglobulins, fatigue, Raynaud's phenomenon, leg ulcers, sicca syndrome
Treatment	Glucocorticoid plus cytotoxic agent	Glucocorticoid. Add cyclophosphamide if life-threatening disease.	Glucocorticoid. Add cyclophosphamide if life-threatening disease	Glucocorticoid plus cytotoxic agent, such as cyclophosphamide	Glucocorticoid. Add cyclophosphamide if life-threatening vasculitis or if not responsive to steroids alone.	Pegylated interferon-α +/− ribavirin. Plasma exchange in fulminent cases. Monitor for interferon alpha-associated exacerbation of vasculitis.
Viral association?			Sometimes associated with hepatitis B, hepatitis C, or HIV. If so, antiviral agent or plasmapheresis should be considered.			Hepatitis C >80%

Modified and reprinted from Langford CA. Vasculitis. J Allergy Clin Immunol 2003;111:S602–12; with permission.

Wegener's granulomatosis

Classically a disease of the upper and lower airways, Wegener's granulomatosis involves mainly capillaries, arterioles, and venules. Peripheral nerve involvement is reported in 14% to 40% of cases [45,46] (see Table 1), usually presenting as painful multiple mononeuropathies or asymmetric polyneuropathy, although cranial neuropathies may occur less commonly [31].

Clinical features of secondary systemic vasculitis

The following are examples of vasculitis triggered by a known underlying cause, such as collagen vascular disease, viral infection, or paraneoplastic disorder.

Rheumatoid vasculitis

As in PAN, rheumatoid vasculitis affects small- to medium-sized arteries, usually sparing the arterioles, capillaries, and venules [47]. Rheumatoid vasculitis usually occurs as a late manifestation of severe seropositive disease. With more modern rheumatoid therapies, the incidence of rheumatoid vasculitis is declining and is less common than the ANCA-related syndromes (see Table 1). Because this complication of RA is seen primarily in established disease, physicians should consider other causes of vasculitis in patients who are positive for rheumatoid factor who do not have an established RA diagnosis, such as cryoglobulinemia, Wegener's granulomatosis, or extraglandular Sjögren's syndrome.

In contradistinction to rheumatoid vasculitic neuropathy, many patients who have RA develop an insidious, mild, symmetric, distal sensory, or sensorimotor polyneuropathy that is not caused by vasculitis [48]. Median neuropathy at the wrist (carpal tunnel syndrome) and other compression neuropathies also are common in RA, and electrophysiologic studies in patients who have RA often are abnormal even without clinical symptoms [49]. When present at multiple sites, these compression neuropathies rarely, at least superficially, can mimic a mononeuritis multiplex [50,51].

Much of the understanding about the pathologic damage of nerve in large arteriole necrotizing vasculitis stems from a detailed autopsy case of a patient who died from vasculitis from RA [36]. More than 10,000 serial skip peripheral nerve sections were performed from her root level, through the lumbosacral plexus, and sciatic nerves distally to her peroneal and tibial nerves. Necrotizing vasculitis of small arteries and large arterioles was found at all levels. Nerve infarction was not observed, however, until the mid thigh (mid sciatic nerve) level, the level that was the end of two vascular distributions (the watershed zone). Initially, central fascicular fiber degeneration was seen. As the nerve was examined progressively more distally, greater degrees of axonal fiber degeneration and multifocal fiber loss were observed.

Hepatitis C and mixed cryoglobulinemia

Elevated serum cryoglobulins may be secondary to chronic infection or autoimmune or hematologic diseases. Type II cryoglobulinemia, containing monoclonal and polyclonal immunoglobulins, shows a strong association with hepatitis C virus infection [52–54]. Neuropathy occurs in type II cryoglobulinemia and is observed in 30% to 70% of cryoglobulinemic vasculitis [55,56]. Arterioles, capillaries, and venules are affected [57,58]. The neuropathy typically presents as a painful, asymmetric, sensorimotor polyneuropathy or multiple mononeuropathies [54,59–62].

HIV and cytomegalovirus

SVN secondary to HIV infection is believed to occur in less than 1% of patients who have HIV and typically occurs in those who have CD4 cell counts between 200 and 500 cells/μl [63]. The inflammatory process is believed the result of immune-complex deposition rather than direct HIV infection. Moreover, HIV infection increases the risk of other forms of secondary vasculitis, including hepatitis B–associated PAN and MPA [64]. SVN also can occur in patients who have HIV in association with lymphoma [41]. In more advanced stages of HIV, particularly in patients who have CD4 counts below 50 cells/μL, a cytomegalovirus-associated vasculitic neuropathy may occur [65].

Paraneoplastic vasculitic neuropathy

Paraneoplastic vasculitic neuropathy is reported. The tumors associated most commonly with vasculitic neuropathy are small cell lung cancer, lymphoma, leukemia, renal cell carcinoma, and other adenocarcinomas. Serum antineuronal nuclear antigen (ANNA-1 or anti-Hu) and anti–CRMP-5 (also known as anti-CV2) autoantibodies are reported in some patients who have cancer, in particular small cell lung cancer and SVN [66].

Clinical features of nonsystemic vasculitic neuropathy

As with SVN, NSVN presents most commonly as multiple mononeuropathies, and an asymmetric neuropathy or sensory/sensorimotor polyneuropathy presentation is less common [17,67,68]. In general, the overall tempo of disease progression in NSVN is slower than in SVN in that the individual attacks of mononeuropathy are less frequent. After a static period, a slow, gradual return of function typically occurs for a given nerve, with most nerves eventually making a good recovery. In general, there are fewer attacks of mononeuropathy in NSVN compared with SVN. Unlike SVN, untreated NSVN usually is not fatal, and long-term follow-up studies show most patients ambulate without assistance and are independent in activities of daily living [17,68].

Clinical features of lumbosacral and cervical radiculoplexus neuropathies

Diabetic and nondiabetic LRPN are unique forms of vasculitic neuropathy because of the stereotypic presentation, relatively confined distribution of nerve injury, frequent weight loss, and monophasic course. Both forms of LRPN present with acute or subacute pain followed by weakness in the lower extremities (proximal and distal segments), typically beginning unilaterally but often spreading to the other lower extremity. Pain is severe and includes aching, sharp stabbing, burning, and contact allodynia. A concomitant thoracic radiculopathy is common, which presents with a band and pain in the abdomen or chest and weakness of abdominal wall musculature. A cervical BPN may accompany LRPN in up to 15% of cases, although upper-extremity manifestations are overshadowed by the lower-extremity neuropathic symptoms, impairments, and disability [69]. The LRPNs are monophasic illnesses—in contrast to most other cases of NSVN—with progression lasting weeks, months, and, rarely, years and with slow but incomplete recovery of motor function. Although it seems that this disorder is more prevalent in diabetes mellitus, glycemic exposure does not seem to be the direct metabolic cause. The frequently associated weight loss may perhaps provide an indication of systemic involvement. The authors question whether or not circulating cytokines might be the possible explanation for the weight loss and have shown that they are increased in this disorder [70]. Although motor predominant, the LRPNs also involve sensory and autonomic nerves and symptoms, and findings in these systems are frequent. The pathologic findings of DLRPN and LRPN are ischemic injury (multifocal fiber loss, injury neuroma, neovascularization, perineurial thickening, and hemosiderin laden macrophages) from microvasculitis (focal disruption of the muscle layers of small epineurial blood vessels by mononuclear inflammatory cells) (see Fig. 2). In contrast, the pathologic basis of noninherited and inherited immune BPN (a cervical RPN) has not been studied as extensively as LRPN, but inflammation and nerve microvasculitis are demonstrated in some cases [23]. Some cases of hereditary BPN (also called hereditary neuralgic amyotrophy) are caused by a mutation in the SEPT9 gene [71]. It is of considerable interest that this inherited neuropathy seems to be triggered by endocrine or immune-mediated factors. Within hours of parturition, when the immune system changes to a less tolerant state, patients who have the mutant gene may develop an acute BPN. Biopsy of a superficial radial nerve during an attack has shown changes suggestive of microvasculitis [72].

Treatment—general comments

An important role of neurologists in vasculitic neuropathy management is the assessment of clinical response, especially in terms of neuropathic impairment. For the assessment of response to treatment, it is important to follow predetermined neurologic endpoints. Reliable endpoints include routine examination of muscle power, deep-tendon reflexes, and sensory thresholds, functional rating scores, and electrodiagnostic testing, whereas worsening pain seems to be a less reliable endpoint. If, in the course of treatment, new neurologic deficits develop, more aggressive therapy is indicated. Treatment decisions should be made in consultation with a rheumatologist or internist and are based, in part, on the form of systemic vasculitis, extent and degree of organ involvement, prior responsiveness to any treatments, and presence or absence of viral infection [8]. For example, chronic immunosuppressive agents, which may be first-line therapy for nonviral vasculitis, often are relatively contraindicated in viral-associated SVN.

Treatment of systemic vasculitic neuropathy

Vasculitic neuropathy not associated with virus

For nonviral SVN, corticosteroids are the initial therapy. Damage from systemic vasculitis appears and accumulates early. Treatment strategies have been developed to stop inflammatory damage (induction) rapidly, followed by safer long-term suppression (maintenance). Corticosteroids plus an additional immunosuppressant, such as cyclophosphamide, usually are required to treat MPA or Wegener's granulomatosis [73]. In PAN and Churg-Strauss syndrome, cyclophosphamide should be added in life-threatening cases (Table 2), such as those with cardiac, gastrointestinal, or CNS involvement. The addition of plasma exchange in severe cases does not seem to improve survival [43]. Some patients who have Wegener's granulomatosis or MPA require long-term immunosuppression because of relapsing disease [74,75].

Corticosteroids

In general, corticosteroids remain first-line therapy for systemic vasculitis (see Table 2), either alone or combined with other immunosuppressants [74,75]. Steroids have been used for systemic vasculitis since the 1960s, yet controlled trials and consensus statements on dosing regimens are lacking. Dosage titration should be based on patients' disease severity and response to treatment [34]. Most investigators recommend starting oral prednisone (1 to 2 mg/kg per day) [7,20,34,73,74]. In severe cases, intravenous (IV) methylprednisolone may be appropriate for initial therapy (eg, 1000 mg IV daily for 3 to 5 days followed by daily oral prednisone). Daily oral steroids should be continued until patients show a clear response. During the subacute phase of treatment, usually after 6 to 8 weeks [20], patients may be transitioned to alternate-day dosing, either at the same or at a lower averaged daily dose. At this time or after another 1 to 2 months of observation, physicians should begin tapering the steroid dose, for example by 5 to 10 mg per day per month, perhaps with lesser decrements occurring near the end of the taper. Table 2 lists the potential adverse effects of steroid therapy.

Table 2
Treatment options, potential side effects, and suggested measures to monitor for and manage side effects for nonviral systemic vasculitic neuropathy

Drug	Partial list of potential side effects	Management of potential side effects
Steroids (Prednisone)		
Initially daily 1–1.5 mg/kg, subsequent transition to alternate day dosing and gradual taper	Acute: Increased susceptibility to infections, hyperglycemia, increased appetite and weight gain, anxiety, confusion, insomnia, impaired wound healing, electrolyte disturbances. Chronic: Avascular necrosis of the femoral heads, hyperlipoproteinemia, accelerated atherosclerosis, osteoporosis, myopathy, alteration in fat deposition, peptic ulcer disease, cataracts.	Patients should start or continue an exercise program, monitoring their diet and weight. Blood glucose monitoring periodically during treatment. Bone mineral density testing baseline and annually. Consider bisphosphonates for prophylaxis of steroid-induced osteoporosis (avoid during pregnancy).
Cyclophosphamide		
Oral cyclophosphamide at 2 mg/kg as a once-daily dose	Hemorrhagic cystitis, TCCA of the bladder, oncogenicity, bone marrow suppression, gonadal toxicity, teratogenicity. Approximately one half of patients develop hematuria, usually resulting from cystitis.	Hematuria is a sensitive marker for cyclophosphamide-induced bladder injury. Injury is due to acrolein, a toxic metabolite, which is excreted into the urine. Shortening the duration of acrolein exposure to the bladder epithelium may minimize the risk of toxicity. Hence, oral administration should be every day, usually in the morning, followed by a large amount of fluids. TCCA, when it develops, almost always does so after episodes of hematuria. Urinalyses every 3 to 6 months, even after discontinuation, as TCCA may develop decades after cyclophosphamide is stopped. In cases of hematuria, discontinuation and referral to a urologist is necessary.

	Dose-related bone marrow suppression is common, with an increased risk of infection associated with leucopenia.	CBC with platelets weekly the irst month, then every month while on treatment. Total leukocyte counts below 3500/mL or absolute neutrophil counts below 1500/mL mandate titration or suspension of the drug. Lower neutrophil counts may warrant admission to the hospital and perhaps treatment with broad-spectrum antibiotics. A precipitous drop in cell counts also warrants more aggressive intervention, including cessation of cyclophosphamide.
	Nausea and vomiting.	Taking oral cyclophosphamide with or after a meal lessons the likelihood of nausea and vomiting. Consider anti-nausea medications. IV monthly cyclophosphamide also shortens the time patients experience nausea.
	Increased risk of Pneumocystis carinii pneumonia, especially with combined steroids and cytotoxic therapy.	Patients not allergic to sulfa who are on combination therapy may be treated with "low-dose" oral trimethoprim (160 mg) and sulfamethoxazole (800 mg) 3 times per week.
	Potential increased risk of other malignancies, including myelo- and lymphoproliferative disorders, years after its discontinuation. Permanent infertility may also occur because of its ability to interfere with spermatogenesis and oogenesis, which is related to its cumulative dose. Teratogenicity may occur.	Counseling and birth-control measures.
Methotrexate Often used for maintenance therapy, once SVN is in remission.	Bone marrow toxicity	Baseline CBC with platelets should be obtained prior to initiation (usually done as part of vasculitic neuropathy evaluation) and every 3 months thereafter. Repeat testing with fever, rash, or mouth ulcers.

(*continued on next page*)

Table 2 (*continued*)

Drug	Partial list of potential side effects	Management of potential side effects
In patients who have SVN, starting dose is 0.3 mg/kg orally (not exceeding 15 mg orally) per week. If tolerated, the dose can be increased gradually to 20–25 mg/week.	Hepatic fibrosis and cirrhosis; elevated LFTs	Baseline LFTs should be obtained prior to initiation of therapy and at least every 3 months. Repeat testing with fever, rash, or jaundice, especially within the first 3 months of treatment. Consider other adjuvant therapy in patients who have hepatitis or frequent alcohol consumption.
	Nephrotoxicity	Relatively uncommon, but extra caution should be used in patients who have baseline renal impairment. A baseline serum urea nitrogen and creatinine probably is sufficient, provided the vasculitis itself does not involve the kidneys.
	Increased risk for opportunistic infections	Prophylactic trimethoprim/ sulfamethoxazole (160 mg/800 mg) 3 times per week is recommended.
	Stevens-Johnson syndrome, erythema multiforme, and toxic epidermal necrolysis	Discontinue the drug in suspected rash secondary to methotrexate.
	Pulmonary fibrosis (rare)	Baseline PFTs in those who have rheumatoid vasculopathy may be helpful for comparison if symptoms develop; PFTs not helpful for subclinical detection. Discontinue drug in cases of new or worsening pulmonary function.
	Lowers seizure threshold	Consider other adjuvant therapies in patients who have seizures.
Azathioprine		
May be used for maintenance, once SVN is in remission.		

Reprinted from Schaublin GA, Michet CR Jr, Dyck PJ, et al. An update on the classification and treatment of vasculitis neuropathy. Lancet Neurol 2005;4:853–65; with permission.

Immunosuppressant adjuvant therapies

An important decision in the treatment of SVN is whether or not to add a cytotoxic or corticosteroid-sparing agent, such as cyclophosphamide, methotrexate, azathioprine, mycophenolate mofetil, or leflunomide. Most investigators recommend starting a cytotoxic agent, such as cyclophosphamide, in cases of Wegener's granulomatosis or MPA [7,74]. Cytotoxic agents also are indicated in patients who have other forms of systemic vasculitis who progress despite corticosteroid therapy or who have severe multiorgan involvement, such as pulmonary-renal syndrome, rapidly progressive necrotizing glomerulonephritis, central nervous system involvement, or other life-threatening organ involvement. Physicians must keep in mind that adjuvant therapies have a delayed onset of action, often weeks to months.

Regardless of the treatment, it is important that physicians monitor for and promptly identify any life-threatening organ involvement, including of the gastrointestinal tract, heart, or central nervous system [7,74,75]. The involvement of these systems should prompt physicians to add an adjuvant therapy, if not yet done, or to escalate the doses of existing therapy. Worsening subjective constitutional symptoms may not signify relapse reliably, however, so objective clinical and laboratory parameters must be followed closely. This includes a thorough general and neurologic examination and surveillance CBC, chemistries, ESR, and urinalysis at least every 3 months and chest radiograph at least annually [75]. Physicians also must monitor for potential drug side effects; recommendations for each therapy are in Table 2.

Cyclophosphamide seems to be the most effective drug for remission induction and prolonging survival in the nonviral systemic vasculitides [74,76]. Patients usually require between 3 and 12 months of cyclophosphomide induction therapy before they can be switched to a maintenance immunosuppressant [7,73]. Oral cyclophosphamide typically is dosed at 2 mg/kg per day. There is debate as to whether or not IV pulse-dose cyclophosphamide with prednisone is as safe and effective as the oral continuous-dose combination. Current available data do suggest that pulse-dosing cyclophosphamide results in fewer adverse effects but carries an increased risk for relapses compared with oral cyclophosphamide [29].

Cyclophosphamide is known to cause hemorrhagic cystitis and transitional cell carcinoma (TCCA) of the bladder (see Table 2). Hydration and frequent voiding should be emphasized. A urinalysis is indicated every 3 to 6 months. The development of hematuria should prompt discontinuation of the drug and patient referral to a urologist. Recommendations for surveillance and prophylaxis of other potential cyclophosphamide-associated complications are listed in Table 2.

Methotrexate has been used most commonly for remission maintenance after cyclophosphamide induction [75]. A common approach is to use cyclophosphamide as the adjuvant agent until remission, then to switch to methotrexate or azathioprine for maintenance. Once the vasculitis is in remission, it is reasonable to continue maintenance therapy for at least a year before attempting to taper the methotrexate or azathioprine. Methotrexate dosing, in the range of 15 to 25 mg once weekly, is used for systemic vasculitis [7,73,74]. Methotrexate also is associated with an acute interstitial pneumonitis, and checking pulmonary function tests (PFTs) is indicated in patients who are symptomatic (see Table 2).

Azathioprine may be considered for patients unable to tolerate cyclophosphamide therapy [7,74]. Azathioprine is a purine derivative that inhibits T-cell activation and antibody-mediated responses. Azathioprine may be as effective as cyclophosphamide in maintaining remission in Wegener's granulomatosis or MPA [77]. Azathioprine initially is dosed at 50 to 100 mg or 1 mg/kg orally, usually divided into two daily doses. The dose then is increased, by 50 mg per day every 4 weeks, to a goal dose, 2 to 2.5 mg/kg per day divided into two daily doses. An idiosyncratic hypersensitivity reaction can occur, usually within the first few weeks of therapy (see Table 2); symptoms often include nausea, diarrhea, malaise, myalgias, and rash. Liver function tests (LFTs) may be elevated. The symptoms are reversible with discontinuation, but even a single-dose rechallenge can reinitiate the syndrome.

Mycophenolate mofetil and leflunomide are reported in pilot studies as potentially useful for maintaining remission after cyclophosphamide induction in Wegener's granulomatosis [78,79].

Other agents

IV immunoglobulin (IVIg) has been used in nonvasculitic, immune-mediated neuropathies and generally has a benign safety profile, making it an attractive consideration as adjuvant therapy. Small, open-label trials of IVIg in SVN suggest clinical benefit, although randomized, controlled trials have not been performed [80–82]. Rituximab, a chimeric anti-CD20 antibody, shows promise in the treatment of cryoglobulinemic vasculitis and RA [83,84]. Randomized controlled trials of rituximab for vasculitis, however, have not been performed.

Vasculitic neuropathy associated with hepatitis B or hepatitis C

It is necessary to determine whether or not the vasculitic neuropathy is associated with a virus, such as hepatitis B or C or HIV. A detailed discussion of treatment of viral-associated vasculitis is beyond the scope of this review. Physicians experienced in treating viral hepatitis, for example, hepatologists, should make the treatment decisions and manage such patients. In general, chronic immunosuppression is relatively contraindicated in viral-associated vasculitides because such treatment may increase viremia. Shorter courses of immunosuppression, however, still are used for PAN associated with hepatitis B. Corticosteroids typically are followed by a 6-month course of an antiviral agent (either interferon-α2b or the nucleoside analog lamivudine), often with concomitant plasma exchange [85–90]. Treatment of hepatitis C typically involves pegylated interferon (pegIFN)-α2a or -α2b, often with ribavirin [91,92]. Interferon-α treatment is associated with clinical improvement in patients who have hepatitis C–cryoglobulinemic vasculitic neuropathy [93–96]. Neurologists must be aware, however, that exacerbation of vasculitic neuropathy subsequent to initiation of pegIFN-α is an infrequent but well-reported complication of treatment [95,97,98]. In such cases, drug discontinuation may lead to improvement and should be considered [97]. Rituximab may hold promise for treatment of patients who have hepatitis C–cryoglobulinemic vasculitic neuropathy, although randomized, controlled trials are needed [99,100]. Plasma exchange should be considered in fulminant cases, although no randomized, controlled trials have been performed.

Treatment of nonsystemic vasculitic neuropathy, diabetic lumbosacral radiculoplexus neuropathy, and lumbosacral radiculoplexus neuropathy

NSVN, DLRPN, and LRPN generally are not fatal and, thus, differ from that of untreated systemic vasculitis. DLRPN and LRPN usually are monophasic, whereas other forms of NSVN often are chronic. Furthermore, the neurologic deficits seen with NSVN often resolve gradually without treatment and NSVN disease activity may remit for years or even decades before relapsing. All of these factors should be considered when arriving at treatment decisions for these microvasculitides. Immunosuppressive treatment may not be indicated for patients who have NSVN and who have either mild or improving neuropathy. For more fulminant disease, treatment clearly is indicated. Patients who have active and severe DLRPN or LRPN often are treated with either IV immunoglobulin or IV methylprednisolone. As in SVN, when immunotherapy is initiated, objective endpoints should be predetermined and followed.

Corticosteroids for nonsystemic vasculitic neuropathy

For cases of NSVN warranting treatment, oral prednisone therapy is the usual first-line agent. Most investigators recommend either 40 to 60 mg per day or 1 mg/kg per day [19,34] for 2 to 3 months followed by steroid taper and transition to alternate-day dosing if patients respond clinicially, although others believe that smaller doses suffice [8,34]. See Table 2 for a list of potential side effects.

Cytotoxic adjuvant therapies for nonsystemic vasculitic neuropathy

A detailed discussion of cyclophosphamide dosing and side effects is discussed previously (see Table 2). A recent retrospective study [68] for NSVN (not DLRPN or LRPN) argues for both corticosteroids and cytotoxic adjuvant therapy, based on statistically significant better response rates and disability scores. Patients exposed to immunosuppressant therapy, however, also experience significantly more episodes of pneumonia, *Varicella zoster*, and sepsis. A prospective, randomized trial would be ideal but seems impractical given the infrequency of NSVN.

Another option in the adjuvant treatment of NSVN is weekly methotrexate [8,34]. It probably is not necessary to use the higher doses often required in SVN. A starting dose (7.5 mg orally per week), increasing gradually (to 15to 20 mg per week), is one option. See Table 2 for more details.

Azathioprine is another option in the adjuvant therapy of NSVN, one probably better suited for patients who have infrequent mononeuropathies, as its therapeutic onset is delayed up to 8 months after initiating therapy [8]. Delayed onset should be considered when tapering corticosteroids. For dosing, side effect, and management details, see Table 2.

Treatment of diabetic lumbosacral radiculoplexus neuropathy and lumbosacral radiculoplexus neuropathy

There is no proved course-altering therapy for DLRPN or LRPN and only one randomized, controlled trial [24,69]. Based on anecdotal case reports, however, patients who have DLRPN or LRPN often are treated with IV corticosteroids or IVIg [101,102]. One noncontrolled study of a series of patients who had LRPN and were treated with IV corticosteroids showed that they all improved, many to a marked degree, but the investigators warn that the results should be viewed with caution, because the disease improves spontaneously [103]. Treatment should be considered for patients in the acute phase or for those in the subacute phase who do not seem to be improving. The authors tend to treat with IV methylprednisolone because steroids have been first-line therapy for other forms of microvasculitis. Patients treated with steroids—especially patients who have DLRPN—must be monitored closely for hyperglycemia. A randomized, controlled trial comparing IV methylprednisolone with IV placebo in DLRPN is completed but all of the data have not yet been analyzed [24]. Preliminary results suggest that sensory symptoms and pain are helped by IV methylprednisolone [24].

Summary

Because neurologists play an integral role in the diagnosis and management of patients who have vasculitis involving the peripheral nerves, they need to understand the classification and treatment options and indications for these diseases. Provision of care for patients who have vasculitic neuropathy also includes patient counseling, monitoring for potential complications of treatments, and response to treatments. Corticosteroids remain the mainstay of therapy for SVN unassociated with virus, often with adjuvant immunosuppressive therapy. In many instances (eg, systemic vasculitis), neurologists should team up with a rheumatologist or internist to provide care. For the microvasculitides of nerve, such as NSVN, DLRPN, and LRPN, treatment decisions and management often are performed solely by a neurologist.

References

[1] Jennette JC, Falk RJ, Andrassy K, et al. Nomenclature of systemic vasculitides. Proposal of an international consensus conference. Arthritis Rheum 1994;37:187–92.

[2] Zeek PM. Periarteritis nodosa; a critical review. Am J Clin Pathol 1952;22:777–90.

[3] Lie JT. Nomenclature and classification of vasculitis: plus ca change, plus c'est la meme chose. Arthritis Rheum 1994;37:181–6.

[4] Dyck PJB, Engelstad J, Dyck PJ. Microvasculitis. In: Dyck PJ, Thomas PK, editors. Peripheral neuropathy. 4th edition. Philadelphia: Elsevier; 2005.

[5] Sugiura M, Koike H, Iijima M, et al. Clinicopathologic features of nonsystemic vasculitic neuropathy and microscopic polyangiitis-associated neuropathy: a comparative study. J Neurol Sci 2006;241:31–7.

[6] Moore PM, Richardson B. Neurology of the vasculitides and connective tissue diseases. J Neurol Neurosurg Psychiatry 1998;65:10–22.

[7] Langford CA. Vasculitis. J Allergy Clin Immunol 2003;111:S602–12.

[8] Schaublin GA, Michet CJ Jr, Dyck PJ, et al. An update on the classification and treatment of vasculitic neuropathy. Lancet Neurol 2005;4:853–65.

[9] Saleh A, Stone JH. Classification and diagnostic criteria in systemic vasculitis. Best Pract Res Clin Rheumatol 2005;19:209–21.

[10] Vital C, Canron M-H, Jaffre A. Combined nerve and muscle biopsy in the diagnosis of vasculitic neuropathy. A 16-year retrospective sutdy of 202 cases. J Peripher Nerv Syst 2006;11: 20–9.

[11] Moore PM. Vasculitic neuropathies. J Neurol Neurosurg Psychiatry 2000;68:271–4.

[12] Puechal X, Said G, Hilliquin P, et al. Peripheral neuropathy with necrotizing vasculitis in rheumatoid arthritis. A clinicopathologic and prognostic study of thirty-two patients. Arthritis Rheum 1995;38:1618–29.

[13] Vollertsen RS, Conn DL, Ballard DJ, et al. Rheumatoid vasculitis: survival and associated risk factors. Medicine (Baltimore) 1986;65:365–75.

[14] Turesson C, O'Fallon WM, Crowson CS, et al. Extra-articular disease manifestations in rheumatoid arthritis: incidence trends and risk factors over 46 years. Ann Rheum Dis 2003;62:722–7.

[15] Said G, Lacroix C, Plante-Bordeneuve V, et al. Nerve granulomas and vasculitis in sarcoid peripheral neuropathy: a clinicopathological study of 11 patients. Brain 2002;125:264–75.

[16] Burns TM, Dyck PJ, Aksamit AJ. The natural history and long-term outcome of 57 limb sarcoidosis neuropathy cases. J Neurol Sci 2006;244:77–87.

[17] Dyck PJ, Benstead TJ, Conn DL, et al. Nonsystemic vasculitic neuropathy. Brain 1987;110: 843–54.

[18] Burns TM. Vasculitic neuropathy. Continuum (N Y) 2003;9:146–59.

[19] Collins MP, Periquet MI. Non-systemic vasculitic neuropathy. Curr Opin Neurol 2004;17: 587–98.

[20] Said G, Lacroix C. Primary and secondary vasculitic neuropathy. J Neurol 2005;252: 633–41.

[21] Hawke SH, Davies L, Pamphlett R, et al. Vasculitic neuropathy. A clinical and pathological study. Brain 1991;114:2175–90.

[22] Suarez GA, Giannini C, Bosch EP, et al. Immune brachial plexus neuropathy: Suggestive evidence for an inflammatory immune pathogenesis. Neurology 1996;46:559–61.

[23] Dyck PJB, Engelstad J, Suarez GA, et al. Biopsied upper limb nerves provide information about distribution and mechanism in immune brachial plexus neuropathy. Neurology 2001; 56:A395.
[24] Dyck PJB, O'Brien P, Bosch EP, et al. The multi-center, double-blind controlled trial of IV methylprednisolone in diabetic lumbosacral radiculoplexus neuropathy. Neurology 2006; 66(5, Suppl 2):A191.
[25] Kissel JT, Mendell JR. Vasculitic neuropathy. Neurol Clin 1992;10:761–81.
[26] Kissel JT, Slivka AP, Warmolts JR, et al. The clinical spectrum of necrotizing angiopathy of the peripheral nervous system. Ann Neurol 1985;18:251–7.
[27] Sehgal M, Swanson JW, DeRemee RA, et al. Neurologic manifestations of Churg-Strauss syndrome. Mayo Clin Proc 1995;70:337–41.
[28] Guillevin L, Le Thi Huong D, Godeau P, et al. Clinical findings and prognosis of polyarteritis nodosa and Churg-Strauss angiitis: a study in 165 patients. Br J Rheumatol 1988;27: 258–64.
[29] de Groot K, Schmidt DK, Arlt AC, et al. Standardized neurologic evaluations of 128 patients with Wegener granulomatosis. Arch Neurol 2001;58:1215–21.
[30] Said G, Lacroix-Ciaudo C, Fugimura H, et al. The peripheral neuropathy of necrotizing arteritis: a clinico-pathological study. Ann Neurol 1988;23:461–5.
[31] Nishino H, Rubino FA, DeRemee RA, et al. Neurological involvement in Wegener's granulomatosis: an analysis of 324 consecutive patients at the Mayo Clinic. Ann Neurol 1993;33:4–9.
[32] Hattori N, Ichimura M, Nagamatsu M, et al. Clinicopathological features of Churg-Strauss syndrome-associated neuropathy. Brain 1999;122(Pt 3):427–39.
[33] Greenberg SA. P-ANCA vasculitic neuropathy with 12-year latency between onset of neuropathy and systemic symptoms. BMC Neurol 2002;2:10.
[34] Burns TM, Dyck PJB. Treatment of vasculitic neuropathy. In: Johnson RT, Griffin JW, McArthur JC, editors. Current therapy in neurologic disease. 6th ed. St. Louis: Mosby; 2002. p. 390–4.
[35] Collins MP, Mendell JR, Periquet MI, et al. Superficial peroneal nerve/peroneus brevis muscle biopsy in vasculitic neuropathy. Neurology 2000;55:636–43.
[36] Dyck PJ, Conn DL, Okazaki H. Necrotizing angiopathic neuropathy: three-dimensional morphology of fiber degeneration related to sites of occluded vessels. Mayo Clin Proc 1972;47:461–75.
[37] Nukada H, Dyck PJ. Microsphere embolization of nerve capillaries and fiber degeneration. Am J Pathol 1984;115:275–87.
[38] Nukada H, Dyck PJ, Karnes JL. Spatial distribution of capillaries in rat nerves: correlation of ischemic damage. Exp Neurol 1985;87:369–76.
[39] Benstead TJ, Dyck PJ, Sangalang V. Inner perineurial cell vulnerability in ischemia. Brain Res 1989;489:177–81.
[40] Stone JH. Polyarteritis nodosa. JAMA 2002;288:1632–9.
[41] Younger DS. Vasculitis of the nervous system. Curr Opin Neurol 2004;17:317–36.
[42] Lane SE, Watts RA, Shepstone L, et al. Primary systemic vasculitis: clinical features and mortality. Q J Med 2005;98:97–111.
[43] Guillevin L, Lhote F, Cohen P, et al. Corticosteroids plus pulse cyclophosphamide and plasma exchanges versus corticosteroids plus pulse cyclophosphamide alone in the treatment of polyarteritis nodosa and Churg-Strauss syndrome patients with factors predicting poor prognosis. A prospective, randomized trial in sixty-two patients. Arthritis Rheum 1995;38:1638–45.
[44] Noth I, Strek ME, Leff AR. Churg-Strauss syndrome [comment]. Lancet 2003;361:587–94.
[45] Reinhold-Keller E, Beuge N, Latza U, et al. An interdisciplinary approach to the care of patients with Wegener's granulomatosis: long-term outcome in 155 patients. Arthritis Rheum 2000;43:1021–32.
[46] Hoffman GS, Kerr GS, Leavitt RY, et al. Wegener granulomatosis: an analysis of 158 patients. Ann Intern Med 1992;116:488–98.

[47] Scott DG, Bacon PA, Tribe CR. Systemic rheumatoid vasculitis: a clinical and laboratory study of 50 cases. Medicine (Baltimore) 1981;60:288–97.
[48] Good AE, Christopher RP, Koepke GH, et al. peripheral neuropathy associated with rheumatoid arthritis. a clinical and electrodiagnostic study of 70 consecutive rheumatoid arthritis patients. Ann Intern Med 1965;63:87–99.
[49] Lanzillo B, Pappone N, Crisci C, et al. Subclinical peripheral nerve involvement in patients with rheumatoid arthritis. Arthritis Rheum 1998;41:1196–202.
[50] Herbison GJ, Teng C, Martin JH, et al. Carpal tunnel syndrome in rheumatoid arthritis. Am J Phys Med 1973;52:68–74.
[51] Rosenbaum R. Neuromuscular complications of connective tissue diseases. Muscle Nerve 2001;24:154–69.
[52] Agnello V, Chung RT, Kaplan LM. A role for hepatitis C virus infection in type II cryoglobulinemia. N Engl J Med 1992;327:1490–5.
[53] Ferri C, Greco F, Longombardo G, et al. Association between hepatitis C virus and mixed cryoglobulinemia. Clin Exp Rheumatol 1991;9:621–4.
[54] Trejo O, Ramos-Casals M, Garcia-Carrasco M, et al. Cryoglobulinemia: study of etiologic factors and clinical and immunologic features in 443 patients from a single center. Medicine 2001;80:252–62.
[55] Zaltron S, Puoti M, Liberini P, et al. High prevalence of peripheral neuropathy in hepatitis C virus infected patients with symptomatic and asymptomatic cryoglobulinaemia. Ital J Gastroenterol Hepatol 1998;30:391–5.
[56] Lamprecht P, Gause A, Gross WL. Cryoglobulinemic vasculitis. Arthritis Rheum 1999;42: 2507–16.
[57] Nemni R, Corbo M, Fazio R, et al. Cryoglobulinaemic neuropathy. A clinical, morphological and immunocytochemical study of 8 cases. Brain 1988;111:541–52.
[58] Chad D, Pariser K, Bradley WG, et al. The pathogenesis of cryoglobulinemic neuropathy. Neurology 1982;32:725–9.
[59] Steck AJ. Neurological manifestations of malignant and non-malignant dysglobulinaemias. J Neurol 1998;245:634–9.
[60] Simmons Z. Paraproteinemia and neuropathy. Curr Opin Neurol 1999;12:589–95.
[61] Tembl JI, Ferrer JM, Sevilla MT, et al. Neurologic complications associated with hepatitis C virus infection. Neurology 1999;53:861–4.
[62] David WS, Peine C, Schlesinger P, et al. Nonsystemic vasculitic mononeuropathy multiplex, cryoglobulinemia, and hepatitis C. Muscle Nerve 1996;19:1596–602.
[63] Brew BJ. The peripheral nerve complications of human immunodeficiency virus (HIV) infection. Muscle Nerve 2003;28:542–52.
[64] Johnson RM, Barbarini G, Barbaro G. Kawasaki-like syndromes and other vasculitic syndromes in HIV-infected patients. AIDS 2003;17(Suppl 1):S77–82.
[65] Meyer MF, Hellmich B, Kotterba S, et al. Cytomegalovirus infection in systemic necrotizing vasculitis: causative agent or opportunistic infection? Rheumatol Int 2000;20:35–8.
[66] Rudnicki SA, Dalmau J. Paraneoplastic syndromes of the peripheral nerves. Curr Opin Neurol 2005;18:598–603.
[67] Davies L, Spies JM, Pollard JD, et al. Vasculitis confined to peripheral nerves. Brain 1996; 119:1441–8.
[68] Collins MP, Periquet MI, Mendell JR, et al. Nonsystemic vasculitic neuropathy: insights from a clinical cohort. Neurology 2003;61:623–30.
[69] Dyck PJB, Windebank AJ. Diabetic and non-diabetic lumbosacral radiculoplexus neuropathies: New insights into pathophysiology and treatment. Muscle Nerve 2002;25: 477–91.
[70] Dyck PJB, Norell JE, Dyck PJ. Microvasculitis and ischemia in diabetic lumbosacral radiculoplexus neuropathy. Neurology 1999;53:2113–21.
[71] Kuhlenbaumer G, Hannibal MC, Nelis E, et al. Mutations in SEPT9 cause hereditary neuralgic amyotrophy. Nat Genet 2005;37:1044–6.

[72] Klein CJ, Dyck PJ, Friedenberg SM, et al. Inflammation and neuropathic attacks in hereditary brachial plexus neuropathy. J Neurol Neurosurg Psychiatry 2002;73:45–50.
[73] Gold R, Fontana A, Zierz S. Therapy of neurological disorders in systemic vasculitis. Semin Neurol 2003;23:207–14.
[74] Kamesh L, Harper L, Savage CO. ANCA-positive vasculitis. J Am Soc Nephrol 2002;13:1953–60.
[75] Langford CA. How can relapses be detected and prevented in primary systemic small-vessel vasculitides? Best PractRes ClinRheumatol 2005;19:307–20.
[76] Adu D, Pall A, Luqmani RA, et al. Controlled trial of pulse versus continuous prednisolone and cyclophosphamide in the treatment of systemic vasculitis. Q J Med 1997;90:401–9.
[77] Jayne D, Rasmussen N, Andrassy K, et al. A randomized trial of maintenance therapy for vasculitis associated with antineutrophil cytoplasmic autoantibodies [comment]. N Engl J Med 2003;349:36–44.
[78] Langford CA, Talar-Williams C, Sneller MC. Mycophenolate mofetil for remission maintenance in the treatment of Wegener's granulomatosis. Arthritis Rheum 2004;51:278–83.
[79] Metzler C, Fink C, Lamprecht P, et al. Maintenance of remission with leflunomide in Wegener's granulomatosis. Rheumatology 2004;43:315–20.
[80] Levy Y, Uziel Y, Zandman GG, et al. Intravenous immunoglobulins in peripheral neuropathy associated with vasculitis. Ann Rheum Dis 2003;62:1221–3.
[81] Jayne DR, Davies MJ, Fox CJ, et al. Treatment of systemic vasculitis with pooled intravenous immunoglobulin. Lancet 1991;337:1137–9.
[82] Jayne DR, Chapel H, Adu D, et al. Intravenous immunoglobulin for ANCA-associated systemic vasculitis with persistent disease activity. Q J Med 2000;93:433–9.
[83] Keogh KA, Yttergerg SR, Fervenza FC, et al. Rituximab for remission induction in severe ANCA-associated vasculitis: report of a prospective open-label pilot trial in 10 patients. Arthritis Rheum 2004;50:S270.
[84] Lamprecht P, Lerin-Lozano C, Merz H, et al. Rituximab induces remission in refractory HCV associated cryoglobulinaemic vasculitis. Ann Rheum Dis 2003;62:1230–3.
[85] Guillevin L, Lhote F, Leon A, et al. Treatment of polyarteritis nodosa related to hepatitis B virus with short term steroid therapy associated with antiviral agents and plasma exchanges. A prospective trial in 33 patients. J Rheumatol 1993;20:289–98.
[86] Guillevin L, Lhote F, Cohen P, et al. Polyarteritis nodosa related to hepatitis B virus. A prospective study with long-term observation of 41 patients. Medicine (Baltimore) 1995;74:238–53.
[87] Erhardt A, Sagir A, Guillevin L, et al. Successful treatment of hepatitis B virus associated polyarteritis nodosa with a combination of prednisolone, alpha-interferon and lamivudine. J Hepatol 2000;33:677–83.
[88] Lau CF, Hui PK, Chan WM, et al. Hepatitis B associated fulminant polyarteritis nodosa: successful treatment with pulse cyclophosphamide, prednisolone and lamivudine following emergency surgery. Eur J Gastroenterol Hepatol 2002;14:563–6.
[89] Deeren DH, De Backer AI, Malbrain ML, et al. Treatment of hepatitis B virus-related polyarteritis nodosa: two case reports and a review of the literature. Clin Rheumatol 2004;23:172–6.
[90] Guillevin L, Mahr A, Cohen P, et al. Short-term corticosteroids then lamivudine and plasma exchanges to treat hepatitis B virus-related polyarteritis nodosa [comment]. Arthritis Rheum 2004;51:482–7.
[91] Zeuzem S, Feinman SV, Rasenack J, et al. Peginterferon alfa-2a in patients with chronic hepatitis C [comment]. N Engl J Med 2000;343:1666–72.
[92] Cacoub P, Lidove O, Maisonobe T, et al. Interferon-alpha and ribavirin treatment in patients with hepatitis C virus-related systemic vasculitis. Arthritis Rheum 2002;46:3317–26.
[93] Khella SL, Frost S, Hermann GA, et al. Hepatitis C infection, cryoglobulinemia, and vasculitic neuropathy. Treatment with interferon alfa: case report and literature review. Neurology 1995;45:407–11.

[94] Ghini M, Mascia MT, Gentilini M, et al. Treatment of cryoglobulinemic neuropathy with alpha-interferon. Neurology 1996;46:588–9.
[95] Irioka T, Yamada M, Yamawaki M, et al. Acute autonomic and sensory neuropathy after interferon alpha-2b therapy for chronic hepatitis C. J Neurol Neurosurg Psychiatry 2001; 70:408–10.
[96] Scelsa SN, Herskovitz S, Reichler B. Treatment of mononeuropathy multiplex in hepatitis C virus and cryoglobulinemia. Muscle Nerve 1998;21:1526–9.
[97] Boonyapisit K, Katirji B. Severe exacerbation of hepatitis C-associated vasculitic neuropathy following treatment with interferon alpha: a case report and literature review. Muscle Nerve 2002;25:909–13.
[98] LaCivita L, Pasero G, Ferri C. Axonal neuropathy in a patient receiving interferon-alpha therapy for chronic Hepatic C. J Rheumatol 1997;24:1656.
[99] Zaja F, De Vita S, Mazzaro C, et al. Efficacy and safety of rituximab in type II mixed cryoglobulinemia. Blood 2003;101:3827–34.
[100] Sansonno D, De Re V, Lauletta G, et al. Monoclonal antibody treatment of mixed cryoglobulinemia resistant to interferon alpha with an anti-CD20. Blood 2003;101:3818–26.
[101] Triggs WJ, Young MS, Eskin T, et al. Treatment of idiopathic lumbosacral plexopathy with intravenous immunoglobulin. Muscle Nerve 1997;20:244–6.
[102] Verma A, Bradley WG. High-dose intravenous immunoglobulin therapy in chronic progressive lumbosacral plexopathy. Neurology 1994;44:248–50.
[103] Dyck PJB, Norell JE, Dyck PJ. Methylprednisolone may improve lumbosacral radiculoplexus neuropathy. Can J Neurol Sci 2001;28:224–7.

NEUROLOGIC CLINICS

Neurol Clin 25 (2007) 115–137

Infectious Neuropathies

Gérard Said, MD, FRCP

Service de Neurologie, Hôpital de Bicêtre, Université Paris XI, 94275 Le Kremlin Bicêtre, France

In many patients, inflammatory neuropathies follow infection of the peripheral nervous system (PNS) caused by viruses, bacteria, or parasites, which makes this group of neuropathy the largest group of neuropathies in the world, and, in addition, neuropathies that often are treatable or preventable. In this context, nerve lesions can result from the inflammatory reaction induced by the infective agent or from the immune reaction of the host.

Infection with retroviruses

Peripheral nerve (PN) lesions commonly are associated with human retroviral infection, which includes infection with HIV-1 and -2, the agents of AIDS, and the human T-lymphotropic virus type 1 (HTLV-1), the agent of tropical myeloneuropathy.

Neuropathies in HIV infection

Neuropathy occurs in a variable proportion of patients infected with the HIV [1–11]. Subclinical involvement of the PNS, as detected by systematic electrophysiologic investigations [8,12] or found at autopsy, is common in patients who have HIV, but the nerve lesions remain silent in most cases. In addition, minor alterations of the nerve action potentials or of nerve conduction velocity in patients who do not present signs or symptoms of neuropathy are not predictive of the occurrence of symptomatic neuropathy [13], making systematic electrophysiologic investigations unnecessary in patients who are asymptomatic. The incidence of disabling clinical neuropathy increases with progression of the immunodepression but remains difficult to

E-mail address: gerard.said@bct.aphp.fr

0733-8619/07/$ - see front matter
doi:10.1016/j.ncl.2006.11.004 **neurologic.theclinics.com**

establish. Symptomatic neuropathy affects an estimated 5% to 10% of patients who are HIV infected.

A wide variety of neuropathies occurs in the course of HIV infection, including Guillain-Barré syndrome (GBS), multifocal neuropathy, meningoradiculoneuritis, acute uni- or bilateral facial palsy, and pandysautonomia. All these manifestations can be associated with central nervous system (CNS) involvement or with inflammatory myopathy.

Inflammatory polyneuritis of the Guillain-Barré type

GBS can occur at the time of seroconversion to HIV [13–16]. Mild to severe motor deficit is associated with high fever, diarrhea, rash, adenopathy, and mononucleosic syndrome. Modifications of the cerebrospinal fluid (CSF) content are similar to those observed in classical GBS. The protein content is high and the cell count low, but the cell content often is more elevated than in classical GBS. The outcome of these GBS-like syndromes is not different from classical GBS. Relapsing forms are rare [17]. Recently, GBS has been reported during the immune reconstitution syndrome after treatment of HIV infection in children who are immunodepressed [18].

Nerve biopsy specimens from patients who have HIV-related GBS-like syndrome show the whole range of lesions seen in GBS, including macrophage-mediated demyelination, mixed axonal and demyelinating lesions, or predominantly axonal lesions. The intensity of inflammatory infiltrates vary, but usually it is more pronounced in distal nerves than in non–HIV-related GBS.

Subacute multifocal neuropathy

This is a relatively common pattern of neuropathy observed in patients who have HIV, before the onset of cellular immunosuppression. Sensory or sensorimotor deficit often predominates in the lower limbs. Paresthesiae and spontaneous pain are common. They usually are bilateral but often predominate on one side or can affect the territory of a nerve trunk or of a spinal root. They often progress over a few weeks, affecting the upper limbs. The CSF protein content often is elevated, with mild pleocytosis and normal glucose level, or remains normal. Cranial nerves, especially the facial nerves, can be affected [19–22]. Examination shows sensorimotor deficit of peripheral origin often associated with exaggerated tendon reflexes and sometimes Babinski's sign. The outcome of these neuropathies usually is good. Patients improve spontaneously or after treatment with corticosteroids. Occasionally, a motor neuropathy can mimick motor neuron disease [23,24].

In nerve biopsies of patients who have subacute multifocal neuropathy, mixed axonal and demyelinative lesions of nerve fibers are associated with mild inflammatory infiltrates [25]. In most cases, perivascular cuffing is associated with endoneurial inflammatory infiltrate, mainly made of CD8 T lymphocytes and macrophages. In a few patients, the author has found necrotising arteritis of the type observed in polyarteritis nodosa in nerve

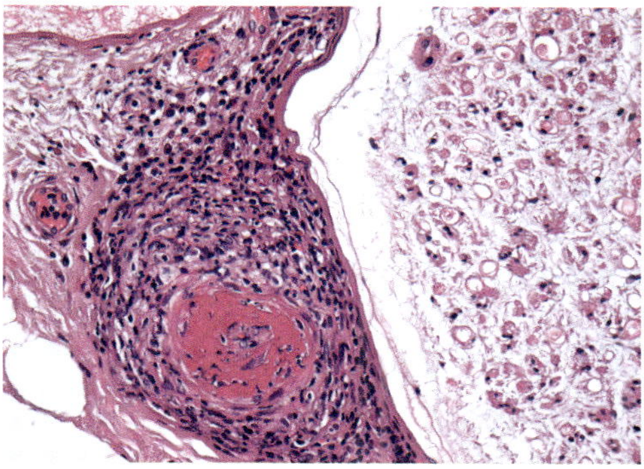

Fig. 1. HIV multifocal neuropathy. Necrotizing arteritis of an epineurial artery of the superficial peroneal nerve biopsy sample. Note axonal degeneration of the nerve fibers of the neighboring fascicle (hematoxylin-eosin staining).

and in muscle specimens (Figs. 1 and 2) [25]. In one patient, demyelinating neuropathy was associated with a spectacular polyclonal proliferation of B lymphocytes that predominated around endoneurial blood vessels, similar to that seen in Liebow's syndrome [26–29].

Distal symmetric polyneuropathy

Distal symmetric neuropathies represent the most common type of peripheral neuropathy in patients who have HIV, especially at a late stage of the HIV infection [1]. Both feet are affected simultaneously by painful sensations, often of the burning type, associated with allodynia, which renders examination difficult. Painful retraction of the calf muscles occurs. Motor involvement usually is absent or moderate. Slight pyramidal tract involvement is common. The ankle reflexes are absent or decreased; the other tendon reflexes often are exaggerated.

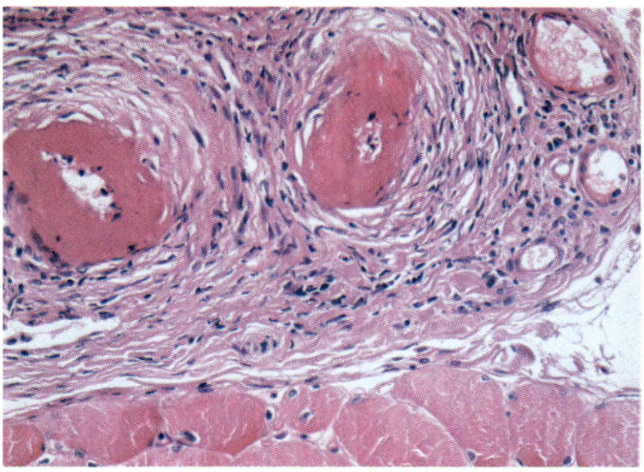

Fig. 2. Peroneus brevis muscle specimen of the same patient as in Fig. 1, who has HIV, to show similar involvement of small arteries in the muscle biopsy specimen (hematoxylin-eosin staining).

Morphologically, axonal lesions markedly predominate in this group. Inflammatory infiltrates are uncommon. In one such case, the author found occasional multinucleated endoneurial cells, which are known to result from fusion of macrophages infected with the HIV. In a recent study of a cohort of 101 subjects who were HIV infected [30], distal sensory polyneuropathy was common and relatively stable over 48 weeks. Previously established risk factors, including CD4 cell count, plasma HIV RNA, and use of dideoxynucleoside antiretrovirals, were not predictive of the progression of distal sensory polyneuropathy.

Dysautonomia in HIV infection

Disabling autonomic manifestations, including postural hypotension and syncopes, paroxysmal arterial hypertension, sphincter disturbances, abnormal pupil reaction to light, and abnormal sweating, are reported in patients who have HIV [31–33]. These autonomic manifestations occur in association with sensorimotor neuropathy, sometimes at each recurrence of a relapsing demyelinative neuropathy [18], or as an isolated manifestation of HIV neuropathy.

Cytomegalovirus neuropathy

Cytomegalovirus (CMV) neuropathy is a treatable neuropathy that occurs at a late stage of immunodepression (Fig. 3) [34–42]. CMV infection represents the most common viral opportunistic infection in AIDS, affecting 15% to 35% of patients who have AIDS. Its most common clinical manifestation is retinitis, with vision loss that often is bilateral. Peripheral neuropathy often is associated with retinitis or with symptomatic CMV infection of other organs (colitis or pancreatitis). The diagnosis of CMV neuropathy should not be missed, because it is accessible to specific treatment by

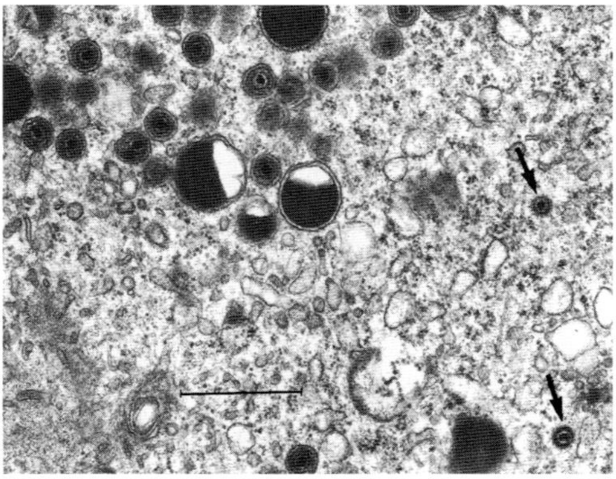

Fig. 3. Electron micrograph of a nerve specimen from a patient who has CMV neuropathy. Viruses (*arrows*) are found in nuclei and cytoplasm of macrophages, Schwann cells, and endothelial cells in PNs (uranyl acetate and lead citrate staining). Bar, 1 μm.

ganciclovir or foscarnet. In most cases, patients who have proved CMV neuropathy have AIDS with opportunistic infections, profound immunodepression, fever, cachexia, a CD4 T-cell count below 50 per mL, and CMV retinitis, but in some of them, CMV neuropathy is the first and only opportunistic infection and occurs in patients who are in relatively good general condition.

The different patterns of CMV neuropathy include (1) the polyradiculopathic pattern—within a few days or weeks, patients develop a sensorimotor deficit of the lower spinal roots or a complete cauda equina syndrome with sphincter disturbances, often associated with signs of CNS involvement and general signs and symptoms; (2) the multifocal pattern, which may include symptomatic lesions of spinal roots, nerve trunks, and sometimes cranial nerve involvement; (3) both patterns of peripheral neuropathy, which may be associated in the same patient; (4) severe CNS manifestations, including necrotic myelitis and encephalitis; and (5) the CSF abnormalities that can be observed in this setting, which include high protein content (more than 10 g/L in one of the author's patients), pleocytosis with polymorphonuclear leucocytes reaction, and decreased CSF glucose [34,40] but CSF that can remain normal.

The range of clinical aspects of CMV neuropathy is in keeping with the potential ubiquity of lesions related to CMV infection of the nervous system. Nerve lesions associated with endoneurial CMV infection in patients who have AIDS range from occasional, scattered, cytomegalic cells with minimal surrounding inflammation to large areas of necrosis. A prominent neutrophilic cell response often is associated with mixed, axonal and demyelinative, multifocal lesions of neighboring nerve fibers [34].

Malignant lymphomas

Malignant lymphomas, which may complicate the immunosuppression of AIDS, seldom can induce focal or multifocal nerve lesions by invading spinal roots or nerve trunks [43].

Toxic neuropathy in AIDS

The antagonist of DNA viral synthesis, 2′,3′-dideoxyinosine, induces a distal symmetric sensory polyneuropathy in 7% of the patients receiving less than 12 mg/kg/day. The symptoms disappear after withdrawal of the drug, which can be started again later at lower doses [44].

Neuropathies in human T-lymphotropic virus type 1–related tropical myeloneuropathy

Although tropical myeloneuropathy primarily is a spinal cord disorder [45,46], PN dysfunction has been noted in various studies. Roman and Roman noted absent ankle jerks in 28% of their patients from Colombia [47]. Electrophysiologic evidence of PND has ranged from negligible to 32%.

Clinical evidence of PN involvement has been found in 16 of their patients by Bhighjee and colleagues [48]. In Brazil, a study of a cohort of 335 HTLV-1 infected individuals who did not have spastic paraparesis evaluated for the presence of PN showed that 45 of them had clinical or electrophysiologic evidence of PNS involvement, including 21 patients who had isolated PN [49].

PN involvement is characterized by mild sensorimotor, bilateral, deficit affecting distal lower limbs in association with sphincter disturbances and spinal cord involvement. In some patients, predominantly motor deficit and pyramidal tract involvement mimicks amyotrophic lateral sclerosis. HTLV-1 infection also often is associated with sicca syndrome.

On nerve biopsy specimens, perineurial and perivascular inflammatory infiltrates with moderate axon loss and mixture of segmental demyelination and axonal degeneration can be observed [50], sometimes without inflammatory infiltrates [51]. Demyelination and irregularity of the myelin sheath occur [52].

Leprous neuropathy

Since the identification in 1874 by Hansen, in Bergen, Norway, of a bacillus, the *Mycobacterium leprae*, as the agent of leprosy, much has been learned about the natural history, the clinical and pathological manifestations, and the treatment of leprosy. Subsequent improvements in the treatment, management, and public health approach all have contributed to a near eradication of the disease in industrialized countries. Yet leprosy remains among the first causes for neuropathy in the world, even though the latest estimate of the number of leprosy cases worldwide decreases. Still, 407,791 new cases were detected in the world during the year 2004, according to World Health Organization (WHO) records. Leprosy is found primarily in tropical and subtropical developing countries. Several features of leprosy are unique and strikingly different from other infectious human diseases, in relation to the nature of the infective agent and the immunologic status of the host. Many of the neurologic aspects of leprous neuropathies have been known for decades [53–56], yet leprosy remains a subject of interest because the form of leprosy depends mainly on the immune reaction of the host to *M leprae* antigens, ranging from the extremity with the lowest cell-mediated immunity to *M leprae*, the lepromatous pole or polybacillar pattern, to that with the highest cell-mediated immunity, the tuberculoid pole [57,58].

Clinical manifestations

Specific cutaneous lesions, including maculae and lepromae, reveal the disease in half or more of the patients, especially in the polybacillar-lepromatous type. In the others, small areas of sensory loss, limited anhydrosis and alopecia zones, paresis of some facial muscles, hypochromic or atrophic cutaneous zones, or painful enlargement of a nerve trunk are the presenting manifestations. Plantar ulcers and other trophic changes occur later in the course of the disease, as a consequence of sensory loss.

Sensory loss

Sensory loss is the most constant finding of leprous neuropathy. Sensory loss, which is the result of mixed dermal nerve and nerve trunk damage, is variable in distribution, ranging from a small skin patch with impaired sensation to severe sensory loss over most of the body surface but avoiding the body folds. Early cutaneous lesions show some preservation of sensation, with impairment of light touch and loss of thermal and pain sense while preserving proprioception, so patients still can use their largely anesthetic limbs effectively, which leads to painless trauma and trophic changes. Loss of dermal pigment in the territory of affected cutaneous nerves leads to development of large anesthetic patches in dark-skinned people, with loss of sweating in corresponding area. Colder areas of the body seem more affected [59], but temperature-linked sensory loss, which is not observed in tuberculoid leprosy, cannot account for all the patterns of nerve lesions in leprosy. In some cases, complete loss of pain and temperature sensations in a certain area contrasts with preservation of tactile sensation. This classical dissociation of sensory loss seldom is complete in leprosy. In most cases, all modalities of superficial sensations are affected. Sensory loss also occurs in the areas corresponding to maculae, demonstrating early involvement of sensory nerve terminals.

The topographic distribution of sensory disturbances is variable. Sensory loss may affect an "insular" pattern, in which anesthetic areas of variable forms, size, and number are found and superpose or not to macular-type cutaneous lesions. These manifestations, which may last for years, usually are associated with other disturbances, such as anhydrosis, alopecia, and vasomotor areflexia [53]. These manifestations are related to lesions of sensory nerve endings or to those of a limited number of nerve fascicles of a nerve trunk. Sensory loss also may affect a nerve trunk pattern or, in some cases, a pseudoradicular pattern, as a consequence of involvement of large nerve trunks. In cases of longstanding evolution, the distal part of the limbs show the greatest sensory loss. This extends proximally to a greater or lesser extent, rarely to the trunk. When the trunk is involved, sensory loss affects an insular pattern. This pattern of sensory loss does not affect the anterior aspect of the trunk in a length-dependent pattern, the way it does in severe diabetic, amyloid, or alcoholic polyneuropathy [60,61]. In individual patients, dissociation between sensations may be found in some areas only. The large nerve trunks affected most commonly are the ulnar and the lateral popliteal nerves, followed by the median, posterior tibial, superficial radial, and peroneal nerves and the greater auricular and facial nerves [62].

Nerve hypertrophy

Nerve trunks are enlarged palpably in an estimated one third of patients who have leprosy [63], sometimes before the onset of sensory loss in the corresponding territory. Superficial nerves, such as the greater auricular nerve in the neck, the supraorbitary branch of the trigeminal nerve or larger nerve trunks (especially the ulnar nerve above the elbow), the peroneal nerve, and the radial cutaneous nerve at the lateral border of the wrist often are enlarged. Nerve hypertrophy sometimes is associated with spontaneous tingling or with painful sensations. Nerve thickening is regular, cylindroid, or sometimes nodular. Palpation of the nerve itself occasionally is painful. Nerve hypertrophy often is difficult to ascertain.

Motor disturbance and amyotrophy

Motor involvement usually is a late event in the course of the disease. Amyotrophy and motor weakness usually progress pari passu; in some cases however, amyotrophy is more marked than weakness, both of which predominate in the ulnar and median nerves territories, with characteristic claw hands. In the lower limbs, the peroneal nerve is affected predominantly. Motor involvement and amyotrophy usually progress slowly in an approximately symmetric way. Preservation of deep tendon reflexes in many cases of leprous neuropathy is characteristic of predominant involvement of the most distal part of the nerves.

Facial palsy with lagophthalmos of one or both eyes, with sparing of the other muscles supplied by the facial nerve, is a classical feature of leprosy. Surgical exploration of the facial nerve showed involvement of one or several branches of division destined to the frontal muscle and to the orbicularis oculi. This involvement often is associated with sensory loss in the malar region and in the cornea of the eye [62].

Trophic disturbances

Trophic plantar ulcers is a common, nonspecific complication of loss of pain sensation over the plantar sole. Severe sensory disturbances always are found in those areas where ulcers occur. Plantar ulcer is subsequent to microtrauma on skin that has lost painful sensation. The absence of protective sensation of limb extremities leads to overuse, accidental self injury, recurrent infections, and gradual development of further deformities as observed in sensory neuropathy of different origin [63] or in congenital indifference to pain [64]. Bone lesions, osteolysis, always are distally located, often are bilateral, and have a centripetal evolution, gradually affecting the phalanges, metacarpal, and metatarsal bones, causing deformities of the limbs. Radiologic examination reveals concentric progressive atrophy of phalanges and metatarsal and metacarpal bones. The process starts in the distal end of phalanges, destroys the joint surfaces, and progresses without causing bone reaction.

The spectrum of clinical manifestations correlates well with the cellular immune responsiveness of patients to *M leprae* antigens, which range from the extremity with the lowest cell-mediated immunity to *M leprae*, the lepromatous pole, to that with the highest cell-mediated immunity, the tuberculoid pole [65,66].

Genetic markers of susceptibility to leprosy are identified in different populations in Asia [67,68].

Immunologic and morphologic aspects

Lepromatous and borderline lepromatous leprosy

Lepromatous and borderline lepromatous leprosy represent the most common types of leprosy in many endemic areas of Africa. In nearly all cases, they are associated with characteristic skin lesions (Figs. 4–6). Occasionally, there is no detectable skin lesion. Skin lesions usually are numerous, consisting of macules, papules, nodules with infiltration, and thickening of the skin, affecting predominantly the cooler areas of the body. Diffuse, bilateral, and generally symmetric nerve damage occurs. In such patients, bacteria can be found in skin lesions, nasal smears, or even in blood smears. In this form, the specific unresponsiveness of the host to antigens of the leprosy bacillus permits unchecked proliferation of bacilli [69]. This unresponsiveness is manifest by negative skin test to lepromin in vivo (Mitsuda reaction). The inflammatory infiltrates of cutaneous lesions of patients who have most of the cells are of the monocyte-macrophage lineage and the remainder predominantly are made of suppressor T lymphocytes [74]. With respect to function, CD4+ T cells seem to be strongly cytolytic for antigen-presenting cells pulsed with antigens.

The more lepromatous the findings, in general, the less marked the symptoms [69]. What seems "early" clinically in leprosy may be late on

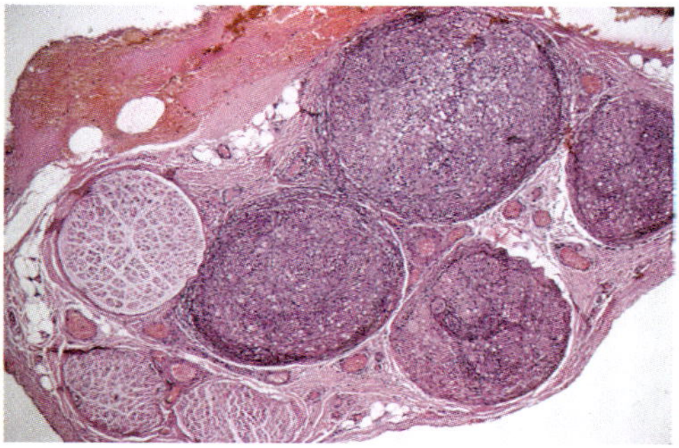

Fig. 4. Superficial peroneal nerve biopsy of a patient who has mononeuritis multiplex resulting from borderline-lepromatous leprous neuropathy. Note the important inflammatory infiltration that spares one fascicle, in keeping with the pattern of sensory loss observed in leprosy (hematoxylin-eosin staining).

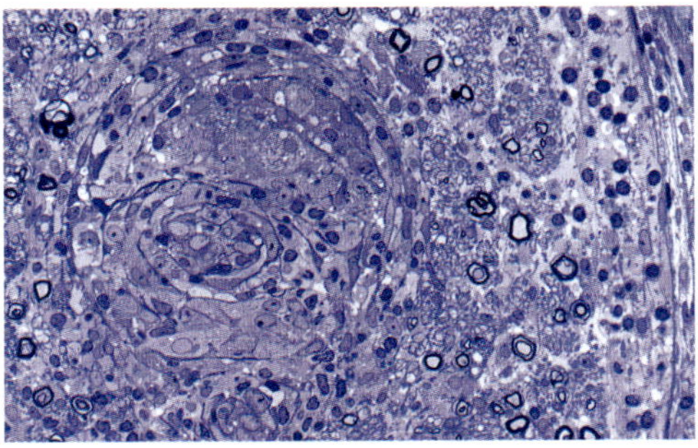

Fig. 5. Superficial peroneal nerve biopsy. Multifocal neuropathy in a patient treated for lepromatous leprosy for several months. Upgrade reversal reaction showing formation of a granuloma inside a nerve fascicle. Epon-embedded specimen (thionin blue staining).

morphologic examination of a nerve biopsy. Palpably enlarged nerves may be functioning well, but they eventually do fail. In a combined clinical, electrophysiologic, and morphologic study of seven patients who had lepromatous leprosy, palpably enlarged cutaneous radial nerves, and preservation of all modalities of sensations in the corresponding territory, the author found that the conduction velocity of the radial cutaneous nerve did not differ significantly from those found in patients who had lepromatous leprosy and hypertrophy of the cutaneous radial nerve with sensory deficit [70]. Conversely, the mean value of the action potential of the radial cutaneous nerve was significantly lower in patients who had sensory loss, suggesting that axon loss, rather than demyelination of nerve fibers, was responsible for sensory deficit. These findings also confirm that nerve conduction velocity may be decreased before any sensory deficit and used for detection of asymptomatic nerve involvement [71].

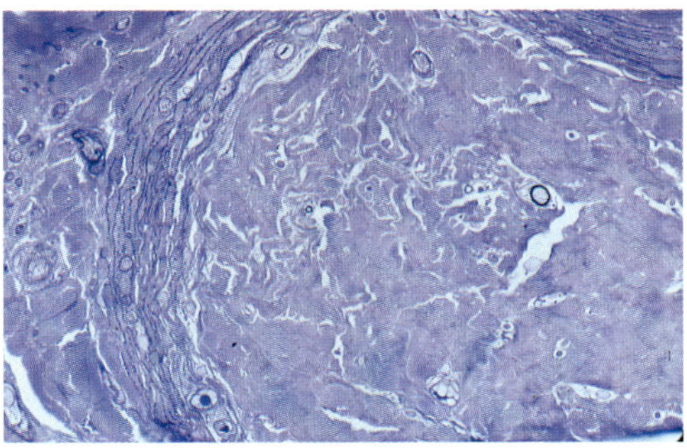

Fig. 6. Complete fibrosis of a nerve fascicle from a patient who presented with osteoarthropathy of the feet caused by leprous neuropathy. A single myelinated fiber is present in the center of the fascicle (thionin blue staining).

Morphologic study in patients who have silent hypertrophy of the radial cutaneous nerve and lepromatous leprosy shows preservation of the overall structure of the nerve and marked asymmetry of the inflammatory lesions between and within individual fascicles; some fascicles are affected massively whereas others look totally preserved, a feature that fits well with the occurrence of partial deficit in a nerve territory. Light microscopic examination of nerve cross-sections shows an enormous inflammatory reaction affecting the epineurium of all nerve specimens and the perineurium of most fascicles. This inflammatory reaction is responsible for the nerve enlargement. Increase in nerve volume may lead to nerve compression in sites of physiologic nerve entrapment and induce additional damage of mechanical origin. Around some fascicles, the perineurium has an onion-skin hypertrophic appearance, as noted by other investigators [72,73]. *M leprae* are numerous in all forms of lepromatous neuropathy; they often are in globus arrangement on Ziehl-stained paraffin-embedded specimens. They are present in all nerve compartments and affect a large variety of cells [74]. *M leprae* are identified easily on electron microscopic examination as dark, osmiophilic inclusions usually located in a cytoplasmic vacuole containing a phenolic glycolipid I (PGL-I) and lipoarabinomannan, both produced in large amounts by *M leprae*. *M leprae* are present in a variety of cells, including perineurial cells, fibroblasts, cells of the macrophage-histiocyte lineage, Schwann cells, and endothelial cells [75]. In some nerve specimens from patients who have nerve hypertrophy, the inflammatory infiltrates and infection of cells seem to follow connective tissue septa and vascular axes, from the perineurium toward the endoneurium. In other cases, infection of endoneurial cells is observed without hypertrophic changes. Axons surrounded by a normal myelin sheath may contain occasional bacilli, but the responsibility of intra-axonal bacilli in nerve lesions is unlikely.

On teased fiber preparations of nerve specimens from patients who have silent hypertrophy of the superficial radial nerve in the setting of lepromatous leprosy [70], segmental abnormalities of the myelin sheath, including segmental demyelination or the presence of short remyelinated internodes, predominate in some. All cases of symptomatic neuropathy are associated with severe axon loss, with average reduction of nerve fiber density to 5% of control values versus 25% to 30% in patients who have silent hypertrophy of the radial nerve [60].

Tuberculoid leprosy

At the other end of the spectrum, tuberculoid leprosy is marked by complete or near-complete nerve destruction. In this form, patients develop high levels of specific cell-mediated immunity that ultimately kill and clear the bacilli in the tissues, inducing concommittent damage to the nerves that harbor the bacilli. Clinically tuberculoid lesions may be single or few and are distributed asymmetrically in the vicinity of typical hypoesthetic or anesthetic hypopigmented skin lesions. There is considerable evidence suggesting that patients who have tuberculoid leprosy have nerve damage caused not by the bacilli but by the cell-mediated immune response to *M leprae* antigens [65].

Histopathologically, the lesion is characterized by epithelioid-cell granulomata with intense lymphocytic infiltrations [73,74]. Normal nerve structure no longer may be identified in many cases and bacilli are not found in the lesions, but *M leprae* antigens have been detected in nerves using anti-BCG antisera, which cross-reacts with *M leprae* antigens [75]. In the skin lesions, the tuberculoid infiltrates contain predominantly helper T cells. The basis for the conspicuous destruction of nerve structure is believed a delayed-type hypersensitivity reaction with specific helper T cells reacting with *M leprae* antigens presented in the endoneurium by macrophages and possibly by Schwann cells expressing the HLA-DR antigen induced by interferon-γ released by helper T cells. Activation of macrophages in this context leads to release of several secretory products that can propagate damage to surrounding cells [76]. It, thus, is conceivable that when a delayed-type hypersensitivity reaction occurs in the endoneurium, it can lead to major damage and even to necrosis and intraneural abcesses.

Reactional states

One of the many concerns in patients undergoing treatment for leprous neuropathy is the occurrence of a sudden alteration of the immunologic status and the development of a reactional state.

The reversal or upgrade form of type 1 reaction, which appears commonly during the first year of therapy or later is characterized by a heightened cell-mediated response occurring mainly in patients who have the borderline-lepromatous form of leprosy. During the first 6 to 12 months of therapy with dapsone alone, 50% of patients have type-1 reaction. Patients who developed type-1 reaction were found to have higher concentration of IgM anti–PGL-I antibodies in the serum [77]. This reaction is identified by swelling and exacerbation of existing skin and nerve lesions in association with general malaise and fever. Painful swelling of nerve trunks is accompanied by sensory and motor deficit in corresponding territory. In some cases, nerves that seem unaffected are heavily damaged. Endoneurial granuloma, multinucleated giant cells, lymphocytic infiltration, vasculitis, and perineuritis are present on morphologic examination. Necrosis of the endoneurial content may lead to nerve abscesses. No *M leprae* are observed in this reaction. Therefore, improvement of the cell-mediated immune response in patients undergoing treatment can lead to further damage of nerve trunks.

Erythema nodosum leprosum (ENL), which corresponds to a downgrade reaction, is seen almost exclusively in the lepromatous pole, is common once the start of effective chemotherapy has resulted in massive death of leprosy bacilli and affects an average 50% of patients by the end of the first year of treatment in some areas. The multiple, acute, tender nodules that characterize ENL frequently are accompanied by fever, arthritis, edema, muscle pains, iridocyclitis, and acute PN damage. The ENL is considered a manifestation of the Arthus phenomenon with complement and immunoglobulin granular deposition around dermal vessels [78]. Tumor necrosis factor α and interleukin 1 serum concentrations are increased greatly in lepromatous leprosy and correlate with the severity of ENL and with the incidence of reactions.

Diagnosis

Nerve biopsies are useful in the diagnosis and management of leprosy. In purely neuropathic forms, which are seen in the tuberculoid form and, less often, in lepromatous leprosy, it is the only way to reach the diagnosis. It is useful especially in countries where leprosy is not common. In such countries, leprous neuropathy may become symptomatic years or decades after the patients are moved from endemic areas. In countries where leprosy is endemic, nerve biopsy may be useful in differentiating leprous neuropathy from neuropathy of other origin, including diabetic neuropathy, hereditary sensory neuropathies, or amyloid neuropathy, which can lead to sensory and trophic manifestations that may be mistaken for leprous neuropathy. Ziehl's staining of paraffin embedded sections permits viusalization of bacilli in the pluribacillar forms of the disease. Bacilli are scarce or absent from nerves with tuberculoid leprosy and in reactional states. In such forms, identification of *M leprae* antigens using anti-BCG and MLO4 monoclonal antibodies in paraffin sections, with immunoperoxidase, may be positive even when *M leprae* can not be found on histology. When there is no evidence of infection with *M leprae*, it may be impossible to differentiate a neuropathy resulting from tuberculoid leprosy from sarcoid neuropathy. On the basis of cross-sectional studies, it seems that testing for PGL-I serum antibodies has high sensitivity for multibacillary cases but only moderate sensitivity for paucibacillary cases. Detection of sequences of *M leprae* DNA by polymerase chain reaction techniques [79] may prove helpful in the diagnosis of paucibacillary leprous neuropathy and in the follow-up of patients who are undertreated.

Treatment

Enormous progress has been made in chemotherapy of leprosy thanks to control programs of the WHO. Leprologists advised to treat patients who have paucibacillary leprosy, which include the tuberculoid and borderline tuberculoid forms, for 6 months only, with daily unsupervised dapsone (100 mg) and monthly supervised rifampicin (600 mg); all treatment then stops and patients remain under observation for 2 years. Multibacillary patients require a minimum of 2 years' treatment, but should continue preferably until skin smears are negative; they are treated with daily dapsone (100 mg) together with clofamizine (300 mg), both supervised. On completion, multibacillary patients should remain under observation for 5 years.

Corticosteroids are useful in the treatment of reversal reaction. Contact tracing and disability prevention are other aspects of treatment of leprosy.

Lyme disease

The first descriptions of tick bite–associated paralysis and meningitis were made in Europe [79–83] but the recognition of Lyme disease as a separate entity occurred in 1977 [84] because of a geographic clustering in Lyme, Connecticut. Lyme disease is a multisystem illness that affects the skin, joints, heart, and nervous system, caused by a tick-transmitted spirochetae, *Borrelia burgdorferi* [85]. Certain differences are noted between American and European isolates of *B burgdorferi* in morphology, outer surface proteins, plasmids, and DNA homology [86].

Ixodic ticks are the usual vectors. Ticks feed once during the three stages of their usual 2-year life. Larval ticks take one blood meal in late summer, nymphs feed during the following spring and early summer, and adults during that autumn [87]. In the United States, the preferred host for the larval and nympheal stages of *Ixodes dammini* is the white-footed mouse, whereas the white-tailed deer are the preferred host for adult *I dammini.*

In Europe, thousands of new cases of Lyme borreliosis occur each summer, particularly in Germany, Austria, Switzerland, France, and Sweden. In the United States, Lyme borreliosis is reported mainly from Massachussets to Maryland in the northeast, Wisconsin and Minnesota in the midwest, and California and Oregon in the West [86].

Clinical manifestations

The course of the disease follows three stages.

Stage 1: Typical patients first have erythema migrans, sometimes followed several weeks or months later by meningitis or facial palsy and, often, months later by arthritis. Localized erythema migrans results from local spreading of *B burgdorferi* in the skin. It starts as a red macule or papule at the site of the bite and expands to form a large red ring with central clearing. It is accompanied by fever, minor constitutional symptoms, or regional lymphadenopathy.

Stage 2: Within days or weeks after inoculation, the spirochete may spread in patients' blood to many sites and has been recovered from blood during this stage and from many organs. Secondary annular lesions, which resemble the primary erythema migrans, occur in approximately half of patients in association with migratory musculoskeletal and joint pain [87]. Widely disseminated symptoms seem to be more common in the United states than in Europe. By this time, the host starts to develop a strong immune response to *B burgdorferi* antigens that result in destruction of spirochetes by complement activation through immune complexes [88]. Polymorphonuclear leukocytes and monocytes phagocytose the spirochete readily and histologically lymphocytic infiltration is observed in all affected tissues with plentiful plasma cells and mild vasculitis.

After several weeks or months, 15% to 20% of patients develop neurologic signs. The first neurologic sign usually is radicular pain, often of the burning type, associated or not with weakness, with little or no clinical signs of meningitis. Meningitis is the most common neurologic abnormality in Lyme disease. It can be the first symptom but is preceded in most cases by erythema migrans, then usually begins after the skin lesions resolve. Papilledema and increased CSF pressure can occur. CSF examination reveals a lymphocytic pleocytosis, usually a few tens or hundreds of cells per mL, with mild elevation of protein with a high proportion of oligoclonal bands of immunoglobulins. The CSF glucose usually is normal but can be low [89,90]. The spirochete has been cultured from the CSF on several occasions.

Multifocal spinal root or cranial nerve involvement often develops within a few days or weeks, with uni- or bilateral facial palsy and asymmetric sensorimotor radiculoneuropathy. Cranial neuropathy is present in 50% of patients who have neurologic abnormalities [89–92]. Facial palsy often is bilateral. The cranial nerves can be affected, in association with meningitis. Cranial nerve palsies resolve within weeks or months, sometimes incompletely. Sphincter disturbances occur.

Peripheral neuropathy occurs in approximately half of patients who have meningitis. Focal or multifocal involvement is the most common presentation. Common patterns include painful thoracoabdominal sensory radiculitis, associated with distal involvement. Weakness and sensory loss improve within a few weeks, but recovery may take up to several months and often remains incomplete.

Electrophysiologic testing of patients who have peripheral neuropathy has shown evidence of demyelination and of axonal degeneration, but usually axonal lesions predominate [92,93]. Histologically, the nerve lesions associate lymphoplasmocytic inflammatory infiltrates that predominate in nerve roots with axonal lesions. The presence of *B burgdorferi* has not been documented convincingly in the nerves. The author has had the opportunity to perform a post mortem study on a patient who had multifocal neuropathy and meningitis, who died from pulmonary embolism at this stage of the disease in spite of preventive treatment with low molecular weight heparin. The PNs were normal, although there were important inflammatory infiltrates of the meninges, around spinal roots and cranial nerves, especially around the facial nerves. The CNS was not affected. Stage 2 neurologic abnormalities usually last for weeks or months.

Cardiac involvement occurs in 4% to 8% of patients. They include fluctuating atrioventricular node block, mild left ventricular dysfunction, or, rarely, cardiomegaly or fatal pancarditis. The duration of cardiac abnormalities usually is brief and does not necessitate permanent insertion of a pacemaker [94–96].

Stage 3: Arthritis occurs by transient episodes, a mean of 6 months after the onset of the disease. They affect about 60% of the patients in the United States [87] and are characterized by asymmetric oligoarticular arthritis especially of the knee; one or a few joints are affected. The spirochete occasionally has been cultured from joint fluid. Arthritis seems less common in Europe; the susceptibility to develop Lyme arthritis seem to be determined genetically.

A variety of late syndromes affecting the CNS is described, including spastic paraparesis, ataxia, relapsing multiple sclerosis–like illness, bladder dysfunction, cognitive impairment, dementia, and subacute encephalitis [97,98]. Although patients who had CNS manifestations had serologic evidence of Lyme disease, they did not have intrathecal synthesis of antibody to *B burdorferi* or were not tested for it [87]. Thus, there is no convincing evidence for CNS complications of Lyme disease.

Diagnosis

From a neurologic point of view, presence of a subacute meningoradiculoneuritis with facial palsy and signs and symptoms suggesting a multifocal involvement of the PNS is highly suggestive of Lyme borreliosis. Serology is the only practical laboratory aid in diagnosis, but serologic testing is not yet standardized and the results from different laboratories may vary. Physicians must be aware of false-negative and, more commonly, false-positive results [87]. Titres should increase fourfold or more between the erythema migrans phase and subsequent neurologic involvement. Many patients have asymptomatic *B burgdoferi* infection, and, in addition to that, false-positive results, particularly with IgM, may occur in healthy subjects and in patients who have a variety of other diseases [84]. Refinements of serologic methods may be helpful in the future to differentiate patients who have residual positivity and false-positive patients from those suffering from Lyme disease.

Treatment

Treatment with high doses of penicillin gives good results at stage 1, but the results are not as good in patients who have stage 2 neurologic abnormalities and in patients who have arthritis. *B burgdorferi* seems highly sensitive to tetracycline, ampicilline, and ceftriaxone but only moderately sensitive to penicillin. For early Lyme disease localized stage 1 or disseminated stage 2, oral tetracycline generally is an effective antibiotic [99]. Doxycycline, a long-acting tetracycline that achieves better tissue levels, may be preferable. The treatment should be administered for 10 to 30 days.

Although intravenous penicillin generally is considered effective in the treatment of neurologic disease, ceftriaxone now is used commonly because it crosses the blood-brain barrier more readily and requires only once-a-day administration [100]. Corticosteroids may be associated with antibiotic treatment in some cases. In view of the low risk of Lyme disease after a recognized deer tick bite and uncertain effectiveness of prophylactic antimicrobial agents, routine antimicrobial prophylaxis for persons who have a recognized deer tick bite is not indicated [101].

Chagas' disease

In Chagas' disease, infection is with the trypomastigote form of *Trypanosoma cruzi* by blood-sucking bugs of the *Triatoma* subfamily, *Triatoma infestans*. The metacyclic trypanosome in the bugs' feces penetrates minute skin abrasions, mucous membranes, or the conjunctiva. Other ways of transmission include congenital infection, laboratory accidents, organ transplantation, and blood transfusion. Chagas' disease is widespread in Latin America, where it affects several millions of people. After penetration in the host, the trypomastigote loses its flagellum, transforms into an amastigote, and multiplies in pseudocysts. Some amastigotes eventually may transform back into trypomastigotes and circulate in the blood.

Initial local multiplication of the parasite may result in local inflammation with heat, redness and swelling (chagoma), and enlargement of satellite lymph nodes. During this phase of active parasite multiplication, there is an intense interstitial inflammatory reaction with mononuclear cells. Later on, the parasite multiplication is suppressed by the cellular and humoral immune reaction of the host and becomes increasingly difficult to detect in the tissues. Ninety percent of the patients survive the acute phase but it is doubtful if the infection is ever eradicated. It usually remains asymptomatic throughout life in many of them, whereas others develop manifest symptoms after a period of years.

The neurologic manifestations are characterized mainly by the occurrence of the autonomic neuropathy at the chronic stage of the disease. There is some regional differences in Chagas' disease because of the existence of different strains of *T cruzi*. The autonomic manifestations include cardiac and gastrointestinal involvement which are associated with inflammatory lesions of muscle and autonomic ganglia and nerves [102].

Peripheral neuropathy is not a prominent manifestation of Chagas' disease. It was recognized first in animal models [103–107] before its identification in man. Although peripheral neuropathy seems common at a subclinical level in humans, especially on electrophysiologic examination at the acute and at the chronic phases of the disease [108,109], the electromyogram abnormalities remain subtle. Clinical neuropathy is uncommon [110], yet experimental models of Chagas' disease are useful in understanding the pathophysiology of nerve and muscle lesions. In a series of investigations performed in the mouse model, the author has found that early localization of *T cruzi* occurred at the acute phase, associated with mild lesions. At the chronic stage of the disease, the amastigotes are increasingly difficult to localize but immunostaining clearly shows the presence of *T cruzi* antigens in the nerve and muscle inflammatory infiltrates. Additionnally, the author has been able to show that the endoneurial granulomas were the result of a delayed-type hypersensitivity reaction [111–113]. Nifurtimox and Benznidazole are used at the acute stage but are less active at the chronic stage. Only symptomatic treatment can be offered at the chronic stage [101].

Summary

Peripheral neuropathies can result from several infective agents, ranging from viruses, especially retroviruses, to parasites and bacilli. Leprosy, which often is considered a disorder of the past, is still common in some geographic areas, especially in Africa, South America, and Asia. An increasing number of cases of neuropathies occurs in patients who have HIV or Lyme disease. The important point is that all these neuropathies are treatable and often preventable.

References

[1] Snider WD, Simpson DM, Nielsen S, et al. Neurological complications of human immune-deficiency syndrome. Ann Neurol 1983;14:403–18.

[2] Lipkin WI, Parry G, Kiprov DD, et al. Inflammatory neuropathy in homosexual men with lymphadenopathy. Neurology 1985;35:1479–83.

[3] Levy RM, Bredesen DE, Rosenblum ML. Neurological manifestations of the acquired immunodeficiency syndrome (AIDS): experience at UCSF and review of the literature. J Neurosurg 1985;62:475–95.

[4] Dehen H, Boulu P, Fenelon G, et al. Neuropathie périphérique type polyradiculonévrite inflammatoire au cours d'anomalies immunitaires évoquant le syndrome d'immunodéficit acquis [Polyneuropathy of the Inflammatory polyneuritis type in patient with acquired immunodeficit]. Nouv Press Med 1985;14:226.

[5] Leport C, Chaunu MP, Sicre J, et al. Neuropathie périphérique en relation avec l'infection par le rétrovirus LAV/HTLV-III [Peripheral neuropathy in retroviral infection]. Presse Med (Paris) 1987;16:55–8.

[6] Cornblath DR, McArthur JC, Kennedy PGE, et al. Inflammatory demyelinating peripheral neuropathies associated with human T-cell lymphotropic Virus type III infection. Ann Neurol 1987;21:32–40.

[7] Léger JM, Bouche P, Bolgert F, et al. The spectrum of polyneuropathies in patients infected with HIV. J Neurol Neurosurg Psychiatry 1989;52:1369–74.

[8] Chavanet P, Giroud M, Lancon JP, et al. Neuropathies infracliniques chez les malades HIV + [Subclinical neuropathy in HIV positive patients]. Presse Med 1987;16:1764.

[9] So YT, Holtzman DM, Abrams DI, et al. Peripheral neuropathy associated with acquired immunodeficiency syndrome. Arch Neurol 1988;45:945–8.
[10] Cornblath DR, McArthur JC. Predominantly sensory neuropathy in patients with AIDS and AIDS related complex. Neurology 1988;38:794–6.
[11] Miller RG, Parry GJ, Pfaeffl W, et al. The spectrum of peripheral neuropathy associated with ARC and AIDS. Muscle Nerve 1988;11:857–63.
[12] Gastaut JL, Gastaut JF, Pélissier JF, et al. Neuropathies périphériques au cours de l'infection par le virus de l'immunodéficience humaine [Peripheral neuropathy in the course of infection with the HIV]. Rev Neurol 1989;145:451–9.
[13] Piette AM, Tusseau F, Chapman A. Symptomatologie aiguë contemporaine de la primo-infection par le virus HIV [Acute manifestations during primo-infection with the HIV]. Deux observations. Presse Med 1987;16:346–8.
[14] Vendrell J, Heredia C, Pujol M, et al. Guillain-Barré syndrome associated with seroconversion for anti-HTLV-III. Neurology 1987;37:544.
[15] Persuy PH, Arnott G, Fortier B, et al. Syndrome de Guillain-Barré d'évolution favorable dans un cas d'infection récente par le virus de l'immunodéficience humaine [Guillain-Barré syndrome with favorable outcome in a patient with recent infection with the HIV]. Rev Neurol 1988;144:32–5.
[16] Beytout J, Llory JF, Clavelou P, et al. Méningoradiculite à la phase de primo-infection à VIH. Intérêt de la plasmaphérèse [HIV primoinfection. Usefulness of plasma exchanges]. Presse Med 1989;18:1031–2.
[17] Gibbels E, Diederich N. Human immunodeficiency virus (HIV)-related chronic relapsing inflammatory demyelinating polyneuropathy with multifocal unsusual onion bulbs in sural nerve biopsy. Acta Neuropathol (Berl) 1988;75:529–34.
[18] Puthanakit T, Oberdorfer P, Akarathum N, et al. Immune reconstitution syndrome after highly active antiretroviral therapy in human immunodeficiency virus-infected thai children. Pediatr Infect Dis J 2006;25:53–8.
[19] Follezou JY, Smadja D, Baulac M, et al. Paralysie faciale isolée associée à l'infection HIV [Isolated facial nerve palsy and HIV infection]. Presse Med 1987;16:357–8.
[20] Brown MM, Thompson A, Goh BT, et al. Bell's palsy and HIV infection. J Neurol Neurosurg Psychiatry 1988;51:425–6.
[21] Schielke E, Pfister RHW, Einhäupl KM. Peripheral facial nerve palsy associated with HIV infection. Lancet 1989;i:553–4.
[22] Weschler AF, Ho DD. Bilateral Bell's palsy at time of HIV seroconversion. Neurology 1988;39:747–8.
[23] Verma RK, Ziegler DK, Kepes JJ. HIV-related neuromuscular syndrome simulating motor neuron disease. Neurology 1990;40:544–6.
[24] Berger JR, Espinosa PS, Kissel J. Brachial amyotrophic diplegia in a patient with human immunodeficiency virus infection: widening the spectrum of motor neuron diseases occurring with the human immunodeficiency virus. Arch Neurol 2005;62:817–23.
[25] de la Monte S, Gabudza DH, Ho DD, et al. Peripheral neuropathy in the acquired immunodeficiency syndrome. Ann Neurol 1988;23:485–92.
[26] Said G, Lacroix-Ciaudo C, Fujimura H, et al. The peripheral neuropathy of necrotizing arteritis: A clinicopathological study. Ann Neurol 1988;23:461–5.
[27] Said G, Lacroix C, Chemouilli P. Les neuropathies périphériques au cours de l'infection par le VIH [Peripheral neuropathy and HIV infection]. In: Said G, Saimot G, editors. Manifestations neurologiques et infection rétrovirale [Neurological manifestations of HIV infection]. Paris: Pradel; 1991. p. 123–43.
[28] Liebow AA, Carrington CRB, Friedman PJ. Lymphomatoid granulomatosis. Hum Pathol 1972;3:457–70.
[29] Gherardi RK, Chretien F, Delfau-Larue MH, et al. Neuropathy in diffuse infiltrative lymphocytosis syndrome: an HIV neuropathy, not a lymphoma. Neurology 1998;50:1041–4.

[30] Simpson DM, Kitch D, Evans SR, et al. ACTG A5117 Study Goup. HIV neuropathy natural history cohort study: assessment measures and risk factors. Neurology 2006;66: 1679–87.
[31] Craddock C, Pasvol G, Bull R, et al. Cardiorespiratory arrest and autonomic neuropathy in AIDS. Lancet 1987;2:16–8.
[32] Harle JR, Disdier P, Chouc PY, et al. Hypotension orthostatique dysautonomique au cours d'une infection par le virus de l'immunodéficience humaine [Postural hypotension in HIV infection]. Presse Med 1988;17:917–8.
[33] Freeman R, Roberts MS, Friedman LS, et al. Autonomic function and human immunodeficiency virus infection. Neurology 1990;40:575–80.
[34] Said G, Lacroix C, Chemouilli P, et al. Cytomegalovirus (CMV) neuropathy in AIDS: a clinical and pathological study. Ann Neurol 1991;29:139–46.
[35] Miller RG, Storey J, Greco C. Ganciclovir in the treatment of progressive AIDS-related polyradiculopathy. Neurology 1990;40:569–74.
[36] Eidelberg D, Sotrel A, Vogel H, et al. Progressive polyradiculopathy in acquired immune deficiency syndrome. Neurology 1986;36:912–6.
[37] Behar R, Wiley C, McCutchan JA. Cytomegalovirus polyradiculoneuropathy in acquired immune deficiency syndrome. Neurology 1987;37:557–61.
[38] Singh BM, Levine S, Yarrish RL, et al. Spinal cord syndrome in the acquired immune deficiency syndrome. Acta Neurol Scand 1986;73:590–8.
[39] Mahieux F, Gray F, Fenelon G, et al. Acute myeloradiculitis due to cytomegalovirus as the initial manifestation of AIDS. J Neurol Neurosurg Psychiatry 1989;52:270–4.
[40] Vinters HV, Kwok MK, Ho HW, et al. Cytomegalovirus in the nervous system of patients with the acquired immune deficiency syndrome. Brain 1989;112:245–68.
[41] Small PM, McPhaul LW, Sooy CD, et al. Cytomegalovirus infection of the laryngeal nerve presenting as hoarseness in patients with acquired immunodeficiency syndrome. JAMA 1989;86:108–10.
[42] Moskowitz LB, Gregorios JB, Hensley GT, et al. Cytomegalovirus-induced demyelination associated with acquired immune deficiency syndrome. Arch Pathol Lab Med 1984;108: 873–7.
[43] Gold JE, Jimenez E, Zalusky R. Human immunodeficiency virus-related lymphoreticular malignancies and peripheral neurologic disease. Cancer 1988;61:2318–24.
[44] Lambert JS, Seidlin M, Reichman RC, et al. 2′, 3′-dideoxyinosine (ddI) in patients with the acquired immunodeficiency syndrome or AIDS-related complex. N Engl J Med 1990;322: 1333–40.
[45] Vernant JC, Bellance R, Bucher B. Manifestations neurologiques associées au virus HTLV-1 [Neurological manifestations associated with HTLV-1 infection]. In: Said G, Saimot G, editors. Manifestations neurologiques et infection rétrovirale [Neurological manifestations and retroviral infections]. Paris: Pradel; 1991. p. 193–207.
[46] Gessain A, Goult O. Chronic myelopathy associated with human T-lymphotropic virus type I (HTLV-I). Ann Intern Med 1992;117:933–46.
[47] Roman GC, Roman LN. Tropical spastic paraparesis. A clinical study of 50 patients from Tumaco (Columbia) and review of the worldwide features of the syndrome. J Neurol Sci 1988;87:121–38.
[48] Bighjee AI, Kelbe C, Haribahai HC, et al. Human T-cell lymphotropic virus type 1 (HTLV-1) associated myelopathy in Natal, South Africa. Brain 1990;113:1307–20.
[49] Leite AC, Silva MT, Alamy AH, et al. Peripheral neuropathy in HTLV-I infected individuals without tropical spastic paraparesis/HTLV-I-associated myelopathy. J Neurol 2004; 251:877–81.
[50] Said G, Goulon-Goeau C, Lacroix C, et al. Inflammatory lesion of a peripheral nerve in a patient with human T-lymphotropic virus type 1-associated myelopathy. Ann Neurol 1988;24:275–7.

[51] Nakazato O, Mori T, Okajima T. Sural nerve pathology in HTLV-1 associated myelopathy. Neurology and Neurobiology 1989;51:269–74.
[52] Sugimura K, Takahashi A, Watanabe M, et al. Demyelinating changes in sural nerve biopsy of patients with HTLV-1 associated myelopathy. Neurology 1990;40:1263–6.
[53] Juliao OF, Rotberg A. Neural involvement in leprosy. In: Van Bogaert L, Pereyra Kafer L, Poch GF, editors. Tropical neurology. Buenos Aires: Lopez Libreros Editores; 1963. p. 43–80.
[54] Datsur DK. Leprosy. In: Vinken PJ, GW Bruyn GW, editors. Handbock of clinical neurology, vol. 33. Amsterdam: North Holland Publishing Company; 1978. p. 421–68.
[55] Sabin TD, Swift TR. Leprosy. In: Dyck PJ, Thomas PK, Lambert EH, et al, editors. Peripheral neuropathy, vol. 2. 2nd ed. Philadelphia: WB Saunders; 1984. p. 1955–87.
[56] Monrad-Krohn GH. The neurological aspect of leprosy. Videnskapsselskapets Skrifter. I. Mat-Naturv Klasse 1923;16:1–78.
[57] Ridley DS, Jopling WH. Classification of leprosy according to immunity. A five group system. Int J Lepr 1966;34:255–73.
[58] Ridley DS. Histological classification and the immunological spectrum of leprosy. Bull WHO 1974;51:451–65.
[59] Hastings RC, Brand PW, Mansfield ER, et al. Bacterial density in the skin in lepromatous leprosy as related to temperature. Lepr Rev 1968;39:71–4.
[60] Said G, Slama G, Selva J. Progressive centripetal degeneration of axons in small fibre type diabetic polyneuropathy. A clinical and pathological study. Brain 1983;106:791–807.
[61] Said G, Ropert A, Faux N. Length dependent degeneration of fibers in Portuguese amyloid polyneuropathy. A clinicopathological study. Neurology 1984;34:1025–32.
[62] Datsur DK, Antia NH, Divekar SC. The facial nerve in leprosy. II. Pathology, pathogenesis, electromyography and clinical correlation. Int J Lepr 1966;34:118–38.
[63] Said G. A clinicopathologic study of acrodystrophic neuropathies. Muscle Nerve 1980;3: 491–501.
[64] Landrieu P, Said G, Alaire C. Dominantly transmitted congenital indifference to pain. Ann Neurol 1990;27:574–8.
[65] Bloom BR, Godal T. Selective primary health care: strategies for control of disease in the developing world. V. Leprosy. Rev Infect Dis 1983;5:765–80.
[66] Sansonetti P, Lagrange PH. The immunology of leprosy: speculations on the leprosy spectrum. Rev Infect Dis 1981;3:422–69.
[67] Tosh K, Meisner S, Siddiqui R, et al. A region of chromosome 20 is linked to leprosy susceptibility in south India. J Infect Did 2002;186:1190–3.
[68] Mira MT, Alacïs A, Van Thuc N, et al. Chromosome 6q25 is linked to susceptibility to leprosy in a Vietnamese population. Nat Genet 2003;33:412–5.
[69] Pedley JC, Harman DJ, Waudby H, et al. Leprosy in peripheral nerves: histopathological findings in 119 untreated patients in Nepal. J Neurol Neurosurg Psychiatry 1980;43:198–204.
[70] Tzourio C, Said G, Milan J. Asymptomatic nerve hypertrophy in lepromatous leprosy: a clinical, electrophysiological and morphological study. J Neurol 1992;239:367–74.
[71] Sebille A. Respective imporance of different nerve conduction velocities in leprosy. J Neurol Sci 1978;38:89–95.
[72] Pearson JMH, Weddell AGM. Perineurial changes in untreated leprosy. Lepr Rev 1975;46: 51–67.
[73] Boddingius J. Ultrastructural changes in blood vessels of peripheral nerves in leprosy neuropathy. II. Borderline, borderline lepromatous and lepromatous patients. Acta Neuropathol (Berl) 1977;40:21–39.
[74] Job CK. Mycobacterium leprae in nerve lesions in lepromatous leprosy. An electron microscopic study. Arch Pathol 1970;89:195–207.
[75] Barros V, Shetty VP, Antia NH. Demonstration of Mycobacterium leprae antigen in nerves of tuberculoid leprosy. Acta Neuropathol (Berl) 1987;73:387–92.

[76] Said G, Hontebeyrie M. Nerve lesions induced by macrophage activation. Res Immunol 1992;143:589–99.

[77] Roche P, Theuvenet WJ, Britton WJ. Risk factors for type-1 reactions in borderline leprosy patients. Lancet 1991;338:654–7.

[78] Wemambu SNC, Turk JL, Waters MFR, et al. Erythema nodosum leprosum: a clinical manifestation of Arthus phenomenon. Lancet 1969;2:933–5.

[79] Woods SA, Cole S. A family of dispersed repeats in *Mycobacterium leprae*. Mol Microbiol 1990;4:1745–51.

[80] Afzelius A. Erythema chronicum migrans. Acta Derm Venereol 1921;2:120–5.

[81] Lipschütz B. Weiterer Beitrag zur Kenntis des "Erythema chronicum migrans". Arch Dermatol Syph 1923;143:365–74.

[82] Bannwarth A. Zur Klinik und Pathogenese der "chronischen lymphocytaren Meningitis" [Clinical aspects and pathogenesis of chronic lymphocytic meningitis]. Arch Psychiatr Nervenkr 1944;117:161–85.

[83] Garin C, Bujadoux C. Paralysie par les tiques [Tick paralysis]. J Med Lyon 1922;3:765–7.

[84] Steere AC, Malawista SE, Snydman DR, et al. Lyme arthritis: an epidemic of oligoarticular arthritis in children and adults in three Connecticut communities. Arthritis Rheum 1977;20: 7–17.

[85] Budgrofer W, Barbour AG, Hayes SF, et al. Lyme disease—a tick borne spirochetosis? Science 1982;216:1317–9.

[86] Wilson ML, Spielman A. Seasonal activity of immature Ixodes dammini. J Med Entomol 1985;22:408–14.

[87] Steere AC. Lyme disease. N Engl J Med 1989;321:586–96.

[88] Kochi SK, Johnson RC. Role of immunoglobulin G in killing of Borrelia burgdorferi by the classical complement pathway. Infect Immun 1988;56:314–21.

[89] Reik L, Steere AC, Bartenhagen NH, et al. Neurologic abnormalities of Lyme disease. Medicine (Baltimore) 1979;58:281–94.

[90] Pachner AR, Steere AC. The triad of neurologic manifestations of Lyme disease: meningitis, cranial neuritis, and radiculoneuritis. Neurology 1985;35:47–53.

[91] Reik L Jr, Burgdorfer W, Donaldson JO. Neurologic abnormalities in Lyme disease without erythema chronicum migrans. Am J Med 1986;81:73–8.

[92] Duray PH, Steere AC. Clinical pathologic correlations of Lyme disease by stage. Ann N Y Acad Sci 1988;539:65–79.

[93] Vallat JM, Hugon J, Lubeau M, et al. Tick-bite meningoradiculoneuritis: clinical, electrophysiologic, and histologic findings in 10 cases. Neurology 1987;37:749–53.

[94] Steere AC, Batsford WP, Weinberg M, et al. Lyme carditis: cardiac abnormalities of Lyme disease. Ann Intern Med 1980;93:8–16.

[95] Marcus LC, Steere AC, Duray PH, et al. Fatal pancarditis in a patient with coexistent Lyme disease and babesiosis: demonstration of spirochetes in the myocardium. Ann Intern Med 1985;103:374–6.

[96] Ackermann R, Rehse-Kupper B, Gollmer E, et al. Chronic neurologic manifestations of erythema migrans borreliosis. Ann N Y Acad Sci 1988;539:16–23.

[97] Pachner AR, Duray P, Steere AC. Central nervous system manifestations of Lyme disease. Arch Neurol 1989;46:790–5.

[98] Halperin JJ, Luft BJ, Anand AK, et al. Lyme neuroborreliosis: central nervous system manifestations. Neurology 1989;39:753–9.

[99] Steere AC, Hutchinson GJ, Rahn DW, et al. Treatment of early manifestations of Lyme disease. Ann Intern Med 1983;99:22–6.

[100] Dattwyler RJ, Halperin JJ, Volkman DJ, et al. Treatment of late Lyme borreliosis—randomised comparison of ceftriaxone and penicillin. Lancet 1988;1:1191–4.

[101] Shapiro ED, Gerber MA, Holabird NB, et al. A controlled trial of antimicrobial prophylaxis for Lyme disease after deer-tick bites. N Engl J Med 1992;237:1769–73.

[102] Fernandez A, Hontebeyrie M, Said G. Autonomic neuropathy and immunological abnormalities in Chagas' disease. Clin Auton Res 1992;2:409–12.
[103] Barreira A, Said G, Krettli A. Multifocal demyelinative lesions of peripheral nerves in experimental chronic Chagas disease. Trans R Soc Trop Med Hyg 1981;75:751.
[104] Said G, Joskowicz M, Barreira A, et al. Neuropathy associated with experimental Chagas' disease. Ann Neurol 1985;18:676–83.
[105] Gonzalez Cappa SM, Sanz OP, Müller LA, et al. Peripheral nervous system damage in experimental Chagas' disease. Am J Trop Med Hyg 1987;36:41–5.
[106] Molina HA, Cardoni RL, Rimoldi MT. The neuromuscular pathology of experimental Chagas' disease. J Neurol Sci 1987;81:287–300.
[107] Losavio A, Jones MC, Sanz OP, et al. A sequential study of the peripheral nervous system involvement in experimental Chagas' disease. Am J Trop Med Hyg 1989;41: 539–47.
[108] Benavente OR, Patino Ledesma O, et al. Motor unit involvement in human Chagas' disease. Arq Neuro-Psiquiat (Sao-Paolo) 1989;47:283–6.
[109] Sica REP, Filipini D, Panizza M, et al. Involvement of the peripheral sensory nervous system in human chronic Chagas disease. Medicina (Buenos Aires) 1986;46:662–8.
[110] Nascimento OJM, De Freitas MRG, Chimelli L. Polyneuropathie axonale dans la maladie de Chagas [Axonal polyneuropathy in Chagas' disease]. Rev Neurol 1991;147:679–81.
[111] Hontebeyrie-Joskowicz M, Said G, Milon G, et al. L3T4 + T cells able to mediate parasite-specific delayed type hypersensitivity play a role in the pathology of experimental Chagas' disease. Eur J Immunol 1987;17:1027–33.
[112] Ben Younes-Chennoufi A, Hontebeyrie-Joskowicz M, Tricottet V, et al. Persistence of Trypanosoma cruzi antigens in the inflammatory lesions of chronically infected mice. Trans R Soc Trop Med Hyg 1988;82:77–83.
[113] Ben Younes-Chennoufi A, Said G, Eisen H, et al. Cellular immunity to Trypanosoma cruzi is mediated by helper T cells (CD4 +). Trans R Soc Trop Med Hyg 1988;82:84–9.

ELSEVIER
SAUNDERS

Neurol Clin 25 (2007) 139–171

NEUROLOGIC
CLINICS

Plexopathies

Asa J. Wilbourn, MD[a,b,*]

[a]EMG Laboratory, Cleveland Clinic, Cleveland, OH, USA
[b]Department of Neurology, Case Western Reserve University School of Medicine, 10900 Euclid Avenue, Cleveland, OH 44106, USA

The neural plexuses are intricate networks of nerve fibers interposed between the spinal cord or anterior primary rami (APR) proximally and the most proximal portions of peripheral nerves distally. (The term, plexus, means "interweaving of strands.") Depending on how they are defined, there are three or four neural plexuses: cervical, brachial, and lumbosacral (also known as pelvic) or lumbar and sacral. If the lumbar and sacral plexuses are considered as a single entity, then they constitute the largest peripheral nervous system (PNS) structure. Each of the plexuses varies substantially from the others in its overall vulnerability to injury, the specific types of trauma or disease that most often affects it, and the ease with which it is assessed by the two laboratory diagnostic procedures in current use for doing so: neuroimaging studies and electrodiagnostic (EDX) examinations [1].

The neural plexuses vary substantially in the significance in which they are viewed by clinicians, in part because of the marked differences in the incidence of the lesions that affect them. Cervical plexopathies reportedly are rare. This reputed low incidence may be deceptive, however, because of their being overlooked, with many lesions affecting the neck because of more obvious coexisting injuries to neighboring structures. In contrast, brachial plexopathies unquestionably are the most common plexus lesions encountered. Lumbar plexopathies and sacral plexopathies, considered either alone or as one, are intermediate in this regard. Similarly, the ability of laboratory diagnostic aids, in particular an EDX examination, to assess the various plexuses is variable. (Before discussing the relative value of EDX studies with the various plexopathies, a distinction must be made between EDX procedures that theoretically can be performed—and even are in a limited

* Department of Neurology, Case Western Reserve University School of Medicine, 10900 Euclid Avenue, Cleveland, OH 44106.
E-mail address: asa.wilbourn@case.edu

0733-8619/07/$ - see front matter
doi:10.1016/j.ncl.2006.11.005

number of laboratories—and those that are performed routinely in nearly all laboratories. The following comments pertain solely to the latter.) Only a fragmentary assessment of the cervical plexus can be accomplished in an EDX laboratory. Using surface recording electrodes, just a single motor nerve conduction study (NCS), the phrenic, can be performed, and only one sensory NCS, the great auricular. Unfortunately, even with thin, young patients, the findings on phrenic motor NCSs often are inconclusive, because the compound muscle action potentials (CMAPs) normally are low in amplitude; moreover, the CMAP amplitudes recorded from a normal person may vary substantially in amplitude from one side to another, seriously compromising the value of side-to-side amplitude comparisons to detect axon loss lesions (using a CMAP amplitude change of greater than 50% as a marker of abnormality). No muscles innervated by the cervical plexus, with the occasional exception of the diaphragm, are assessed routinely in most EDX laboratories. Because NCSs and needle electromyography (EMG) are of little value in cervical plexopathy assessment, EDX physicians have little to offer diagnostically with these lesions [1,2].

In contrast to cervical plexopathies, EDX examination is of substantial value in the assessment of brachial plexopathies. Excluding the sensory fibers traversing the C5 APR, virtually all components of the brachial plexus can be assessed with NCSs and with needle EMG. The fact that brachial plexopathies are by far the most common type of plexopathy encountered and that the brachial plexus is, of all plexuses, the most amenable to EDX evaluation, is a source of elation to EDX physicians, because this favorable situation is encountered so seldom. Typically, just the opposite is seen (eg, axon loss polyneuropathies occur far more often in the elderly), and it is exactly persons of that advanced age in whom an EDX examination of the lower limb is most compromised by many confounding factors, especially the "normal" absence of lower limb sensory NCS responses and H responses [3].

EDX assessment of the lumbar plexus usually is suboptimal, not only because there is no reliably obtainable sensory NCS available for evaluating that structure but also because relatively few muscles are innervated by the lumbar plexus, and most of them receive their intermediate innervation via the femoral nerve; moreover, these muscles are situated proximally in the limb and, therefore, are likely to have been reinnervated in the interim with all but very severe axon loss lesions that are studied soon after onset of symptoms. EDX assessment of the sacral plexus requires that it be considered as two separate, distinct portions: the superior portion, derived from the L4-S1 (minimal S2) roots, that has lower limb representation, and the inferior portion, derived from the S2-S4 roots (if the pudendal plexus is considered a component of it), that has only pelvic floor representation. The superior portion of the sacral plexus can be assessed by EDX examination adequately if confounding factors (the most common being bilaterally absent lower limb sensory NCS responses and H-responses in elderly patients) are not present. Assessments of the superior portion of the sacral plexus are second only to assessments of the brachial plexus in regard to the thoroughness obtainable. In contrast, evaluation of the inferior portion of the sacral plexus essentially cannot be performed in an EDX laboratory, with the one exception of needle EMG of the anal sphincter muscle. In this regard, the inferior portion of the sacral plexus is even worse than the cervical plexus [4].

Pathology and pathophysiology

Similar to all other PNS axons, those composing the various plexuses can be injured by a great variety of processes. Nonetheless, how they respond to such injury is limited pathologically and pathophysiologically. In practical terms, two types of focal pathology are produced by injury to myelinated fibers: axon loss and demyelination. These two types of pathology can result in three types of pathophysiology: conduction failure, conduction block, and conduction slowing, which are discussed briefly [1,2].

Axon loss and axon degeneration

Axon loss is the most common pathology seen with plexopathies, regardless of the particular plexus affected. It can result from virtually any type of injurious agent, as long as the latter is of sufficient severity to kill nerve fibers. It can act on axons of all sizes, myelinated and unmyelinated. It can affect any element of any plexus, and for the element so involved, it can involve any percentage of the axons, ranging from 1% to 100%. Axon loss is the underlying pathology with nearly all plexopathies of abrupt onset, which are of more than a few weeks' duration, and in almost all chronic static and chronic progressive plexopathies.

In contrast to focal demyelinating lesions (discussed later), an initially highly localized axon loss lesion involving a plexus element, regardless of how small that segment is, never remains focal, because the entire segment of axon distal to the injury site, being separated from its cell body, undergoes wallerian degeneration. This process extends down to the distal tip of the axon and has substantial adverse effects on the structures to which it is connected (ie, sensory receptors, neuromuscular junctions, or muscle fibers). Axon loss has negative and positive manifestations. The former are related directly to the number of axons injured. Whenever only a small percentage of axons degenerate, there are few, if any, negative symptoms. Conversely, when a substantial number of them degenerate, then weakness, usually followed by atrophy, is present if motor axons are affected, whereas sensory loss, involving all modalities (including pain and temperature) occurs if sensory axons are affected. The positive manifestations of axon loss lesions include pain, resulting from small fiber sensory involvement, and paresthesias, fasciculations, myokymia, and cramps, caused by damage of large fiber sensory and motor axons. Unlike the positive phenomenon, the negative manifestations of axon loss do not have a direct relationship to the severity of axon loss. Thus, a mild sensory axon loss lesion can produce severe pain, just as a mild loss of large sensory and motor axons can result in intense paresthesias and prominent fasciculations. (An exception to this dictum is that the likelihood of avulsion pain developing after brachial plexus root avulsions is related directly to the number of roots avulsed.)

During the initial days after a complete focal axon loss lesion is sustained, pathophysiologically, a conduction block is present at the lesion site: stimulations proximal to it produce no responses, whereas stimulations distal to it generate responses that decrease in amplitude with each succeeding day (after days 2–3 motor fibers and day 5 sensory fibers). This "axon discontinuity conduction block" is seen as long as the distal stump is capable of conducting impulses (6 days for motor fibers and 8–9 days for sensory fibers). From approximately the 11th day onward, however, the distal stump has degenerated sufficiently that solely conduction failure is seen: no responses, motor or sensory, can be elicited on distal recording, regardless of where the nerve is stimulated, either proximal to, at, or distal to the lesion site [1,2,5].

Focal demyelination

The myelinated axons that compose the plexuses have an additional response to those injuries that are insufficient to produce axon degeneration: focal demyelination. This type of pathology differs from axon loss in that, as its name indicates, it affects only myelinated axons at the lesion site, and it remains focal as long as it persists. Thus, it has no effect on the distal (or proximal) segment of nerve.

Focal demyelination, a single type of pathology, produces two distinct types of pathophysiology, depending on its severity: conduction slowing and conduction block. These two processes have different clinical and EDX manifestations. Focal demyelinating conduction slowing is the milder of the two. All the nerve impulses traverse the lesion site, although the speed of impulse transmission is reduced as they do so. This process, per se, does not produce any clinical symptoms. Because all the nerve impulses ultimately reach their intended destinations, slowing along motor fibers does not result in weakness (or atrophy), and slowing along sensory fibers causes no sensory deficits. The same focal demyelinating process that has produced focal slowing, however, independently of the latter, can give rise to the positive phenomena of paresthesias, fasciculations, myokymia, and cramps. Whenever demyelinating conduction slowing affects all axons at the lesion site to the same degree, it has no effect on the formal neurologic examination. If slowing is present along the nerve fibers to different degrees (a process referred to as "differential slowing"), however, it alters those neurologic examination procedures that require nerve impulses to travel in synchronized volleys (eg, deep tendon reflex [DTR] testing) and vibratory, position sense, and light touch assessment. Because demyelinating conduction slowing has no clinical manifestations, except sometimes in formal testing, it is the only type of pathophysiology encountered that is not included in any of the clinical classifications of peripheral nerve injuries, such as those described by Seddon and Sunderland [6,7]. Of the various types of pathophysiology, focal demyelinating conduction slowing is the one encountered least often with plexopathies in EDX laboratories. This is mainly because it produces no symptoms, whereas nearly all plexus lesions are symptomatic. Also, because the plexuses are situated so proximally, detecting such slowing can be difficult [1,2,5].

Although focal demyelinating conduction block shares the same underlying pathology with focal demyelinating conduction slowing, it is a different process pathophysiologically, because it stops nerve impulses from traversing the lesion site rather than merely slowing them. Because the nerve impulses do not reach their targets, in its clinical manifestations this process is more akin to conduction failure, caused by axon degeneration, than it is to focal demyelinating conduction slowing. Most of its clinical manifestations are identical to those seen with conduction failure resulting from axon loss. It can affect any element of any plexus and any percentage of the myelinated axons traversing that element, ranging from 1% to 100%. Whenever it involves a sufficient number of motor axons, it causes clinical weakness that is indistinguishable from that seen when the same number of motor axons undergo degeneration. Similarly, it produces sensory deficits when it involves a sufficient number of sensory axons. There are three major differences, however, between these two processes, one involving motor manifestations, another sensory manifestations, and the third lesion duration. First, demyelinating conduction block rarely causes atrophy, because of its relatively brief duration. When it persists for months, however, as it may be in certain uncommon instances (eg, radiation-induced brachial plexopathy or multifocal motor conduction block), disuse atrophy may be prominent. Second, it causes sensory deficits that, by definition, are restricted to those sensory modalities mediated over large myelinated fibers (ie, position sense, vibration sense, and light touch); it has no effect on pain or temperature, which are conducted over unmyelinated and lightly myelinated axons. Third, generally it varies greatly from axon loss in its duration. Because axon loss causes nerve fibers to degenerate from the lesion site distally, function is restored only after the nerve fibers have regenerated or until axon sprouts have arisen distally to re-establish motor and sensory integrity. This typically is a slow, and sometimes imperfect, process. Conversely, focal demyelinating conduction block causes no abnormalities of the nerve segment distal to the lesion site, so nerve impulse transmission is restored as soon as the myelin at the lesion site is reconstituted. Although this depends on the extensiveness of the underlying pathology, usually it is rather rapid, and it is always complete. The major exception to this rule are the focal demyelinating conduction block lesions that are associated with radiation-induced brachial plexopathy and multifocal motor conduction block. Unlike the short-lived focal demyelinating conduction blocks resulting from mild traction or compression (clinically labeled "neurapraxia"), the demyelinating conduction blocks with these disorders tend to persist indefinitely and, ultimately, to convert gradually to axon loss [1,2,5].

Just as most polyneuropathies are axon loss (rather than demyelinating) in type, most plexopathies, regardless of the particular plexus involved, are the result of axon loss, rather than demyelination. The relatively few exceptions are discussed.

Cervical plexus lesions

The cervical plexus is the smallest of the four PNS plexuses. It is formed from the APR of the C1, C2, C3, and C4 mixed spinal nerves (Fig. 1). The C2, C3, and C4 APR divide into anterior and posterior branches or divisions, which unite to form three anastomotic loops, from which arise sensory and motor (or predominately) motor, nerves. The cervical plexus is situated in the lateral neck, adjacent to the upper four cervical vertebrae, ventrolateral to the levator scapulae and scalenus medius muscles, and

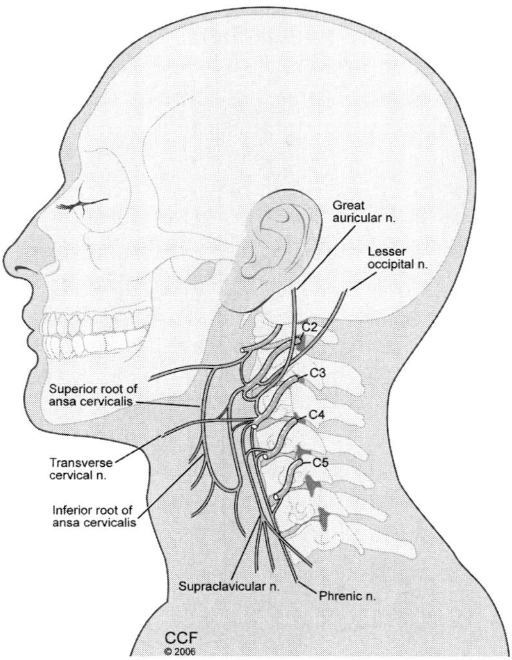

Fig. 1. The cervical plexus (left side). (*Courtesy of* the Cleveland Clinic Foundation, Cleveland, OH.)

deep to the sternocleidomastoid. It has communications with three lower cranial nerves: the vagus, accessory, and hypoglossal. The sensory (cutaneous) nerves that arise from the cervical plexus include the lesser occipital (primarily C2), the great auricular, the anterior cutaneous (transverse cervical) (C2, C3), and the supraclavicular (C3, C4). The motor (deep), or predominately motor, branches that originate from the cervical plexus include those that (1) innervate various paravertebral muscles (eg, the rectus capitis [C1, C2] and the longus capitis [C1-C4]) along with those to the scalenus medius and levator scapulae (C3, C4); (2) join with the spinal accessory nerve to supply portions of the trapezius muscle (C3, C4) and, with the hypoglossal nerve, to innervate various infrahyoid muscles (C1-C3); and (3) form the phrenic nerve (C3, C4, and sometimes C5) that innervates the diaphragm. The phrenic nerve is the most important nerve derived from the cervical plexus. Postganglionic sympathetic nerve fibers that originate in the superior cervical ganglion also traverse the cervical plexus [2,8].

Those who have obtained lists of causes of "cervical plexopathies" by perusing the medical literature or by searching medical databases (such as Medline) soon encounter, while reading them, an unannounced major shift in the topic. Instead of the subject being "cervical plexopathies," it suddenly, without fanfare, becomes "phrenic neuropathies." Although the phrenic nerve is the principal derivative of the cervical plexus, it is a peripheral nerve, not a component of the cervical plexus. The reason for this unacknowledged change in focus is simple: there are surprisingly few articles that discuss cervical plexopathies, presumably because open and closed lesions of this structure are uncommon.

Open lesions of the cervical plexus principally are the result of surgical procedures performed on, or penetrating injuries to, the lateral neck. Surgical causes include radical neck dissections and carotid endarterectomies [9,10]. Penetrating injuries have a variety of causes (eg, bullets, knives, and metal and glass fragments) but are of low frequency, even in wartime [2,11].

Closed lesions of the cervical plexus probably are more common than the open variety. Neoplasms are a major cause. Usually, the cervical plexus is invaded by tumor from neighboring structures. This invasion may be direct, or indirect, via intermediate metastatic spread to regional lymph nodes or bony structures (eg, clavicle, first rib, or cervical vertebral bodies). Primary sources include lymphomas and squamous cell carcinomas of the head and neck, whereas secondary ones include metastatic deposits in lymph nodes and vertebrae, most often from lung or breast adenocarcinomas [12,13]. Closed cervical plexopathies also can result from iatrogenic causes, including radiation therapy for breast carcinoma, and the use of interscapular rolls for positioning during open-heart surgery. Another type of closed cervical plexopathy, which probably is under-reported, results from violent trauma. Most reports concern combined cervical and brachial plexopathies—with the upper trunk always involved with the latter—sustained in motorcycle accidents.

Generally, coexisting sensory loss in a cervical plexus distribution is viewed as an indicator of the severity of an upper plexus or panplexus brachial plexopathy. Often, this means that multiple root avulsions have occurred [2].

The sensory (cutaneous) branches of the cervical plexus, after emerging from the posterior aspect of the sternocleidomastoid muscle, in the posterior triangle of the neck, divide to supply sensation to the head (posterior to the interauricular line), the neck, anterosuperior and lateral regions, and the submandibular area and the cape region [2,8].

Cervical plexopathies may be nearly asymptomatic, because their symptoms are overshadowed by those resulting from damage to other structures (eg, the brachial plexus). Some cervical plexopathies, however, cause pain. This usually is the presenting, and often the most common, complaint with neoplastic lesions. Typically, this pain is described as unrelenting, deep, boring, and located in the neck, throat, or shoulder. It may be in the distribution of any of the sensory branches and may be exaggerated by swallowing, coughing, and neck movements. The involvement of the motor branches often is unapparent. Not only do the partially denervated muscles receive multiple innervations but also they are relatively inaccessible, and their dysfunction may be concealed by the actions of nearby, uninvolved muscles [10,11,14]. Undoubtedly, the most serious motor complication of cervical plexopathies results from injury to those axons that more distally are in the phrenic nerve, which innervates the diaphragm. Unilateral diaphragmatic paralysis frequently is asymptomatic, although patients may experience orthopnea and exertional dyspnea [9,10].

Open injuries of the cervical plexus are readily apparent, whereas closed lesions, particularly when neoplasms are the culprits, may yield surprisingly normal physical examinations, with the positive findings consisting only of unilateral neck tenderness or, less often, a palpable mass or firm cervical or supraclavicular lymph nodes. Jaeckle has emphasized that neoplastic cervical plexus involvement indicates that the tumor is precariously near the cervical spine. If neck movements produce sharp pain or if cervical spine percussion yields tenderness, an impending epidural tumor extension must be excluded promptly by neuroimaging studies [13].

Ancillary diagnostic studies with suspected cervical plexopathies are of variable benefit. As discussed previously, EDX examinations typically are of almost no value in most instances. MRI yields the best anatomic detail and is the preferred neuroimaging procedure. Plain neck radiographs and CT scans may be helpful with some neoplastic plexopathies, particularly if associated bone involvement is suspected. Chest radiographs or fluoroscopy often are of benefit when there is involvement of the fibers that more caudally comprise the phrenic nerve. Positron emission tomography (PET) scans may detect neoplasms, but the value of this procedure has not yet been established [2,13].

Probably the majority of cervical plexopathies are not treated, because of the circumstances under which they occur, the relative insignificance of the particular nerve fibers injured, or both. Although conceivably surgical repair of transected components of the cervical plexus can be attempted, this probably occurs infrequently. Thus, in two standard textbooks dealing with the surgical repair of nerve lesions, cervical plexopathies, per se, are not mentioned in either [15,16]. A variety of treatments is available for neoplastic cervical plexopathies, although most have shortcomings. These are discussed in detail later.

In many instances, cervical plexopathies are of secondary importance and, consequently, a suboptimal recovery is of relatively little consequence. Nonetheless, in situations in which patients survive, there usually are residuals, especially in regard to sensory deficits and diaphragmatic compromise [2].

Brachial plexus lesions

The brachial plexus extends from the axilla distally to either the base of the neck or the spinal cord proximally, depending on how it is defined. It is described as having five components: (1) five roots (C5-T1); (2) three trunks—upper, middle, and lower; (3) six divisions—three anterior and three posterior; (4) three cords—lateral, posterior, and medial; and (5) three to five (depending on the source) terminal nerves, consisting of the median, radial, ulnar, and often the axillary and musculocutaneous (Fig. 2).

What the roots of the brachial plexus consist of is debated. Anatomy books define these as the C5-T1 APRs, thus indicating that the brachial plexus is a purely extraforaminal structure that begins proximally at the external ostea of the intervertebal foramina. Most peripheral nerve surgeons,

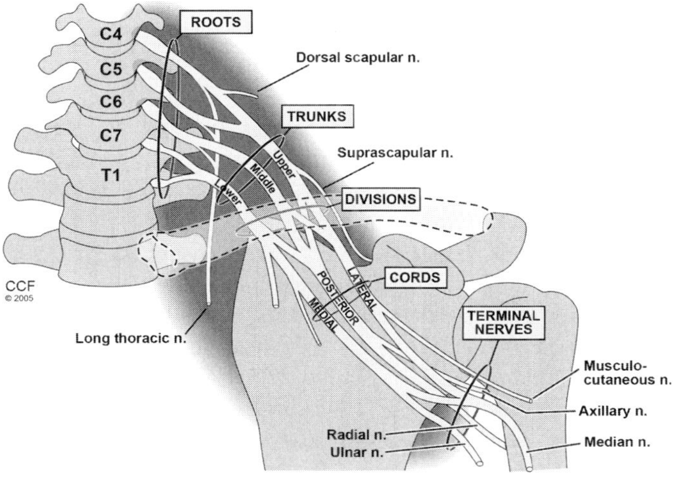

Fig. 2. The brachial plexus (left side). (*Courtesy of* the Cleveland Clinic Foundation, Cleveland, OH.)

however, consider the roots to be more extensive, consisting not only of the APRs but also the mixed spinal nerves and the dorsal and ventral primary roots. Thus, they view the brachial plexus as having not only extraforaminal but also intraforaminal and intraspinal canal components, with its origin at the spinal cord. Using this latter definition, avulsions of the roots of the brachial plexus are just as much brachial plexopathies as are trunk and cord lesions. The APR derived from the C5-T1 mixed spinal nerves are situated deep in the neck, between the scalenus anticus and medius muscles. Two peripheral nerves arise from these APR, the dorsal scapular (C5) and the long thoracic (C5-C7). The APRs terminate as trunks: the C5 and C6 APRs fuse to form the upper trunk, the C7 APR continues as the middle trunk, and the C8 and T1 APRs join to form the lower trunk. The trunks are situated in the anteroinferior portion of the posterior triangle of the neck. The suprascapular nerve, the only significant peripheral nerve arising at the trunk level, originates from the upper trunk near its origin. The divisions consist of three anterior and posterior components, with one anterior and one posterior originating from each trunk. Although no major peripheral nerves arise from the divisions, they are important for two reasons. First, at their level a major internal reorganization of the brachial plexus occurs, with the axons proximally being in a root distribution, whereas the ones distally are in the distribution of one or more peripheral nerves. Second, with the upper limb at the side, the divisions are situated behind the clavicle. Consequently, they separate the "supraclavicular" and the "infraclavicular" portions of the brachial plexus (Fig. 3). These designations have important clinical and EDX implications. The cords, named for their positions in relation to the second portion of the axillary artery, are situated in the proximal axilla. Most of the major nerves derived from the plexus originate from them. These include the lateral pectorial, musculocutaneous and median (lateral head) nerves (C5-C7) that arise from the lateral cord; the thoracodorsal, axillary and radial nerves (C5-C8) that originate from the posterior cord; and the medial cutaneous and antebrachial cutaneous, ulnar, and medial head of the median (C8, T1) nerves that arise from the medial cord.

Brachial plexopathies are classified as supraclavicular or infraclavicular, depending on whether or not the lesions are located proximal or distal to the divisions (see Fig. 3). Supraclavicular plexopathies are more common than infraclavicular ones and, for various reasons, they are less prone to recover. Supraclavicular plexopathies are subdivided into upper plexus, middle plexus, and lower plexus lesions. This classification combines abnormalities of the primary roots, mixed spinal nerves, APRs, and trunks together, without attempting to distinguish between them (eg, an upper plexic lesion may involve the C5, C6 primary roots, mixed spinal nerves, or APR and the upper trunk). Supraclavicular plexopathies generally can be assigned to one of five categories, depending on the particular elements they affect: (1) upper plexus alone; (2) upper and middle plexus; (3) middle and lower plexus; (4) lower plexus alone; or (5) diffuse or panplexus.

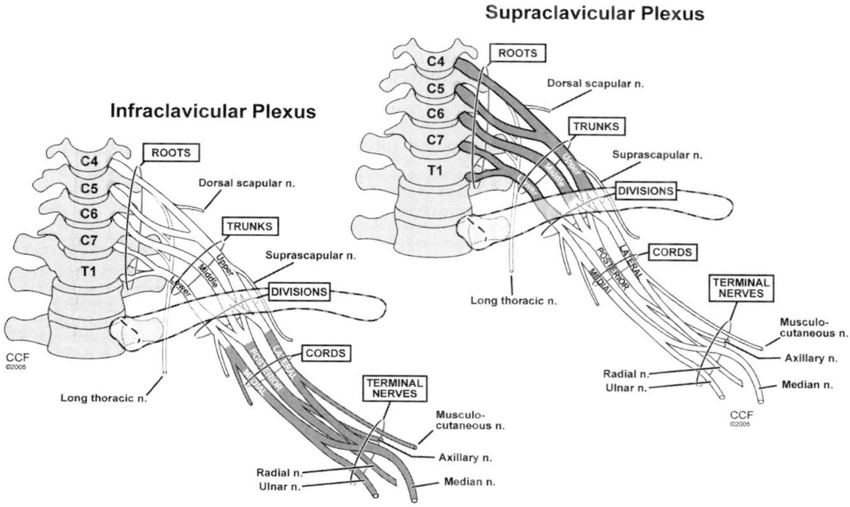

Fig. 3. The two major divisions of the brachial plexus: supraclavicular and infraclavicular. (*Courtesy of* the Cleveland Clinic Foundation, Cleveland OH.)

Infraclavicular plexopathies are divided into cord and terminal peripheral nerve lesions, although at times it is impossible to distinguish between the two (eg, the clinical and EDX features of a posterior cord lesion essentially are identical to those seen with combined thoracodorsal, axillary, and radial nerve lesions). Brachial plexopathies can be characterized further as being either "complete/total" or "incomplete/partial." They also may be subdivided into "open" and "closed"; closed disorders are more common, even during wartime [1,3,17].

Clinically, most brachial plexopathies present with weakness, to varying degrees, in the distribution of the affected plexus elements. Pain is a somewhat less common symptom. Its incidence approaches 100% with brachial plexopathies caused by metastatic neoplasms, multiple root avulsions, and injuries from disputed neurogenic thoracic outlet syndromes (TOS) surgery. In contrast, it usually is absent with classic postoperative paralysis and rucksack paralysis and is seldom substantial with true neurogenic TOS and most radiation-induced lesions. Paresthesias occur less often than pain, because their underlying cause is demyelination. Consequently, they typically are prominent with those relatively few brachial plexopathies in which demyelinating conduction block occurs, such as a minority of closed traction injuries, classic postoperative paralysis, most postmedian sternotomy lesions early in their course, and radiation-induced injuries [3,17].

Lesions of the supraclavicular and infraclavicular plexus can be classified in many ways. A simple classification is traumatic, nontraumatic, and iatrogenic.

Supraclavicular plexopathies

If of more than modest severity, lesions of the supraclavicular plexus manifest as follows. Upper plexus lesions present with weakness, and often wasting, involving the deltoid, biceps, brachialis, brachioradialis, and, frequently, the pronator teres. Depending on the longitudinal location of the lesion along the upper plexus, the spinati, rhomboids, and portions of the serratus anterior also may be involved. Sensory loss and any sensory symptoms that may be present (eg, pain or paresthesias) are in the distribution of the axillary and lateral antebrachial cutaneous nerves and, partially, the median and superficial radial nerves (ie, they are present over the lateral aspect of the shoulder, arm, and forearm, often extending into the thumb). The biceps and brachioradialis DTRs characteristically are decreased or unelicitable. With middle plexus lesions, weakness involves the triceps, pronator teres, flexor carpi radialis, and sometimes more distal radial nerve–innervated extensor forearm muscles. Sensory loss usually is inconstant and is in the distribution of the lower lateral brachial cutaneous, posterior brachial cutaneous, and posterior antebrachial cutaneous nerves (ie, located along the posterior arm and extensor forearm). Pain may occur in the same distribution, although typically in a discontinuous fashion. The triceps DTR is affected. With lower plexus lesions, all the intrinsic hand muscles are weak, and the forearm muscles innervated by the C8 segment via the median, ulnar, and radial nerves (eg, flexor pollicis longus, flexor carpi ulnaris, extensor indicis proprius). Sensory deficits often are present in the distribution of the medial brachial cutaneous, medial antebrachial cutaneous, and ulnar nerves (ie, along the medial aspect of the arm and forearmand the medial hand and fingers) [1,3,18].

Some of the more common disorders that affect the supraclavicular brachial plexus now are discussed.

Closed traction injuries, caused by trauma, are by far the most common lesions that the brachial plexus sustains. Most result from vehicular accidents, in particular motorcycle accidents. Less common causes include industrial accidents, falls (particularly from a height), objects falling on a shoulder, and a few athletic endeavors (eg, skiing, mountain or rock climbing, and occasionally contact sports [especially football]). The underlying pathology with these lesions varies from predominantly demyelinating conduction block to solely axon loss, but the latter is far more common. A particularly disabling type of supraclavicular closed traction injury is root avulsion. Here the primary roots are torn from the spinal cord by high-energy traction. Root avulsions are especially disabling for several reasons: (1) frequently, more than one root is avulsed, producing extensive damage; (2) because axons do not regenerate with these types of lesions and surgical repair essentially is impossible, the motor and sensory deficits that result are permanent; (3) many patients, especially those who have multiple roots avulsed, develop avulsion pain, which is one of the worse types of pain that affects humans; and (4) often, the patients are young and not well educated, so being functionally one-armed is extremely handicapping for them.

One key point regarding closed traction injuries is that the actual extent and severity of the lesion cannot be determined accurately until 3 to 6 weeks have passed after injury. During this time, any demyelinating conduction block component usually resolves. Alternatively, motor NCSs performed more than 1 week after onset can demonstrate accurately the degree of axon loss that the various recorded muscles had sustained [1–3].

Open traumatic injuries of the supraclavicular brachial plexus occur less frequently than the closed variety. The causes of open injuries include gunshot wounds, lacerations (eg, from knives, glass, or moving metal objects), and animal bites. A major difference between closed and open traumatic supraclavicular lesions is that damage to nearby structures, in particular blood vessels and lung, are common with open injuries; frequently, these are of immediate, overriding concern. Moreover, in many instances, the brachial plexus fibers are not injured directly by the penetrating object but, rather, secondarily, as a result of primary damage to the blood vessels that causes pseudoaneurysms, arteriovenous fistulas, and expanding hematomas [1,15,16].

The burner syndrome is a relatively mild type of traumatic axon loss lesion that affects the upper plexus. It occurs almost solely in athletes, in particular young male athletes who engage in contact sports (eg, football). Initiated by sudden forceful depression of the shoulder, it consists of a brief bout of sudden, intense burning dysesthesia and anesthesia affecting one entire upper limb, usually accompanied by equally short-lived, but generalized, weakness of the limb. Multiple episodes may occur during a single sporting event. Between episodes, the affected limb most often is asymptomatic. When the process is severe, however, some mild (often just subjective) weakness, restricted to an upper plexus distribution, is present [1,2,5].

Rucksack paralysis (pack palsy) is another type of traumatic upper plexus lesion that usually is mild. It occurs most often in military personnel, but one of the largest reported series concerned mountain climbers. Pertinent factors include pack design, amount of weight carried, length of time worn, type of terrain traversed, and use or nonuse of pack frames and waist belts. It presents with weakness, usually unilateral, that some time later may be accompanied by atrophy and paresthesias but seldom pain. The abnormalities most often are in an upper trunk distribution, but cases presenting solely as long thoracic or spinal accessory neuropathies are reported. The fact that the majority of patients recover within a few months indicates that focal demyelinating conduction block is the principal pathophysiology. The remaining patients, however, show slow and occasionally incomplete recovery, a hallmark of axon loss [3,5].

A nontraumatic cause for supraclavicular plexopathies is neoplasms. Primary neoplasms are relatively rare, and most originate from the neural sheath, the most common being neurofibromas. Most malignant neoplasms that affect the brachial plexus, in contrast, are metastatic, usually with the primary sites being the breast or, especially, the lung. Typically, the lower plexus is affected initially. Severe, persistent pain is the cardinal symptom. Progressive weakness usually appears some time later in the course. As expected, these become more extensive with the passing of time. Paresthesias are relatively uncommon. If the cervical sympathetic chain is involved, often Horner's syndrome is present [3,16,17].

Another nontraumatic type of supraclavicular plexopathy is true neurologic TOS (N-TOS), also known as cervical rib and band syndrome. It results from congenital anomalies: either a rudimentary cervical rib or an elongated transverse process arising from the C7 vertebrae, from the tip of which a radiotranslucent taut band extends to the proximal first thoracic rib. The T1 APR or the very proximal lower trunk is stretched and angulated over this band. True N-TOS is a unilateral lesion that dominantly affects women, usually of young to middle age. Because this entity essentially is a motor syndrome, typically patients are not seen until marked hand weakness and wasting is present, involving the lateral thenar eminence, and often, to a lesser extent, all the intrinsic hand muscles and, sometimes, the lower trunk-innervated forearm muscles. Usually, an intermittent aching, typically mild, has been present for years along the medial arm and forearm (in the distribution of the medial brachial cutaneous and medial antebrachial cutaneous nerves), sometimes extending into the medial hand. These sensory symptoms only rarely are severe enough, however, to cause patients to seek medical care. The underlying pathology almost solely is axon loss [1,3,17].

Multifocal motor neuropathy is a nontraumatic disorder that occasionally affects the supraclavicular plexus. Because it can involve any portion of the latter, its symptoms are variable. Typically, however, they consist of progressive weakness and wasting, unaccompanied by sensory complaints, in the distribution of the upper, middle, or lower plexus, or some combination thereof. Similar to true N-TOS, multifocal motor neuropathy involving the brachial plexus is a motor syndrome, so often weakness and wasting is prominent before medical care is sought by patients [3,17].

An iatrogenic cause for supraclavicular plexopathies is classic postoperative paralysis. These lesions actually develop intraoperatively as a result of patients being malpositioned on an operating table. Most often, the operations are performed at a distance from the brachial plexus, so that there is no question of direct surgical injury having occurred. Clinically, these patients present with weakness, sometimes paresthesias, but rarely pain, in an upper plexus distribution. Initially, however, for the first few days after onset, the symptoms often are more widespread, involving the supraclavicular plexus in a diffuse fashion. The underlying pathophysiology characteristically is predominately demyelinating conduction block. For this reason, few patients who have this disorder are assessed in an EDX laboratory, because their symptoms resolve before such studies can be performed. In some instances, however, based on slow and at times incomplete recovery, the pathology is axon loss [1,3]. Classic postoperative paralysis is one of the relatively few types of brachial plexopathy that may be bilateral (obstetric palsy is another).

Obstetric paralysis (congenital brachial plexus palsy) is an iatrogenic type of closed traction injury; it is attributed principally to excessive lateral traction applied by clinicians on the fetal head during the third stage of delivery, usually because of dystocia (ie, difficulty in delivering the shoulder after head delivery, resulting from impaction of the anterior shoulder of the fetus on the mother's pubic symphysis). Nonetheless, it is pertinent to point out that this can occur when medical personnel are not even in attendance, and many instances of obstetric paralysis seem to be the result of other than the extraction efforts of the attending physicians. Predisposing factors include maternal weight gain, diabetes, multiparity, fetal macrosomia, high birth weight, and breech presentation. Most lesions are unilateral, and males and females are affected in approximately equal numbers. The right side is involved somewhat more often than the left. Vertex presentations cause a great majority of these cases, whereas breech presentations, in particular cesarean deliveries, are responsible for only a small portion.

Similar to all other closed traction injuries, obstetric paralysis can manifest any degree of nerve fiber injury, from demyelinating conduction block to root avulsions. It can affect any portion of the supraclavicular plexus, but three presentations are dominant: upper plexus, combined upper and middle plexus, and panplexus. Although Klumpke's paralysis—isolated involvement of the lower plexus—has been linked to obstetric paralysis for more than 100 years, some of the most experienced surgeons dealing with this type of brachial plexopathy report never encountering one and, consequently, doubt that they occur. Most upper and middle plexus lesions consist of a mixture of demyelinating conduction block and axon loss, the latter the result of extraforaminal ruptures of the APR or trunks. In contrast, most lower plexus lesions, which characteristically occur with concomitant involvement of the middle plexus or middle and upper plexus, indicate root avulsions have occurred [2,3,5,15].

Another type of iatrogenic lesion that affects the supraclavicular plexus is postmedian sternotomy brachial plexopathy. This results from open-heart surgery, in which access to the heart is achieved by vertical splitting of the sternum. Their cause is in some dispute, but the most plausible theory is that they are traction injuries involving the C8 APR (rather than the lower trunk per se), resulting from fracture or upward displacement of the very proximal portion of the first thoracic rib, secondary to the sternal retraction. Similar to true N-TOS, this disorder clinically seems to affect only a portion of the lower trunk. In this case, however, it is the C8, rather than the T1, APR. This preferential involvement explains why the hand weakness, along with the paresthesias and sometimes pain in the fourth and fifth fingers, are in very predominantly an ulnar nerve distribution. Nonetheless, C8/radial nerve and median nerve–innervated muscle (eg, extensor indicis proprius, extensor pollicis brevis, and flexor pollicis longus) also are weak. The underlying pathophysiology with these lesions usually is a mixture of demyelinating conduction block and conduction failure caused by axon loss, with the former predominating. Consequently, the hand weakness present often improves substantially within just a few weeks of onset [3,17].

An iatrogenic injury of the supraclavicular plexus, most often the C8 or T1 APR, or the lower trunk, sometimes is sustained during disputed N-TOS surgery. An enormous number of normal first thoracic ribs and scalene muscles are removed yearly to treat a controversial type of reputed neurologic disorder, labeled "disputed" neurogenic TOS. Unlike all other brachial plexopathies, this disorder, according to its proponents—most of whom are neither trained nor experienced in diagnosing PNS disease—is extremely common, often bilateral, and affects women more than men, in particular young to middle-aged women. Although its proponents debate its underlying pathogenesis, most agree that it usually is traumatic in origin, caused by either a single episode of trauma (eg, whiplash injury sustained during a minor vehicular accident) or by repetitive use of the upper limb, producing a cumulative strain–type lesion. Typically, the only symptom is pain, most often in a lower plexus distribution. All skeptics and even most proponents of disputed N-TOS contend that there are no objective findings detectable on clinical, EDX, or neuroimaging examinations. Nonetheless, many patients labeled with this diagnosis undergo a variety of brachial plexus decompression surgical treatments, most often either transaxillary first rib resection or supraclavicular scalenectomies, or sometimes both. During these operations, some patients sustain an iatrogenic brachial plexopathy. Typically, this involves the lower plexus. Hand weakness, or sensory deficit, and severe pain are the typical findings. Although the hand weakness usually is permanent, causing some disability, the persistent pain is the major problem for many patients. This type of supraclavicular plexopathy is very predominately axon loss in nature [2,3].

Infraclavicular plexopathies

The infraclavicular plexus consists of the cords and the terminal nerves.

Lateral cord lesions affect the motor and sensory axons that more distally compose the musculocutaneous nerve and the lateral head of the median nerve. Consequently, these lesions manifest weakness of the biceps, brachialis, pronator teres, and flexor carpi radialis along with a sensory disturbance in the distribution of the lateral antebrachial cutaneous nerve and the cutaneous portion of the lateral head of the median nerve (eg, along the lateral aspect of the forearm, the hand, and the volar aspects of the lateral three or four lateral digits). With lateral cord lesions, the biceps DTR is reduced or absent.

Posterior cord lesions affect the motor and sensory axons that more distally constitute the thoracodorsal, axillary, and radial nerves. They manifest as weakness and sometimes wasting of the subscapularis, latissimus dorsi, deltoid, teres minor, and all muscles innervated by the radial nerve in the arm and forearm and by the postinterosseous nerve. Generally, sensory disturbances with posterior cord lesions are much less extensive than the motor deficits; they appear in a discontinuous fashion in the distributions of the lower lateral brachial cutaneous, posterior brachial cutaneous, and posterior antebrachial cutaneous nerves (ie, along the lateral surface of the arm, the posterior surface of the forearm, and the dorsum of the hand—radial aspect). The triceps and brachioradialis DTRs usually are diminished or absent.

Medial cord lesions affect principally the motor and sensory axons composing the ulnar nerve and the medial head of the median nerve. The most typical findings are weakness and usually wasting of the intrinsic hand muscles, with similar changes in the ulnar nerve–innervated and median nerve–innervated forearm muscles. Sensory abnormalities nearly always are present in the distribution of the ulnar nerve, and sometimes in the distribution of the medial brachial cutaneous and also medial antebrachial cutaneous nerve (ie, along the medial aspect of the hand and fingers, sometimes extending along the medial forearm and arm). The sensory changes above the wrist are variable, because the medial brachial cutaneous and medial antebrachial cutaneous nerves originate from the proximal portion of the medial cord, so they are not necessarily affected by lesions involving the mid or distal portions. On clinical and EDX examinations, assessment of the C8/radial nerve–innervated muscles (eg, extensor indicis proprius and extensor pollicis brevis) is the principal means of distinguishing these lesions from those of the lower trunk. These muscles are normal with medial cord lesions because the radial nerve derives from the posterior cord [3,17].

Each of the five terminal nerves that compose the fifth and most distal portion of the brachial plexus has well-defined motor and sensory distributions. Consequently, these are not discussed in detail. There is, however, no well-defined external demarcation along the distal ends of the terminal nerves, marking the boundary between them and the very proximal portions of the major peripheral nerve trunks that arise from them. Nonetheless, lesions of the terminal nerves are considered brachial plexopathies, whereas the latter are not. For practical purposes, any damage that occurs to these nerve fibers while they are within the axilla should be classified as terminal nerve lesions and, therefore, infraclavicular plexopathies [3,17].

Traumatic infraclavicular plexopathies have two major causes: falls and vehicular accidents. Most are closed lesions. Nonetheless, with high-energy trauma, often there is primary damage of the axillary blood vessels, in particular the artery (thrombosis, ruptures, or tears), leading to secondary involvement of the brachial plexus elements.

Another cause of traumatic infraclavicular plexopathies is fractures or dislocations of the humeral neck. Patient age and coexisting injury to nearby structures play major roles. Older patients are twice as likely as younger patients to sustain brachial plexopathies with these fractures or dislocations. Similarly, patients who have hematomas resulting from associated arterial injuries are twice as likely to have brachial plexus lesions as are those who do not have them. The specific elements of the infraclavicular plexus damaged depends on the position and displacement of the upper limb at the moment when the trauma occurs. Most often, the terminal nerves are injured, especially the axillary. Others affected include the suprascapular and, less often, the musculocutaneous, radial, and ulnar terminal nerves. The predominate pathophysiology with the majority of these lesions is demyelinating conduction block [3,17].

Traumatic TOS is an infraclavicular plexopathy that results most often, directly or indirectly, from clavicular fractures. The latter are the most common fractures sustained by humans; most result from vehicular accidents or falls, and most involve the midportion of the clavicle. This disorder is limited essentially to adults and probably affects more men than women. Although the neurovascular structures are located between the midportion of the clavicle and the first thoracic rib, they usually are unharmed by these bony lesions. When nerve fibers are injured, they typically are in the proximal cords, especially the medial cord. The cords may be injured at the time of the fracture or soon afterwards because of displacement of fracture fragments or to fracture manipulation or initial damage to the blood vessels, with secondary compression of the nerve fibers by hematoma or arteriovenous fistula. These plexus lesions also may appear weeks to months after the fracture, caused by figure-of-eight bandages (which are effective in children but not in adults), allowing movement of fracture fragments at the lesion site or the formation of hypertrophic calluses. Clinically, sensory symptoms (paresthesias and pain) are the most common neurologic complaints. Typically, these radiate down the limb, especially when it is held outstretched or overhead. Less often, limb weakness occurs that usually involves the intrinsic hand muscles. In addition, pain and tenderness characteristically are present at the fracture site. With coexisting vascular injury, ecchymosis and swelling may be noted at the base of the neck [3,17].

The most common causes of nontraumatic infraclavicular brachial plexopathies are neoplasms, primary and secondary. (The pertinent symptoms of these are discussed earlier.) The infraclavicular plexus also can be injured by nontraumatic hematomas or aneurysms that develop spontaneously. Another cause is multifocal motor neuropathy, which can affect any elements of the infraclavicular plexus. These are easier to localize with EDX studies, specifically motor NCSs, than their supraclavicular counterparts, because they can be bracketed with supraclavicular and axilla stimulations [3,17].

Radiation-induced brachial plexopathies usually are initially infraclavicular in location and characteristically unilateral. Three types have been described but by far the most common is a progressive motor and sensory disorder, delayed in onset, caused by radiation fibrosis [3]. Most patients are women who were treated for breast carcinoma, although patients of both genders may develop this disorder after receiving radiation therapy for such neoplasms as lung cancer or lymphoma. The latent period between radiation therapy and onset of symptoms is broad, ranging from a few months to more than 30 years. The four major interrelated factors responsible for radiation-induced brachial plexopathies are (1) total dose given, (2) field intersection (overlapping fields, resulting in "hot spots"), (3) hypofractionation (fewer, larger doses), and (4) simultaneous delivery of chemotherapy. The pathophysiology is very predominately demyelinating conduction block initially. As time passes, however, this gradually converts to axon loss. The initial symptom almost always is persistent paresthesias, usually affecting one of the lateral cord/median nerve–innervated fingers. Soon, weakness appears in the same distribution, often evident first in a forearm muscle. These symptoms spread gradually, encompassing progressively more of the limb. In contrast to the paresthesias, pain is an inconstant symptom and, if present, varies substantially in severity. On clinical examination, these patients often lose their DTRs fairly early in their course because of the involvement of the large myelinated sensory fibers [3,17].

Another iatrogenic infraclavicular brachial plexopathy is the medial brachial fascial compartment (MBFC) syndrome. The MBFC extends from the axilla to the elbow and is formed by the tough medial intramuscular septum dividing near the surface of the arm to enclose the neurovascular bundle. Whenever the axillary artery is punctured during various procedures (ie, axillary arteriograms or axillary regional anesthetic blocks) blood can leak slowly into the MBFC, pool there, and eventually compress one or more of the terminal nerves, resulting in a compartment syndrome: the MBFC syndrome. This unilateral infraclavicular disorder affects almost solely adults and probably has no gender predominance. It first becomes symptomatic anywhere from immediately after the procedure to more than 2 weeks later. Predisposing factors include anticoagulation, bleeding disorders, and uncontrolled hypertension. Clinically, the initial symptoms are sensory in nature—pain, paresthesias, and sometimes sensory deficits—almost invariably in a terminal median nerve distribution. Subsequently, progressive weakness develops in the same distribution. Other terminal nerves also may be affected, either almost simultaneously or more often sequentially with the median, especially the ulnar, terminal nerve. There are reports of all five terminal nerves being involved. On physical examination, an axillary ecchymosis may be seen, or a hematoma palpable in the proximal arm or axilla. As with all compartment syndromes, the distal pulses remain normal, because the elevated pressure at the lesion site is far below mean arterial pressure, although it is sufficient to collapse the vasa nervorem of the terminal nerves [3,19,20].

The elements of the infraclavicular plexus can be injured by a variety of orthopedic procedures performed on the shoulder girdle region for diagnostic and therapeutic reasons. Several series of such plexopathies are described after shoulder arthroscopies. Also, many reports cite these injuries occurring after many operative procedures, including those performed to repair torn rotator cuffs, to treat anterior instability, and for total shoulder replacement. Most of the infraclavicular plexopathies caused by shoulder arthroscopy are transient in nature, indicating the underlying pathophysiology is demyelinating conduction block. Those resulting from therapeutic surgery vary in their underlying pathology, however, ranging from almost solely demyelination to complete axon loss. The brachial plexus elements injured also vary, ranging from a single terminal nerve to extensive, diffuse infraclavicular lesions [1,3,17].

Iatrogenic infraclavicular lesions also result from attempted shoulder reductions. The structure affected most commonly is the axillary terminal nerve, but occasionally the damage is more extensive. The underlying pathology varies from demyelination to axon loss [3,17].

Most gunshot wounds and stab wounds about the shoulder that damage PNS structures involve the infraclavicular plexus. High-velocity trauma (eg, gunshot wounds) usually produce combinations of demyelinating conduction block and axon loss. In contrast, low-velocity trauma (eg, stab wounds) almost always cause solely axon loss [2,3,6].

In addition, a few nonsurgical and surgical iatrogenic infraclavicular brachial plexopathies are reported. Examples of the former include combined use of vest and wrist restraints to manage agitated or combative patients and the intra-arterial injections of drugs, whereas examples of the latter are nerve injuries occurring during breast operations and surgical procedures performed in the axilla [2,3].

Diagnosis

Accurately diagnosing a brachial plexus lesion frequently requires a combination of clinical history, neurologic examination, neuroimaging studies, and EDX examination.

The particular neuroimaging studies used depend on several factors. Plain radiographs are useful with those brachial plexopathies, among others, caused by violent trauma, neoplasms, true N-TOS, radiation, and humeral fractures and dislocations. Plain radiographs of the chest, shoulder, humerus, clavicle, and spine often reveal concomitant injuries to other structures with traumatic lesions. Foreign bodies also may be visualized. Plain CT scanning of the brachial plexus has substantial limitations. It is useful, however, for detecting evidence of hematomas, because it can identify blood. Moreover, when combined with myelography (ie, CT myelography), it is considered by many to be the best neuroimaging procedure for visualizing the structures within the cervical intraspinal canal (ie, primary dorsal and ventral roots). At present, MRI is considered the best neuroimaging technique for assessing the extraforaminal brachial plexus. There are several reasons for this, one of the most important being that it can differentiate one soft tissue element from another. Magnetic resonance myelography, magnetic resonance neurography, and PET scanning all are procedures that limited studies suggest may be helpful in brachial plexus assessment. The value of them, however, has not yet been determined [2,3].

EDX examination is a valuable adjunctive procedure in assessing brachial plexopathies. The studies must be extensive and, therefore, time consuming. On NCSs, usually several additional studies must be performed, because the routine ones are focused so heavily on the lower trunk and medial cord. Certainly, on needle EMG, many other muscles must be assessed than what usually is done during routine situations. Typically, the only helpful component of the NCSs in brachial plexopathy assessment is the amplitudes of the responses. The sensory nerve action potential (SNAP) amplitudes are valuable especially because they are the most sensitive of all the NCS components to axon loss, including those situated along the brachial plexus fibers at or distal to the DRG. The CMAP amplitudes have a twofold purpose. First, they can directly demonstrate conduction blocks located distal to the midtrunk level, using a combination of supraclavicular and distal axillary stimulations. Moreover, they can inferentially reveal conduction blocks that are situated even more proximally when they are combined with needle EMG of the recorded muscle. (A relatively preserved motor NCS amplitude recorded from a muscle that, on needle EMG, shows profound motor unit potential [MUP] dropout, is indicative of a conduction block situated proximal to the most proximal stimulation site.) Second, with established axon loss lesions, they can demonstrate the degree of denervation of the recorded muscle accurately, especially rather early in the course, before substantial collateral sprouting occurs. Regardless of how diligently an EDX examination is performed, however, it has certain inherent limitations, a principal one being that, with axon loss lesions, it cannot distinguish one grade of axon loss from another. Consequently, it provides no useful information regarding the likelihood of nerve fibers being able to grow through the lesion site. In general, EDX examination findings are not specific for a particular supraclavicular or infraclavicular plexopathy, but there are a few exceptions. EDX findings with postmedian sternotomy lesions and true N-TOS are so distinctive—the former with its heavy C8 APR involvement, the latter with its predominate T1 APR emphasis—to be almost pathognomonic. Also, the combination of conduction blocks on NCSs and myokymic discharges on needle EMG are almost pathognomonic for plexopathies resulting from radiation or multifocal motor neuropathy [1,3,17].

Somatosensory evoked potentials (SEPs) are performed routinely, via percutaneous stimulation, and intraoperatively, by stimulating above or below an exposed plexus lesion. Routine SEPs are of no appreciable benefit in brachial plexus assessment, because they provide no more information than the sensory NCSs do, and not enough SEPs are done to assess the C6-T1 DRG-derived sensory fibers. Intraoperative SEPs, however, can be valuable, because they can assess the C5 sensory fibers, and they also can determine whether or not an additional lesion is present proximal to one affecting the extraforaminal plexus elements [1,3,17].

Treatment and prognosis

How brachial plexopathies are treated varies with the specific disorder and depends on such factors as etiology, pathophysiology, severity, and duration. The twin goals are restoring motor and sensory function and alleviating pain if it is present. Unfortunately, with some plexopathies, neither of these goals can be achieved, and sometimes only one is obtainable, often not completely. All abrupt-onset brachial plexopathies, supraclavicular or infraclavicular, in which demyelinating conduction block is the predominate pathophysiology are treated conservatively, because recovery typically is relatively rapid and complete. Classic postoperative paralysis, rucksack paralysis, and postmedian sternotomy lesions generally fall into this category. The major exception is gunshot wounds. Even though they frequently are a mixture of demyelinating conduction block and axon loss, the latter often necessitates surgical repair. The burner syndrome also is treated conservatively because, even though it is an axon loss lesion, the amount of axon loss present is mild [3,16,17].

In supraclavicular brachial plexopathies of all types associated with traumatic axon loss, it must first be determined whether or not a lesion is within the intraspinal canal or extraforaminal. The former most often are avulsion injuries, and no surgical treatment is available to restore function, motor or sensory. The pain associated with avulsion injuries, however, often responds well to cauterization of the dorsal entry zones of the avulsed roots (DREZ, or Nashold, procedure). Traumatic extraforaminal lesions at the trunk level, if axon loss is severe (eg, ruptures; substantial internal scarring with the elements in continuity) are treated with surgical repair; usually this includes placement of cable grafts. Less severe axon loss trunk lesions generally are managed conservatively, unless severe pain is present, which may require neurolysis. Severe axon loss lesions affecting elements of the infraclavicular plexus are explored surgically most often at 3 to 4 months after onset, with operative repair performed at that time, if necessary. Conversely, mild to moderate axon loss lesions of the infraclavicular brachial plexus are treated conservatively [3,17].

Surgery frequently is necessary when cord lesions result from midshaft clavicular fractures. Multiple surgical specialties may be required to treat these injuries, including neurosurgery, orthopedic, and vascular. Most infraclavicular brachial plexopathies resulting from humeral fractures and dislocations manifest predominately demyelinating conduction block and recover with conservative treatment alone. If the injured plexus elements are ruptured or consist of a severe lesion in continuity, however, surgery is required. Many gunshot wounds require surgical exploration with plexus repair. Although the pathology along many of the axons is demyelination, and those affected by axon loss in most instances remain in continuity, the degree, or grade, of axon loss often is so severe that cable grafting is necessary. This procedure usually is delayed 3 to 4 months, even if surgical exploration had been necessary soon after the injury because of vascular damage. Stab wounds most often require prompt surgical exploration and nerve repair, as required. The chance of vascular damage is high, and complete and incomplete lesions of the plexus elements most likely result from actual separation of the axons; this latter type of injury not only requires surgery but also often can be undertaken soon after the injury is sustained. The MBFC syndrome demands almost immediate surgery if permanent deficits are to be avoided. Presumably, ischemic conduction block produces the initial sensory and then motor symptoms, but axon loss supervenes within only 2 to 4 hours after motor deficits first appear. Consequently, these lesions are one of the few actual PNS surgical emergencies. Because of this, promptly operating to reduce pressure in the MBFC is more important than obtaining any laboratory diagnostic procedures (eg, neuroimaging studies) [3,19,20].

Primary neoplasms sometimes can be removed surgically, but metastatic ones generally are incurable. As a result, treatment characteristically is directed at pain relief. The treatment used most commonly is radiotherapy. Regrettably, this helps only a minority of patients, and typically the responses are short-lived. Chemotherapy, including regional intra-arterial chemotherapy, also is of limited value. Other modalities used for pain relief include continuous infusion pumps, local and regional blocks, sympathectomy, rhizotomy, and various medications, including opium analgesics and a variety of antidepressants and antiepileptic drugs. On occasion, surgical neurolysis proves effective [13].

The appropriate treatment for true N-TOS is sectioning of the band via a supraclavicular operative approach [3].

For radiation-induced brachial plexopathies, there is, unfortunately, no effective treatment, either surgical or nonsurgical. Nonetheless, neurolysis is performed occasionally in an attempt to decrease the intensity of severe, unremitting pain, if it is present. The other nontraumatic brachial plexopathy in which the underlying pathology almost solely is demyelinating block, at least for an initial long period, is multifocal neuropathy. This acquired immune-mediated disorder is best treated with intravenous immunoglobulin (IVIg). Sometimes the degree of recovery is striking, and often this can be maintained [3,17].

The prognosis with specific brachial plexus lesions varies strikingly from one to another type, but, overall, the outcome is less satisfactory with supraclavicular lesions than infraclavicular ones. Avulsion injuries never recover, and, excluding their pain component, cannot be treated successfully. Hence, their prognosis usually is poor, because the patients are left more or less functionally one armed. With extraforaminal traction lesions, the prognosis depends on the underlying pathology and, if it is axon loss, on the specific plexus elements and the severity of injury. Neurapraxia, the demyelinating conduction block caused by relatively mild trauma, resolves promptly and completely in almost all instances, so plexopathies with this type of pathophysiology have an excellent outcome. Partial axon loss trunk lesions generally have a good prognosis, because substantial reinnervation can occur, either through proximodistal regeneration for the upper and middle trunks and lateral cord or by collateral sprouting for the lower trunk or medial cord. With complete axon loss trunk lesions, however, the degree of recovery depends on the particular plexus that fibers have damaged. Upper and middle plexus lesions and lateral cord lesions often recover satisfactorily, even in older patients, because of either spontaneous proximodistal regeneration or, if required, operative repair with cable grafting. Total or near total axon loss lesions of the lower plexus and median cord, in contrast, invariably result in permanent residuals. In particular, the intrinsic hand muscles never are reinnervated, because of the adverse time-distance factor for progressive proximodistal regeneration combined with the lack of viable, surviving axons in the intrinsic hand muscles to provide collateral reinnervation [1,3,17].

Classic postoperative paralysis and the burner syndrome usually have excellent prognoses, whereas with postmedian sternotomy lesions and rucksack palsy, the prognosis is more variable, depending principally on the amount of axon loss present. With true N-TOS, there always are substantial permanent residuals. Although operation arrests the progressive hand weakness and wasting and promptly relieves or markedly reduces the hand cramping with use and the intermittent forearm aching, the hand muscle wasting already present persists. The brachial plexopathies resulting from disputed N-TOS surgery nearly always result in severe permanent residuals, most often consisting of a weak wasted hand and causalgic pain, which may prove difficult to treat satisfactorily [3,11,17].

Primary neoplasms have a variable prognosis, but often it is satisfactory. Metastatic neoplasms, in contrast, have a poor prognosis: progression generally occurs, pain control is difficult, and typically other organs are seeded by metastases from the primary source, leading to death [3,11,17].

Radiation-induced brachial plexopathies have a dismal prognosis because the process generally is slowly progressive, ultimately results in axon loss, and cannot be treated. Multifocal motor neuropathy has a variable, but often good, prognosis, because striking improvement may be seen after IVIg therapy [3,17].

Gunshot wounds, laceration injuries, and traumatic TOS (if it produced substantial axon loss cord lesions) always are marred by permanent residuals to some degree. Similarly, the MBFC syndrome, if not recognized and treated promptly, always leaves permanent residuals. Most often these consist of total denervation in the distribution of the median nerve resulting in, among other deficits, permanent sensory loss in the index finger and thumb [3,19,20].

Partial traumatic and iatrogenic axon loss lesions involving any element of the infraclavicular plexus typically have a good prognosis. In contrast, the prognosis with total axon loss lesions involving the same plexus elements is variable, depending on the particular element injured and whether or not surgical repair was performed at the proper time, if it was indicated [3,11,17].

Lumbosacral plexopathies

The lumbar and sacral plexuses, although separate structures, most often are considered as a single entity: the lumbosacral, or pelvis, plexus. This structure is less complicated in its external anatomy than the brachial plexus, consisting of APRs, branches, divisions, and terminal nerves.

The lumbar plexus originates with the L1, L2, L3, and L4 (in part) APR, and frequently receives a contribution from T12. The remaining portion of the L4 APR fuses with the L5 APR to form the lumbosacral trunk (furcal nerve), which then contributes to the formation of the sacral plexus. Arising from these APR are short motor branches, which innervate some of the contiguous muscles (eg, the psoas). The APR of L1, L2, and L4 then divide into upper and lower branches. The upper branch of L1 terminates as the iliohypogastric and ilioinguinal nerves, with the T12 also sometimes contributing to the formation of the iliohypogastric nerve. The lower branch of L1 joins with the upper branch of L2 to form the genitofemoral nerve. The lower branch of L2 and all of L3 and the upper branch of L4 each terminate by dividing into smaller anterior and larger posterior divisions. The anterior divisions fuse to form the obturator nerve, whereas the posterior divisions combine to form the femoral nerve. The L2 and L3 posterior divisions contribute small branches that join to form the lateral femoral cutaneous nerve (Fig. 4) [8].

The lumbar plexus is located within the posteior aspect of the superior and middle portions of the psoas major muscle, anterior to the transverse processes of the lumbar vertebrae. Its divisions extend caudally enough to lie slightly within the greater, or false, pelvis, but they are within the psoas fascia and, therefore, external to the pelvis fascia. The lumbar plexus supplies sensation to the skin overlying the pubic symphysis, some of the external genitalia, the anterior, medial, and posterior medial thigh, and the medial and anteromedial portions of the leg, extending as far distally as the ankle. Its motor components innervate the iliacus and psoas mucles and all the muscles of the anterior and medial thigh [2,5,8,18].

The sacral plexus originates with the lower branch of the L4, APR, and the L5-S4 APR. Each of these divides into an anterior and posterior division. Whereas the anterior divisions fuse to form the tibial nerve, the upper four posterior divisions join to compose the common peroneal nerve. These two nerves are enclosed within a common sheath, thereby constituting the sciatic nerve. Three major collateral branches arise from the divisions, including (1) the superior gluteal nerve (L4, L5, and S1 posterior divisions);

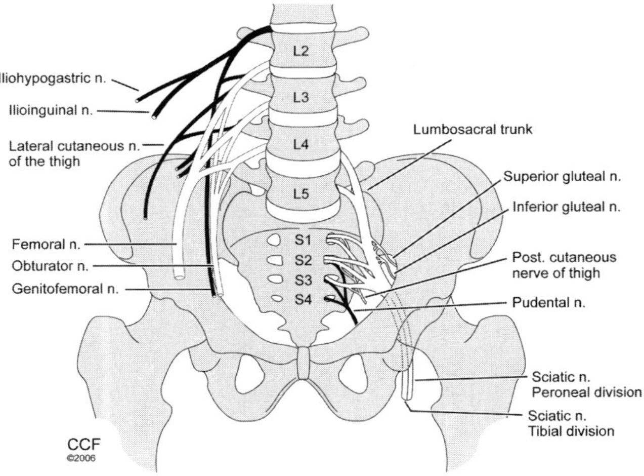

Fig. 4. The lumbosacral plexus (the lumbar plexus to viewer's right the sacral plexus to the viewer's left. (*Courtesy of* the Cleveland Clinic Foundation, Cleveland, OH.)

(2) the inferior gluteal nerve (L5, S1, and S2 posterior divisions); (3) and the posterior femoral cutaneous nerve (S1 and S2 posterior divisions; S1-S3 anterior divisions) (see Fig. 4) [2,8].

The sacral plexus is situated in the posterior aspect of the true pelvis, where it rests on the anterior surface of the piriformis muscle. Structures that are contiguous to or near it include the hypogastric arteries and veins, the lateral rectum, the pelvic colon, and the ureters. The sacral plexus provides sensation to the gluteal regions, some of the external genitalia, and virtually all of the lower limb, except for the anterolateral aspect of the thigh, which is supplied by the lateral femoral cutaneous nerve and the longitudinal strip along the medial leg innervated by the femoral and obturator nerves. The sacral plexus innervates most of the pelvic floor muscles, the glutei and tensor fascia lata (via the gluteal nerves), and the hamstrings and all the muscles of the leg and foot (via the sciatic nerve).

Lumbosacral plexus (or pelvic) plexopathies are less common than are brachial plexopathies, principally because traumatic injuries of them occur so infrequently. Consequently, the majority of lumbosacral plexopathies are nontraumatic in origin. This was illustrated by a report of 86 cases of lumbar plexopathies: less than 6% were caused by trauma, whereas more than 50% were the result of neoplasms [21].

Traumatic closed injuries of the lumbosacral plexus are relatively rare (as discussed previously) because the nerve fibers that compose them are protected by muscle or bone and are not situated near highly mobile structures, as is the brachial plexus. Nearly all lumbosacral plexopathies of this type are the result of exceptionally violent trauma (eg, high-speed vehicular accidents, pedestrians struck by moving vehicles, falls from heights, and various types of industrial accidents). In most instances, these are associated with bony fractures of the pelvic ring and acetabulum or dislocations of the sacroiliac joint.

The two major functions of the bony pelvis are weight bearing and protection of the structures it contains. It is viewed as a pelvic ring, formed by three bones linked together by ligaments. The two innominate bones articulate posteriorly with the sacrum and anteriorly with each other at the pubic symphysis. Because the anterior third of the pelvic ring does not bear weight, fractures of it are usually stable and, if isolated, seldom damage PNS structures. The posterolateral two thirds of the pelvic ring, in contrast, serves as an arch connecting the trunk with the lower limbs, through which the weight load is transmitted. When fractures or dislocations involving this portion of pelvic ring occur, its weight-bearing and protective properties can be compromised severely. Fractures in this area often are unstable and frequently damage structures near or adjacent to it (eg, blood vessels, lumbosacral nerves, genitourinary tract, and rectum). With high-speed traffic accidents, pelvic fractures are one of the markers of injury severity. They are found in only 2% to 4.5% of nonfatal accidents, in 22% of fatal accidents in general, and in 45% of fatal accidents involving pedestrians. Most pelvic fractures are associated with fractures of other bones and with soft tissue injuries. Hemorrhage with subsequent shock and genitourinary damage is the most common and the most devastating complication. Conversely, the incidence of PNS injuries with pelvic fractures, overall, is relatively low (less than 7.5%). This incidence, however, increases significantly with pelvic dislocations and certain types of pelvic fractures (eg, transverse sacral fractures and double vertical fractures). Transverse sacral fractures are especially likely to cause intraspinal and intraforaminal injury to nerve roots. Double vertical pelvic fractures consist of combined separation injuries of the posterior and anterior pelvic ring. The former may be a vertical sacral fracture, a vertical fracture through the adjacent ilium, or rupture of the sacroiliac joint. The anterior ring injury most often is a rupture of the pubic symphysis. Sacroiliac joint ruptures occur most commonly in young adults and are particularly likely to injure the lumbosacral trunk, which is contiguous with the joint. Even severe injuries to the lumbosacral plexus usually are overshadowed by concomitant, frequently severe, injuries of other pelvic structures [5,22].

Clinically, patients who have closed traumatic lumbosacral plexopathies present with weakness, sensory loss, and frequently pain in the distribution of the involved neural structures, which may be the lumbosacral roots, the lumbosacral plexus, or nerves derived from the lumbosacral plexus (eg, obturator). Definite localization to one these neural structures can prove difficult principally because associated bony abnormalities, which almost invariably are present, place limitations on a neurologic examination. In these instances, the differential diagnosis, depending on the specific portions of the lumbosacral plexus damaged, includes lesions located at three different levels: root, plexus, and proximal peripheral nerve [5]. This same diagnostic dilemma is encountered with lumbosacral plexopathies of almost all types. Thus, a review of 171 cases assessed in the author's EDX laboratory, in which a sacral plexopathy was considered in the differential diagnosis, demonstrated that only in approximately one third of instances could the lesions be localized unequivocally to that neural structure. Final diagnoses in the remaining two thirds of patients were indeterminate, in that EDX localization was to the sacral plexus or the L4-S1 roots, the sacral plexus or sciatic nerve, or the L4-S1 roots, sacral plexus, or sciatic nerve. Thus, EDX assessments of sacral plexopathies often yield complex findings, which are difficult to localize to a specific site. Confounding factors include duration of lesion, the bilateral absence of lower limb SNAPs and prior lumbar surgeries [23].

The open types of traumatic lumbosacral plexopathies are less common than the closed variety. Nonetheless, similar to the latter, they also typically coexist with damage to internal organs, major blood vessels, and various bony structures, in particular those composing the pelvic ring. The majority of these are the result ofgunshot wounds and low-velocity puncture wounds [5,16].

Nontraumatic lesions are the most common cause of lumbosacral plexopathies, and the most common of these, by far, are neoplasms. Although occasionally a primary neoplasm (eg, neurofibroma) originates in the lumbosacral plexus, malignant neoplasms occur more frequently. Of these, approximately three fourths invade the plexus by direct extension, the major source for these being the terminal gastrointestinal tract, the genitourinary system (especially the cervix in women), and lymphomas and sarcomas. Approximately one fourth of malignant tumors reach the lumbosacral plexus by metastases, the majority arising from breast carcinomas. (These are responsible for the majority of bilateral lumbosacral plexopathies.) Overall, approximately 50% of malignant neoplasms involve the sacral plexus, 33% the lumbar plexus, and 17% both plexuses. Usually, in these instances, plexus involvement becomes evident only after the primary malignancy is diagnosed and treated [2,12,13].

Clinically, pain usually is the first symptom with neoplastic lumbosacral plexopathies. With lumbar plexus involvement, it is located in the low back, hip, and thigh, whereas with sacral plexus involvement, it is experienced in the posterolateral thigh, leg, and foot. Although they may be delayed for months, paresthesias, especially weakness, ultimately appear. Gait abnormalities and lower extremity edema may be seen, especially with bilateral lesions. Rectal masses may be palpated in more than one third of patients who have neoplastic sacral plexopathies, although rectal incontinence is uncommon [2,12,13].

Another type of nontraumatic lumbosacral plexopathy is termed, intrapartum maternal lumbosacral plexopathy or maternal paralysis. This occurs during the latter stages of pregnancy and during delivery when the lumbosacral trunk, and sometimes the superior gluteal and obturator nerves, are compressed between the maternal pelvic rim and the fetal head. Predisposing factors include mothers who are relatively small and labor that is prolonged. Typically, intermittent pain is the first symptom, which radiates from the buttock into the limb in an L5 distribution. As it increases in intensity, it often becomes continuous in nature. Motor deficits ultimately appear; characteristically, the most obvious of these is a foot drop. Demyelinating conduction block is the predominate pathophysiology, although it characteristically is accompanied by varying amounts of axon loss. Usually the pain subsides promptly at or soon after delivery, whereas the motor deficits may be more persistent. Nonetheless, because they usually are the result of conduction block, typically they resolve within a few weeks of delivery [1,2,24].

Diabetic amyotrophy is a syndrome that affects elderly patients, mostly men, who have longstanding type 2 diabetes mellitus. It presents with unilateral or bilateral aching pain, of abrupt or subacute onset, located in the back, buttock, or anterior thigh. Characteristically, the pain is worse at night, raising the question of pelvic neoplasm. Anterior thigh weakness and subsequent atrophy, often marked, coexist with or soon follow the pain. The symptoms persist for months during which depression and substantial weight loss may appear. Frequently, diabetic amyotrophy is superimposed on an existing diabetic polyneuropathy. Clinically, in the advanced stage, patients have weakness and wasting of the anterior and lateral thigh muscles. There often is some sensory deficit over the anterior thigh. The quadriceps DTR usually is absent in the affected limbs. This syndrome probably is to the result of ischemic nerve injury, secondary to a microvasculitis [1,2,25].

A syndrome identical to diabetic amyotrophy, although it occurs in patients who are nondiabetic, is reported. Its names include nondiabetic/diabetic amyotrophy and nondiabetic lumbosacral radiculoplexus neuropathy [26]. The diabetic and nondiabetic varieties of this disorder are considered immune-mediated lesions [25,26].

Retroperitoneal infections are stated in review articles to cause lumbosacral plexopathies, with the latter developing secondary to psoas muscle abscesses. Nonetheless, convincing case reports of these lesions are not found in the literature, suggesting they are rare. There has been one patient who had HIV and documented bilateral lumbosacral plexopathies caused by pelvic cellulitis that followed a perirectal abscess [2].

Lumbosacral plexopathies are one of the many complications of aortic aneurysms and their surgical repair. Portions of the lumbosacral plexus can be injured via direct compression by aneurysms and by ischemia when their feeding vessels are occluded by emboli or thrombosis. Usually the neurologic symptoms, consisting of pain, sensory loss, and weakness, are restricted to one limb, even though there may be unilateral or bilateral evidence of vascular insufficiency in the lower limbs. Common iliac and internal iliac artery aneurysms can compress the L5-S2 APR, which lie directly posterior to those vessels. Axon loss is the underlying pathology with lumbosacral plexopathies caused by aneurysms [27].

Retroperitoneal hemorrhage, caused by nontraumatic (eg, hemophilia, leukemia, or disseminated intravascular coagulation) and iatrogenic (eg, anticoagulation) causes can, via the development of compartment syndromes, compromise the femoral nerve, the lumbar plexus, and simultaneously the lumbar and sacral plexuses. With the iliacus syndrome, a relatively small amount of bleeding within the iliacus muscle proximally, or within the intermuscular groove between the iliacus and psoas muscles more distally, produces a femoral neuropathy. With the psoas compartment syndrome, more extensive bleeding within the psoas muscle itself causes a lumbar plexopathy. A widespread retroperitoneal hemorrhage can cause compartment syndromes that affect the lumbar and sacral plexuses. All of these lesions usually are unilateral and present with pain of acute or subacute onset localized to the lower abdominal region or groin that radiates into the anterior thigh and medical leg. Soon, motor and sensory deficits appear in the appropriate distribution. The lesions usually are visualized by MRI. EDX examination typically reveals substantial axon loss in the distribution of the femoral nerve, lumbar plexus, or, less often, the lumbosacral plexus [2,10,27].

Radiation-induced lumbosacral plexopathies are iatrogenic lesions that result from radiotherapy directed to the pelvis to treat various neoplasms, especially testicular cancer in men, gynecologic cancers in women, and lymphomas in both genders. As with radiation-induced brachial plexopathies, the latent period between radiation therapy and the onset of symptoms is markedly variable, ranging from a few months to more than 3 decades. Regardless of the time that elapses between radiation therapy being given and the appearance of a lumbosacral plexopathy, a radiation-induced lesion cannot be excluded. The initial symptom of this disorder usually is painless weakness, often bilateral but frequently asymmetric, in the distribution of the lumbar plexus, the sacral plexus, or both. Limb paresthesias commonly appear somewhat later; limb pain is reported in approximately half the patients, but it seldom is prominent. Even with sacral plexus involvement, bowel and bladder disturbances are uncommon [1,2].

Postoperative lumbosacral plexopathies are surprisingly uncommon, compared with the high incidence of postoperative brachial plexopathies. There are few convincing reports of lumbosacral plexus lesions sustained during surgery. Typically, the latter was pelvic surgery, and the plexopathies resulted from direct instrumentation or ischemia. Although there are reports of hip surgery causing lumbosacral plexopathies, these more likely are instances of multiple mononeuropathies (sciatic or femoral) that are mislocalized [1,2].

Diagnosis

EDX examination with lumbar and sacral plexopathies often yields suboptimal results (for reasons discussed previously). Nonetheless, at times it provides some useful information. Thus, with closed and open traction injuries, any motor NCSs that can be performed demonstrate the amount of motor axon loss present (via the amplitudes of the responses). Similarly, fibrillation potentials can be visualized in denervated muscles on needle EMG, even if the strength of those muscles cannot be assessed on clinical examination because of associated pelvic (and sometimes long bone) fractures. Neuroimaging studies, consisting of plain radiograph, MRI, and CT, always reveal abnormalities, but these often pertain solely to the bony changes that almost invariably are present. At times, specialized neuroimaging studies (eg, pyelograms or pelvic arteriograms) are of major benefit. With neoplastic disease, EDX examination usually is abnormal, although the findings may be relatively minimal, particularly if pain (rather than weakness) is the sole symptom. Even if EDX examination is abnormal, localization may be unsatisfactory (reasons discussed previously). Many neoplastic lesions can be visualized with MRI, particularly if they are presenting as discrete mass lesions. They may be difficult to distinguish from postradiation changes in many instances. With intrapartum maternal lumbosacral plexopathies, EDX examination typically reveals a demyelinating conduction block, located proximal to the popliteal fossa stimulation site, along the motor fibers supplying the muscles of the anterior and lateral compartments of the leg (eg, the tibialis anterior). The needle EMG shows abnormalities in an L5 distribution in the limb, but usually the paraspinal muscles appear normal. Neuroimaging studies, in contrast, are of no value with this disorder Diabetic amyotrophy and nondiabetic lumbosacral radiculoplexus neuropathy always manifest EDX abnormalities, the most characteristic being low amplitude or absent femoral motor NCS responses in the symptomatic limbs and severe denervation, on needle EMG, in the medial (obturator nerve–innervated) and the anterior (femoral nerve–innervated) thigh muscles; the former exclude a "diabetic femoral neuropathy." In addition, in most cases of diabetic amyotrophy, there is EDX evidence of an axon loss polyneuropathy. The lesions with these disorders generally cannot be visualized with neuroimaging studies. When aortic aneurysms, or their surgical repair, cause proximal PNS lesions, EDX examination invariably demonstrates axon loss, but the localization characteristically is poor. Frequently, neuroimaging studies (eg, MRI) reveal an extensive lesion, which, similar to EDX studies, renders accurate localization problematic. With retroperitoneal hemorrhages, EDX examination shows substantial axon loss in the distribution of the femoral nerve, lumbar plexus, or, less often, the lumbosacral plexus. The needle EMG is useful particularly in these patients, because, by demonstrating the presence or absence of fibrillation potentials and MUP dropout in the thigh adductor muscles, it allows localization to be made either to the proximal femoral nerve or lumbar plexus, with a relatively high degree of accuracy. Neuroimaging studies usually are equally helpful in these situations, revealing the mass. CT scans may be especially useful, because they can identify blood. With radiation-induced lumbosacral plexopathies, in all but far advanced cases EDX examination demonstrates inferential evidence of demyelinating conduction block (ie, relatively preserved CMAP reported on motor NCSs from a weak muscle compared with the substantial dropout of MUPs seen on needle EMG of the same muscle). In addition, needle EMG, especially with rather longstanding lesions, shows prominent chronic neurogenic MUPs along with some fibrillation potentials and often fasciculation potentials and myokymic potentials. In the author's experience, myokymic potentials are found more often with lumbar than with sacral plexopathies, and they are seen bilaterally with surprising frequency. Neuroimaging studies almost always are abnormal, but distinguishing radiation-induced lesions from neoplastic ones is difficult at times. Moreover, neuroimaging studies may show incidental abnormalities in the lumbosacral spine, to which patients' symptoms may be attributed incorrectly [2].

Treatment

The optimal treatment of lumbosacral plexopathies depends on a variety of factors, including the cause, location, severity, and duration of the lesions. Most traumatic plexopathies improve spontaneously, at least to some extent, and, therefore, they usually are treated conservatively. Occasionally surgical repair is attempted, which tends to yield better results with lumbar, as opposed to sacral, plexus lesions [2,15]. One group of peripheral nerve surgeons notes that these injuries are difficult to diagnose and treat, and the technical problems associated with the latter are "forbidding" [9]. Few reports of operative treatment of open injuries involving the lumbosacral plexus are available. In general, if surgery is performed on these patients, it is to treat damage to blood vessels or soft tissues, rather than to the neural elements [2,18].

The treatment of neoplastic lumbosacral plexopathies is discussed previously. Intrapartum maternal lumbosacral plexopathy is treated conservatively, because demyelinating conduction block characteristically is the pathophysiology responsible for most, if not all, of the symptoms. Diabetic amyotrophy and nondiabetic radiculoplexoneuropathy are treated conservatively with analgesics and antiepileptics, because the long-term prognosis with these entities is excellent. Even though they are assumed to be immune mediated, typical patients who have this disorder have so many contraindications, relative or absolute, to immune therapy, that it is seldom used. Retroperitoneal hemorrhages generally are treated conservatively, with analgesics, limb immobilization, and, if necessary, blood transfusions. Probably this is the only major compartment syndrome in which surgical decompression is not recommended. There is, unfortunately, no satisfactory treatment for radiation-induced lumbosacral plexopathy. Nonetheless, preventing unnecessary surgical root decompressive procedures from being performed is of benefit [2,10,17,24–26].

References

[1] Ferrante MA, Wilbourn AJ. Plexopathies. In: Levin KH, Luders HO, editors. Comprehensive clinical neurophysiology. Philadelphia: WB Saunders; 2000. p. 201–14.
[2] Wilbourn AJ, Ferrante MA. Plexopathies. In: Pourmand R, editor. Neuromuscular disease: expert clinicians' views. Woburn AMA: Butterworth-Heinemann; 2002. p. 703–15.
[3] Wilbourn AJ. Brachial plexus lesions. In: Dyck PJ, Thomas PK, editors. Peripheral neuropathy, vol. 2. 4th ed. Philadelphia: Saunders; 2005. p. 1339–73.
[4] Wilbourn AJ. Lumbosacral plexopathies. In: Daube JR, Maugierre F, editors. In: Kimura J, editor. Clinical neurophysiology of peripheral nerves. Handbook of clinical neurophysiology, vol. 7. Elsevier; 2005. p. 631–45.
[5] Wilbourn AJ. Plexus injuries. In: Evans RW, editor. Neurology and trauma. 2nd ed. New York: Oxford Press; 2006.
[6] Seddon HJ. Three types of nerve injury. Brain 1943;66:237–81.
[7] Sunderland S. Nerve and nerve injuries. 2nd ed. London: Churchill-Livingstone; 1978.
[8] Clemente CD. Grey's anatomy. 30th ed (Amer). Philadelphia: Lea and Febiger; 1985.
[9] Brazis PW, Masden JC, Briller J. Localization in clinical neurology. 2nd ed. Boston: Little Brown; 1990.
[10] Stewart JD. Focal peripheral neuropathies. 3rd ed. Philadelphia: Lippincott, Williams & Wilkins; 2000.
[11] Haymaker W, Woodhall B. Peripheral nerve injuries. 2nd ed. Philadelphia: WB Saunders; 1953.
[12] Jaeckle KA. Nerve plexus metastasis. Neurol Clin 1991;9:857–66.
[13] Jaeckle KA. Neurological manifestations of neoplastic and radiation-induced plexopathies. Semin Neurol 2004;24:385–93.
[14] Schaafsma. Plexus injuries. In: Vinken PJ, Bruyn GS, editors. Handbook of clinical neurology, vol. 7. Diseases of nerves, part 1. Amsterdam: Elsevier; 1987. p. 402–29.
[15] Birch R, Bonney G, Wynn-Parry CB. Surgical disorders of peripheral nerves. Edinburgh: Churchill-Livingstone; 1998.
[16] Kline DG, Hudson AR. Nerve injuries. Philadelphia: WB Saunders; 1995.
[17] Wilbourn AJ. Brachial plexopathies. In: Brown WF, Bolton CF, Aminoff MA, editors. Neuromuscular function and disease. Philadelphia: WB Saunders; 2002. p. 831–51.
[18] Wilbourn AJ. Evaluation and treatment of the patient with brachial or lumbosacral plexopathy. In: Batjer HH, Loftus CM, editors. Textbook of neurological surgery, vol. 1. Philadelphia: Lippincott, Williams & Wilkins; 2003. p. 599–612.
[19] Tsao B, Wilbourn AJ. Infraclavicular brachial plexus following axillary regional block. Muscle Nerve 2005;30:44–8.
[20] Tsao BE, Wilbourn AJ. The medial brachial fascial compartment syndrome following axillary arteriography. Neurology 2003;61:1037–41.
[21] Mumenthaler M, Schliak H. Peripheral nerve lesions. New York: Thieme Medical; 1991.
[22] Huittinen VM, Slatis P. Nerve injury in double vertical pelvic fractures. Acta Chir Scand 1972;138:571–5.
[23] Tavee J, Mays MA, Wilbourn AJ. Pitfalls in the electrodiagnostic studies of sacral plexopathy, in press.
[24] Katirji B, Wilbourn AJ, Scarberry JL, et al. Intrapartum maternal lumbosacral plexopathy. Muscle Nerve 1998;21:3–7.
[25] Llewelyn JG, Tomilson DR, Thomas PK. Diabetic neuropathies. In: Dyck PJ, Thomas PK, editors. Peripheral neuropathy, vol. 2. 4th ed. Philadelphia: WB Saunders; 2005. p. 1951–91.
[26] Dyck PJB. Radiculoplexus neuropathies: diabetic and nondiabetic varieties. In: Dyck PA, Thomas PK, editors. Peripheral neuropathy, vol. 2. 4th ed. Philadelphia: WB Saunders; 2005. p. 1993–2015.
[27] Wilbourn AJ. Peripheral neuropathies associated with vascular diseases and the vasculitides. In: Brown WF, Bolton CF, Aminoff MA, editors. Neuromuscular function and disease, vol. 2. Philadelphia: WB Saunders; 2002. p. 1229–9.

ELSEVIER
SAUNDERS

Neurol Clin 25 (2007) 173–207

NEUROLOGIC
CLINICS

The Inherited Neuropathies

Christopher J. Klein, MD*

Department of Neurology, Division of Peripheral Nerve Diseases, Mayo Clinic, Rochester, MN, USA

Neuropathy is one of the most common referrals to neurologic clinics. Affected patients often undergo extensive testing for acquired etiologies (ie, diabetes, immune inflammatory, and others) without a specific cause found. Within this group, inherited cause is common. Increasingly, genetic causes are becoming known and commercial testing available. The rate of recent discovery has been rapid and relates to (1) the extent of single gene disorders of nerve; (2) the ease of peripheral nervous system functional examination, including bedside and electrophysiologic testing; and (3) readily accessible pathologic tissue. Foremost, however, in the rate of recent discoveries is the work and tools of, collectively termed, the human genome project. Normal and pathologically affected proteins have been chromosomally mapped, cloned, and functionally characterized in nerve. Many other proteins influencing nerve have been identified using the same molecular techniques. The rapidity of ongoing discovery requires clinicians to be familiar with molecular biologic discoveries and consider wisely which testing be performed, if any. Publicly sponsored internationally available and continually updated Web information is available via (1) certified laboratory contact information; (2) clinically relevant reviews for doctors and patients; (3) and research opportunities that are emphasized collectively in the Web sites for GENE TESTS, OMIM, and IPNMDB [1–3].

Inherited neuropathies are common

Inherited neuropathies present with varied symptoms, signs, and temporal course. In one large prospective study, inherited cause was the diagnosis found most commonly in individuals who were previously

* 200 First Street, SW, Rochester, MN 55905.
E-mail address: klein.christopher@mayo.edu

doi:10.1016/j.ncl.2006.12.001

unclassified and undergoing extensive evaluation [4]. Kindred evaluations were essential in the identification of those individuals. Neurologists greatly underappreciate this group of disorders. The reason inherited forms often are overlooked is complex. The apparent paradox that stagnant gene defects can produce illness in mid to late life likely is contributory. Painless indolent course in many also obscures earlier identification. Specifically, mild neurologic impairments often exist in childhood but handicaps may not be apparent until adulthood. Because patients link their handicaps to clinical onset, subacute course often is described, thereby leading to major consideration of acquired neuropathies. For similar reasons, other affected family members often are not known. Meeting with and examining families considered unaffected often is helpful. Conversely, because pain commonly is found in acquired neuropathies, extensive laboratory searches are performed without adequate consideration of painful inherited conditions. Positive testing for causes of acquired entities should not exclude consideration of inherited disease. Laboratory results must be reviewed critically, as inherited illness may be the primary neuropathic process or additive of impairments. High arches, hammer toes of the feet, subluxed hips, foot ulcers, and various bony abnormalities are nonspecific clues of inherited neuropathy. Other features may include refractory treatment of "acquired" disease, doctor-identified foot drop previously not apparent to patients and often associated with frequent ankle sprains, and sometimes the label of being "clumsy."

Complex pathogenesis in inherited neuropathies

Nerve is susceptible to diverse pathologic insults. In part, these susceptibilities relate to the length of axons. Single-celled axons and their cytoplasm may extend greater than 1 meter in humans, necessitating complex structural, metabolic, and dynamic interactions to preserve function. Consideration of the normal architecture of nerve and its molecular interactions is important in understanding pathogenesis. Subspecialized myelin axonal proteins have been localized and interact at various regions of nerve: (1) adaxonal membranes (K^+ channels and Caspr); (2) paranodal myelin loops (NF155 and NF186); and (3) microvilli or perinodal astrocytes (NF155, NF-186, Nr-CAM, tenascin-C, actin, ezrin, radixin, moesin, spectrin $\beta IV\sum 1$, ankyrin, and Na^+ channels) [5]. Proteins at the basal lamina interacting with myelin at juxtaparanodal areas also have been identified and include F-actin, L-periaxin, laminin-2, utrophin, Dp116, and dystrophin-related protein 2 [DRP2]). Such proteins are essential in nerve integrity and regeneration and provide important scaffolding function for axonal growth cones. Further necessitated by the axons' length are important transport proteins, some of which are known and associated with disease: anterograde transport (dynactin); (2) fast transport (kinesin family member 1B [KIF1B] and heat shock protein 22 [HSP22]); (3) neurofilament scaffolding (filamin 1, neurofilament light [NFL], and gigaxonin [GAN]); (3) mictotubule interacting (spastin and spartin); (4) vesicular transport (ras-associated protein [RAB7]) and others (reviewed elsewhere) [6–8].

Some of the earliest pathogenic discoveries occurred within individuals classified as having Charcot-Marie-Tooth disease (CMT), also known as hereditary motor and sensory neuropathy (HMSN) (discussed later). Identified earliest were defects within structural proteins of myelin (peripheral myelin protein 22 [*PMP22*] and myelin protein zero [*MPZ*]). Now, however, many identified defects have been found in ubiquitously expressed proteins present in multiple extraneural tissues and are important in such basic cell maintenance as transcription (early growth response 2 [EGR2]), translation (glycine tRNA synthetase [GARS]), DNA maintenance (tyrosyl DNA phosphodiesterase 1 [TDP1]), mitochondrial fusion (mitofusin [MFN2]), apoptosis (serine palmitoyltransferase [SPTLC1]), and many others. The discoveries emphasize the susceptibility or fidelity of nerve to defects tolerated by other systems. Different pathologic localization is summarized in Box 1.

Box 1. Molecular pathogenesis of inherited neuropathies

- Myelin structure (*MPZ* and *PMP22*)
- Myelin gap junction transport (connexin 32 [gap junction beta-1 (*GJB1*)])
- Axonal transport (*NFL, KIFIB,* and *GAN*)
- Signaling proteins (ganglioside-induced differentiation-associated protein [*GDAP1*])
- Axonal osmotic homeostasis (potassium chloride cotransporter 3 [*KCC3*])
- tRNA synthetase (*GARS*)
- Mitochondrial fusion (*MFN2*)
- DNA replication (*TDP1*)
- Basal lamina stability (lamin A/C [*LMNA*])
- Glycolipid processing (α-galactosidase deficiency, α-galactosidase)
- Apoptosis (*SPTLC1, RAB7*)
- Nerve trophism (tyrosine receptor kinase A [*TrkA*])
- Na channel hyperexcitabilty (Nav 1.7 mutation)
- Actin cytoskeletal function (septin-like molecule [*SEPT9*])
- Others

Molecular anatomy and clinical disability

Clinical disabilities arising in the peripheral nervous system relate most directly to axonal protein degenerations, malformations, or disturbances. Early clinical studies using histopathologic and phenotypic correlates of nerve conductions suggested the important, clinically relevant interactions between Schwann cell products (myelin) and axons [9,10]. Patients who have demyelinating hereditary phenotypes, such as occur in HMSN type 1 (HMSN1) and Dejerine-Sottas syndrome (DSS), are noted to have axonal atrophy, despite primary myelin protein defect [9]. Longitudinal study (15 years) of patients later identified as having *PMP22* duplication and *MPZ* missense mutations show conduction velocity follows an independent course (slowly improving during maturation, plateauing, and then worsening). Greater reductions in motor nerve conduction velocities correlated with more rapid progression of declines in the amplitudes of compound muscle action potentials (CMAP) and neurologic disabilities [10]. The findings are consistent with the essential role of specific myelin proteins in sustaining axonal health through the identified molecular interactions (described previously). This information has relevance to many acquired neuropathies where more rapid disabilities are accrued with primary axonal injury: (1) systemic and nonsystemic vasculitis [11,12]; (2) forms of axonal Guillain-Barré with periaxonal macrophage invasion (ie, acute motor axonal neuropathy) [13–15]; and (3) many toxic forms [16].

Inherited system atrophies affecting nerve (HMSN, HSAN, HSP, SCA)

Recognizing that many inherited neuropathies are system atrophies is helpful in diagnosis, classification, and management. For instance, patients who have small sensory fiber abnormalities may be at greater risk for mutilating foot injuries, and early aggressive prophylactic foot care and occupational council are emphasized. Chronic symmetric progression of motor, sensory, or mixed deficits initially in lower extremities is the hallmark of presentation in most system atrophy neuropathies. Classes of neurons (or nerve fibers) are affected selectively and fail to develop or degenerate or have supporting cells that undergo similar process. The population of neurons or axons affected and the names of the disorders are: lower motor, primary sensory, and autonomic neurons (HMSN) and primary sensory and autonomic neurons (hereditary sensory and autonomic neuropathy [HSAN]). Other system degenerations include corticospinal tract (spastic paraplegia), lower motor neurons (progressive muscular atrophy) or hereditary motor neuropathy, and large-diameter primary sensory neurons and cerebellum (spinocerebellar degeneration). Other less common inherited neuropathies affect multiple tissues, whereas even rarer forms, such as hereditary brachial plexus neuropathy, affect asymmetric upper extremities without evidence of a more generalized process.

HMSN

The understanding of HMSN has evolved with each new technologic discovery; Fig. 1 summarizes the proper genetic testing. The earliest clinical descriptions include those of Virchow [17] and Eichorst [18]. The subsequent work of Charcot and Marie in France [19] and Tooth in England [20] provides phenotypic understanding: (1) progressive muscular atrophy involving the feet and legs first; second, after many years, affecting the hands; and, later still, affecting the forearms; (2) contractions of atrophic muscles; (3) vasomotor abnormalities; (4) lack of joint contractures; (5) normal sensation (now known not typical [ie, most with sensory loss, but often mild]); (6) frequent cramps; (7) degenerations in atrophic muscles; (8) frequent onset in infancy (symptomatic onsets at later ages in most patients); and (9) occurrence of the disorder in the same generation and in succeeding generation. Additional descriptions included Achilles tendons exuberance, pes cavus, atrophy of leg and thigh muscles so that the lower limbs resembled an "inverted champagne bottle," hammertoes and clawhand, steppage gait, and, in some persons, constant shuffling of feet when standing in one place to maintain balance. Davidenkow provided more elaborate descriptions of the patterns of inheritance [21].

More recent classifications of Dyck and Lambert [22] provide a framework for the current incorporation of molecular data with previous electrophysiologic and histopathologic descriptions that include (1) clinical

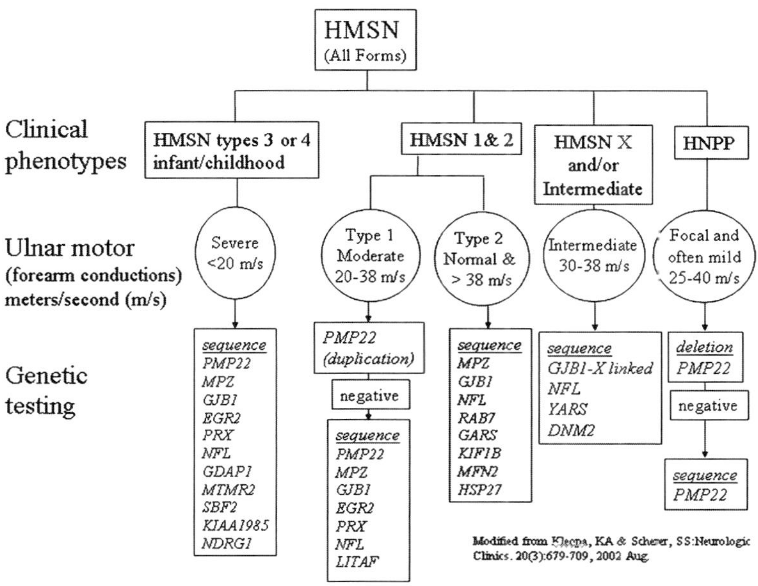

Fig. 1. Algorithm for considering genetic cause. (*Adapted from* Kleopa KA, Scherer SS. Inherited neuropathies. Neurol Clin N Am 2002;20:679–709.)

features, (2) mode of inheritance, and (3) molecular localization. The terminology reflects the hereditary nature, localization, and system involvement (ie, HMSN). The first, dominantly inherited, was a hypertrophic neuropathy (HMSN1), which was associated with slow nerve conduction velocities (typically 20 m per second or less in ulnar forearm) with complex Schwann cell processes forming lamellae separated by longitudinally directed collagen fibrils (onion bulbs) on nerve biopsy. Although the symptoms predominately affected motor nerves, sensory and autonomic fibers also were affected. The second (HMSN2) also affected predominately motor nerves but with normal to borderline slow nerve conduction velocities with axonal atrophy on nerve biopsy. The third (HMSN3) now known with dominant inheritance is present in childhood or infancy with loss of ambulatory milestones and more generalized neurologic deficit (especially proximal and upper distal involvement of upper and lower limbs) and has extremely slow nerve conductions (typically in the single digits to low teens, ulnar forearm) and characteristic exaggerated generalized onion bulbs and axonal fiber degenerations early in disease. The fourth type (HMSN 4), initially described with phytanic acid disease (Refsum), does not include those patients currently but rather refers to those who have autosomal recessive inheritance where demyelinating nerve conductions are most common but not exclusive. Many in this group have childhood onset and often are from consanguineous marriages with extraneural features that include facial dysmorphism and scoliosis. Other initially described forms with spasticity (HMSN 5) have been overshadowed by detailed work in hereditary spastic paraparesis (discussed later). Lastly, two additional categories were created out of observation of patients who had peripheral neuronal degenerations with optic atrophy (HMSN 6) and retinitis pigmentosa (HMSN 7) without clear molecular discovery to date.

Complex observations from the molecular biologic discoveries emphasize the need for incorporation of the clinical expression and molecular localization in the classification. Considering whether or not molecular defects are positioned in myelin or neuronal elements is, in itself, inadequate in classification, as mutations in neuronal elements, such as *NFL*, may disrupt saltatory conduction and cause slow nerve conduction velocities and damaged axons. Other examples include myelin genes, such as *PMP22* and *MPZ*, which can cause either HMSN 1 phenotype or severe congenital onset HMSN 3. Furthermore, abnormalities in *GJB1* and *MPZ* produce variable nerve conductions and pathologic description with apparent primary axonal atrophy. Other examples, however, emphasize the genetic cause over clinical features in the diagnosis. For example, rare *PMP22* micromutations may cause recessive inheritance compared with most mutations in this gene, which are dominantly inherited. By considering the clinical features and genetic mutations, the classification has been improved and is promoting better clinical practice and basic science discovery.

HMSN demyelinating forms (HMSN types I, III, IV, and X-linked)

Motor greater then sensory fibers are affected in this demyelinating group with diverse inheritance patterns, severity, and associated clinical features. Associated with these varieties are different pathologic and specific electrophysiologic features: (1) HMSN1A-C and HMSN4A-F; (2) DSS, also referred to as congenital hypomyelinating neuropathies (CHN); and (4) hereditary neuropathy with pressure palsies (HNPP). Identified genes or specific chromosomal loci are known (summarized in Table 1).

Genetic mutations in demyelinating HMSN

Peripheal myelin protein 22 (HMSN type 1A, hereditary neuropathy with pressure palsies, and Dejerine-Sottas syndrome)

Aberrant interaction between Schwann cells and their axons likely explain clinical progressions with mutation of PMP22. Worsening impairments correlate with severity of electromyograms and nerve conduction abnormality with resultant evolving axonal injury [7]. PMP22 provides 2% to 5% of the total protein content of compact myelin [23]. Its complete function remains unclear, but it may have a role in structural myelin development and neural cell growth and differentiation [24,25].

Diverse phenotypes exist with PMP22 mutations, including, most commonly, HMSN 1A, followed by HNPP, and, rarely, DSS or CHN. All are motor greater than sensory, length-dependent neuropathies with demyelinating nerve conductions. HNPP presents with episodic progressive focal mononeuropathies at sites of compression associated with mild length-dependant neuropathy [26]. CHN and DSS are severe neuropathies that are genetically heterogenous. Abnormalities of developmental milestone in ambulation are the hallmark of the disease. Nerve conduction velocities are often less then 7 m per second with thin myelin surrounded by interposed collagen creating a characteristic onion bulb appearance [27,28].

PMP22 mutations most commonly cause deletions and duplications. The mechanisms leading to duplication mutation explain why the disorder is so common (ie, 60% to 70% of demyelinating forms) [29,30]. Duplications account for HMSN1A phenotype, whereas deletions produce the phenotype of HNPP [31]. Homologous repeat sequences (CMT1A-REP) that flank the region at 17p11.2 are believed to promote misalignment and unequal DNA recombination [32]. Alternate sex-linked mechanisms exist for deletions and duplication at PMP22. Denovo macromutations from paternal origin seem to be duplications alone. Maternal origin mutations, however, produce duplications and deletions. The specific mutation mechanisms at PMP22 during oogenesis include unequal sister chromatid exchange and intrachromatidal loop excision [33]. These sex-dependant mechanisms may in part explain the relative infrequency of HNPP compared with HMSN1A. Ascertainment of the clinical phenotype also may play a role, as HNPP tends to be milder

Table 1
Demyelinating hereditary motor sensory neuropathy

Disease	Locus	Gene	Putative functions	Clinical
Autosomal dominant				
Type 1				
HMSN1A	17p11.2-12	*PMP22*	Myelin structure	Onion bulbs
HMSN1B	1q22-23	*MPZ*	Myelin structure	Onion bulbs
HMSN1C	16p13.1-12.3	*LITAF-SIMPLE*	Possible neuronal apoptosis	Onion bulbs, some with axional phenotypes
HMSN1D	10q21-22	*EGR2*	Transcription regulation	—
HMSN1F	8p21	*NFL*	Myelin stability	—
X-linked dominant				
X1-linked	Xq13.1	*GJB1* (axonal or intermediate conductions)	Myelin gap junctions	±CNS, hearing loss, thenar atrophy, rudimentary onion bulbs
Type 3[a]				
HMSN3A	17p11.2-12	*PMP22*	Myelin structure	Onion bulbs
HMSN3B	1q22-23	*MPZ*	Myelin structure	Onion bulbs
HMSN3C	10q21.1-22.1	*EGR2*	Transcription regulation	Onion bulbs
Autosomal recessive				
Type 4				
HMSN4A	8q13-21.1	*GDAP1*	Neuronal development	±Rare vocal cord paresis
HMSN4B1	11q22	*MTMR2*	Cytoarchitecture	±Focally folded myelin
HMSN4B2	11p15	*SBF2*	Pseudophosphatase	Early-onset glaucoma
HMSN4C	5q32-33	*KIAA1985*	—	±Prominent scoliosis
HMSN4D	8q24.3	*NDRG1*	Transcription regulation	±Deafness
HMSN4E	10q21-22	*EGR2*	Transcription regulation	—
HMSN4F	19q13	*PRX*	Cytoarchitecture	±Prominent sensory, onion bulbs

Abbreviations: KIAA1985, theoretic protein with SH3/TPR domain; *SBF2*, set binding factor 2.

[a] Typically symptomatic onset in infancy, eliminated in some classification schemes when considered severe expression of type 1. *Data from* Michael E, Shy JRL, Phillip F, et al. Hereditary motor and sensory neuropathies: an overview of clinical, genetic, electrophysiologic, and pathologic features. In: Dyck PJ, Thomas PK, editors. Peripheral neuropathy. 4th ed. Philadelphia: Elsevier Saunders; 2005. p. 1623–58.

and, therefore, may not be diagnosed. Rare patients who have frameshift mutations within PMP22 are reported with HNPP phenotype [34,35]. Also rare are missense mutations resulting in the HMSN1A phenotype [36–39]. The existence of autosomal recessive PMP22 point mutation also has been seen [40–42].

PMP22 heterozygous micromutations (typically missense mutations) can produce the severe dysmyelinating phenotype of DSS [43–46]. Factors external to PMP22 may alter clinical expression as identical mutations, even within the same family, with PMP22 duplication producing markedly varied clinical severity [47]. Dosing phenomena are proposed as a possible explanation for the clinical difference between HNPP (deletions) and HMSN1A (duplication) phenotypes. PMP22 mRNA and protein levels are increased in HMSN1A and decreased in HNPP [48,49]. Rare exceptions are noted; for example, patients homozygous for PMP22 duplications are noted for severe and mild phenotypes, suggesting that gene dosing alone is not sufficient to explain clinical variability [50,51].

Despite the understanding of PMP22, treatment remains impractical. Sahenk and colleagues [52] have administered subcutaneous injections of recombinantly generated neurotrophin 3 (NT-3) to promote axonal health and regeneration in the primary Schwann cell disorder, CMT1A. Their work showed pathologic improvements in two different mice models with PMP22 mutation. They then undertook a clinical pilot study in double-blinded placebo-controlled (N = 4 treated, N = 4 placebo) fashion over 28 weeks. Statistical improvements in neuropathy impairments, number of small myelinated fiber regeneration units, and solitary myelinated fibers compared with controls were seen.

Other therapeutic molecular approaches are suggested from animal work, including study of progesterone antagonists and ascorbic acid, whereby rat and mice neuropathies, respectively, have been improved [53,54]. Complex factors are proposed for these benefits, but primary reduction of overexpressed PMP22 remains a potential avenue for targeted therapies.

Myelin protein zero (HMSN type 1B, HMSN type 2, Dejerine-Sottas syndrome, and CH [congenital hypomyelinating])

Mutations of this glycoprotein, *MPZ,* are associated with a great diversity of phenotypes, including (1) most commonly demyelinating nerve conductions (HMSN1B) and axonal forms (HMSN2 I, J) both severe and mild clinically, with (2) Adie's pupil, (3) hemifacial spasm, (4) restless legs, (5) acute onset, (6) hearing loss, and (7) even multiple sclerosis and other CNS manifestations.

MPZ or P-zero (P[0]) is a major structural protein of compact myelin accounting for more than 50% of myelin by weight [55]. It contains one extracellular domain, one transmembrane, and one intracellular domain [56]. It functions as a true myelin adhesion-compacting molecule via homophylic interaction and is expressed only in Schwann cells. Opposed tetramers of P(0) at the membrane surface hold together the intraperiod line, whereas intracellular C-terminals hold by electrostatic interactions the major dense line. MPZ consists of six exons. The extracellar domain has sequence homology with some immunoglobulins [57,58] and antibody directed against P(0) has been observed in chronic inflammatory demyelinating polyneuropathy (CIDP) [59]. Rare patients who have CIDP-like phenotypes are to benefit from immunosuppression [60].

Mutations in the extracelluar domain are noted for extremes of clinical severeity and demyelination and are reviewed elsewhere [61]. More commonly, mutations in the intracellular domain are associated with DSS. DSS phenotypes, however, are associated with all domains. Combinations of these observations have led to speculation that the more deleterious mutations result from a gain of toxic function related to disruption of the P(0) tetramer. Factors external to the loci, however, must influence phenotypic expression.

Consideration of the possibility that inflammatory immune mechanism may influence *MPZ* pathogenesis come from several observations: (1) acute onset cases typical of inflammatory immune mechanism [62,63]; (2) multiple sclerosis, an inflammatory immune disease in two kindreds with MPZ mutation and unusual presentation [63,64]; (3) CIDP-like polyneuropathy responsive to steroids in patients who have MPZ mutations [60]; and (4) heterozygous *Mpz* ± *Mpz*− mice that genetically are unable to generate an immune response develop minimal polyneuropathy compared with immune competent controls [65]. Practical application of this information in care remains distant.

SIMPLE-small integral membrane protein of lysosome or LITAF-Lipopolysaccharide induced tumor necrosis factor alpha or (HMSN1C)

Patients identified as having typical HMSN1 phenotypes may have missense mutations in a gene localizing to 16p13 [66], which was predicted to encode two separate transcripts for lipopolysaccharide-induced tumor necrosis factor α (LITAF) and small integral membrane protein of lysosome (SIMPLE) [67]. Initial reports suggested the defective protein product was the tumor necrosis homolog (ie, LITAF) [67]; however, subsequent work points to the expressed abnormality as SIMPLE [68]. Although SIMPLE protein function is unknown, it may be important in protein degradation given its conserved regions with E3 ubiquitin ligases, which are important proteosome processing proteins. Saifi and collegues [68] suggested mutations in SIMPLE may play a role in demyelinating and axonal phenotypes when a screen of 192 unrelated HMSN cohorts identified base alterations among 16 who had different phenotypes. These changes were not seen in controls and occurred in axonal and demyelinating forms. The tracking of these base alterations with disease phenotypes was not established in most families and, therefore, causative nature remains unclear.

Early growth response 2 (HMSN type 1D, HMSN type 3C, and HMSN type 4E [Dejerine-Sottas syndrome and congenital hypomyelination])

Mutations of EGR2 seem rare and are reported with dominant and recessive inheritance with varied severity and demyelination [69–72]. The protein, EGR2, is a zinc finger transcription factor, which binds DNA, and is encoded by two exons [73]. The pathophysiology probably relates to regulation of peripheral myelin pathways, including PMP22 and MPZ (P[0]). In part, the EGR2 knockout mouse (Krox20) has provided evidence to the pathology, as hypomyelination is noted in the peripheral nervous system of these animals [74,75].

Neurofilament light chain (HMSN type 2E and HMSN type 1F)

This neuron-specific protein, when mutated, has accounted for rare axonal phenotypes [76–78]. One family had saltatory conduction disruption as evidenced by demyelinating nerve conductions [79]. An initially described mutation, Glu528del, in a Bulgarian patient subsequently was found to represent a simple polymorphism in Japanese populations [80]. Expression studies of several mutations leading to this disorder suggest disruption of neurofilament assembly and axonal transport of neurofilaments in cultured mammalian cells and neurons [81]. Neural mitochondrial localization also may be implicated.

GJB1—connexin 32 Charcot-Marie-Tooth X (CMTX1)

The transmembrane protein, connexin 32, is a gap-junction molecule encoded by gene GJB1 and expressed at paranodal regions within the Schmidt-Lanterman incisures of peripheral nerve myelin [82]. In nerve, the protein has two extracelluar loops, one intracellular loop, and two intracellular terminal domains. It seems to form reflexive gap junctions. These pathways probably provide diffusion pathways to transport ions, metabolites, and second messenger molecules through intracellular channels between axons and myelin [83].

Families have an X-linked dominant pattern of inheritance with chromosomal localization to Xq13.2. Males in general tend to be affected more severely, probably the result of gene dosing. Other X-linked forms are described with recessive inheritance and separate localization CMTX2 (Xp22.2) and CMTX3 (Xq26) without gene identification to date [84]. In large kindreds, absence of male-to-male inheritance and disparity in clinical severity between the sexes should raise suspicion as to the diagnosis of CMTX. Affected males may have variably slowed conduction velocities (between HMSN I and II), whereas females may have conduction velocities in the range of HMSN II [85–87]. Other investigators, however, show that the females have intermediate slowing, whereas the men have normal conduction velocities [88]. Still other investigators describe nonuniform slowing when examining multiple nerves [89,90]. Other investigators describe clinical central nervous system (CNS) involvement [91,92]. Using strict electrophysiologic criteria, presenting patients more likely are classified as having an axonal form with mild demyelinating features. Together, the electrophysiology, pathologic description, and animal models [93] suggest that connexin 32 neuropathy is a Schwann cell disorder that leads to axonal loss, with maldevelopment and loss of myelin.

Genetic analysis for connexin 32 mutations has allowed for several important observations. This disorder is not rare and probably accounts for the second most common form of HMSN after HMSN1A [94]. Point mutations are the most common mutation by far, and more than 150 different mutations have been identified in more than 200 unrelated families [95]. These data have provided for speculation about genotype-phenotype correlations. Nonsense mutations (frameshift mutations) tend to produce more severe phenotypes with earlier presentation compared with missense mutations [86,88,94]. Exceptions are noted, however, including the most dramatic case in two male siblings who had complete deletion of the connexin 32 coding sequence [96]. These brothers were affected no more severely than others who have typical missense mutation. Such observations suggest that factors external to the loci influence clinical expression and confuse whether or not connexin mutations exert their affect by a primary loss of function or by a dominant negative affect [97]. Extensive ongoing work is attempting to answer such difficult questions [83].

Ganglioside-induced differentiation-associated protein 1 (HMSN type 4A and HMSN type 2K)

The GDAP1 gene is expressed in brain and spinal cord more than in peripheral nerve [98]. The function of GDAP1 is unknown, but it may be involved in signal transduction pathways in neuronal development. This may suggest primary pathogenesis and the cell bodies. Patients who have this disorder typically accrue deficits in the first decade of life and, as with many recessive disorders, consangunity often is present with varied expression, including peroneal atrophy with or without (1) hand weakness, (2) vocal cord paresis, and (3) optic atrophy [98–102]. Axonal features can be seen rarely in patients, but demyelination is foremost [103].

Myotubularin-related protein 2 (HMSN type 4B1)

By inference from other myotubularin proteins, this protein, myotubularin-related protein 2 (MTMR2), may be important in regulation of RNA transcription in nerve. Specific mutations are noted for reduced phosphatase active in nerve [104]. Patients meet infantile developmental milestones but typically, by 2 years of age, are clinically affected and are wheelchair bound by young adulthood with proximal weakness and abnormal auditory evoked potentials. Death may occur in the fourth to fifth decade from presumed respiratory failure proportionate to the severity of the neuropathy [105,106].

N-myc downstream-regulated gene 1 (HMSN type 4D)

This gene, N-myc downstream-regulated gene 1 (NDRG1), is expressed ubiquitously in nerve with particularly high levels of RNA transcripts in Schwann cells. It has been proposed to function in growth arrest and differentiation of myelinated fibers and perhaps Schwann cell signaling essential in axonal survival [107]. Mutations within this gene have resulted in severe neuropathy inherited in autosomal recessive fashion. Intially, a single mutation producing a premature stop codon at position 148 was believed causative of a founder affect in divergent Romani (Gypsy) groups across Europe [107,108]. Subsequently, different mutations were identified [109]. Clinically, patients have early-onset neuropathy, muscle weakness, and wasting with skeletal and foot deformities, panmodality sensory loss, and marked conduction velocity slowing with axonal degenerations. Patients have neural deafness in the second or third decade of life with conduction slowing in central pathways.

PRX—L-periaxin (HMSN type 4F)

The periaxin protein seems important in myelin development and its localization changes from fetal to adult age. The gene is spliced alternatively to encode L- and S-periaxin and is essential for maintenance of peripheral nerve myelin [110–112]. At the molecular level, L-periaxin associates with DRP2 and dystroglycan at the basal lamina or extracellular membrane and is important for the correct localization of the DRP2-dystroglycan complex in sciatic nerve. In the Schwann cells of embryos, it is found only in the nucleus, but perinatally it localizes to adaxonal or periaxonal space. In contrast, adults show localization away from the axon on the surface of extracellular myelin. Nerve biopsies from patients who have HMSN4F demonstrate paranodal abnormalities characterized by disruption of paranodal loops and separation of myelin stuctures from periaxonal structures. Autosomal recessive point mutations of PRX are demonstrated as causative for severe demyelinating neuropathies characteristic of the dominately inherited Dejerine-Sottas form [112–116].

HMSN axonal forms (HMSN type II and others)

As in the primary demyelinating neuropathies, clinical spectrum and genetic abnormalities are diverse. Because indolent axonal disease may not be determined as easily with electrophysiology, many inherited forms go without gene localization. The varied clinical and pathologic discoveries in this form include (1) the diverse group of HMSN II, (2) rare individuals who have HMSN IV (3) HMSN X, (4) and others, including HMSN V, VI, and VII as ascertained by nerve conduction abnormalities (Table 2).

Kinesin family member 1β (HMSN type 2A)

The kinesin superfamily motor protein isoform, KIF1Bβ, is important in transporting synaptic vesicle precursors. Mutations result in a loss of

Table 2
Axonal and intermediate hereditary motor sensory neuropathy

Disease	Locus	Gene	Putative functions	Clinical
Autosomal dominant (HMSN2 and CMT2)				
A	1p35-36	*KIF1B*	Axonal transport	One Japanese family
A	1p35-36	*MFN2*	Mitochondrial fusion	Multiple different families some with optic atrophy spasticity (ie, HMSN VI)
B	3q13-22	*RAB7*	Axonal transport	±Foot ulcers
C	12q23-24	—	—	±Diaphragm vocal paresis, several with infant onset
D	7p14	*GARS*	tRNA synthetase	Allelic to dSMAV
2E & 1F	8p21	*NFL*	Neurofilament organization	±Hyperkeratosis
F	7q11-21	*HSP27*	Axonal cytoskeleton transport	Young adults
G	12q12	—	—	Allelic to HMSN1B
I & J	1q22	*MPZ*	Myelin structural protein	J = pupillary involvement ± deafness
L	12q24	*HSPB8*	Heat shock protein	Proximal and distal involvement, some
P	3q13.1	—	—	P = proximal involvement, elevated creatine kinase
Autosomal dominant (HMSN DI [intermediate slowed conductions])				
A	10q24	—	—	—
B	19p32	DNM2	Membrane protein	±Neutropenia, primary axonal or demyelinating unclear
C	1p35	YARS	tRNA transferase	Primary axonal or demyelinating unclear
Autosomal recessive and X-linked (HMSN2 and CMT 2)				
G & K	8q21	*GDAP1*	Neuronal development	±Vocal cord involvement
H	8q21	—	—	Pyramidal features
X1-linked	Xq13.1	GJB1 (axonal and demyelinating conductions)	Myelin gap junctions	±CNS, hearing loss, thenar atrophy
X2-linked	Xp22.2	—	—	Infantile onset, ±mental retardation
X3-linked	Xq26	—	—	±Spasticity
2B2		Lamin A/C	Nuclear envelope	Algerian family

Abbreviation: MFN2, mitofusin GTPase.

microtuble binding and altered transport along the axon. A single family is demonstrated with such mutation [117]. Mice with inactivation of KIF1β also have an axonal neuropathy. Other genes also may disrupt axonal transport and, therefore, cause axonal predominant neuropathies, namely *NFL* (see previous discussion) and likely gigaxonin [118]. The latter is associated with a rare autosomal recessive neuropathy not classified as HMSN with characteristic axonal swellings and CNS (mental retardation) and hair (kinky hair) abnormalities. Disorganization of intermediate filaments is noted in this condition, termed giant axonal neuropathy, and gigaxonin localizes to the cytoskeletal.

Mitofusin 2 (HMSN type 2A2 and HMSN type VI)

Some families who have chromosomal localization to 1p36 do not have mutation in KIF1B. Recently, they have been found to have mutation in the gene mitofusin 2 *(MFN2)* localizing to 1p36 [119–121]. Some individuals also have optic atrophy and spastic paraparesis, designated HMSN VI [122,123]. This nuclear-encoded mitochondrial GTPase gene seems to account for most affected individuals who have abnormality colocalizing to 1p36. The gene seems important in the fusion of mitochondrial membranes. Of particular note is the lost ability of mitochondria with mutation in MFN2 to transport along actin or microtubule filaments. This likely is relevant in neuropathy whereby axonal transport is predicted to be defective and, therefore, a plausible specific pathogenesis in distal axonal neuroapthies. The extent of DNA polymorphisms still is being ascertained as are genotype-phenotype correlations. Careful correlation within families is emphasized to better understand expression and varied presentation versus polymorphisms. At the same time, penetrance and extent of variable clinical expression are important to study within and between different families.

RAB7 (HMSN type 2B or HSAN type I)

The extent of sensory involvement in patients affected by mutations of this gene can be so severe as to qualify as a dominant form of HSAN (discussed later). The mutilating foot injuries are accompanied by significant ankle dorsi flexor weakness. The gene seems important in axonal vesicular transport. The protein localizes to endosomes and is important in retrograde tubular extensions. Active RAB7 on phagosomal membranes associates with the effector protein, RAB7-interacting lysosomal protein (RILP), which in turn bridges phagosomes with dynein-dynactin, a microtubule-associated motor complex [124,125]. Activation of RAB7 is important to allow recruitment of RILP and consequent association of phagosomes with microtubule-associated motors [126]. It is predicted, therefore, that mutations of RAB7 ultimately affect axonal transport. Disruption of other specific microtubule motor complex proteins in nerve disease is known. For example, mutations of dynactin are believed to be causative of a motor neuron disease described in one family who had associated vocal cord paralysis and facial and hand predominant weakness [127]. Patients are described who do not have sensory symptoms, but detailed sensory testing is not reported. The described mutation is predicted to distort the folding of dynactins microtubule-binding domain and, thereby, interfere with retrograde axonal transport. Because mutations of this gene are associated with infectious ulcerations of the feet and neuropathy, it is an intriguing possibility that in addition to disruption of axonal transport it has potential defect in the innate immune system through disruption of phagocytosis. Foot insensitivity alone may not be adequate to explain acromutilations with infectious ulceration.

Glycyl tRNA synthetase (HMSN type 2D and dSMAV type V)

Patients who have mutations in this gene, glycyl tRNA synthetase (GARS), may or may not have sensory involvement. Those who do not have sensory loss are labeled as having distal spinal muscular atrophy type V (dSMAV) whereas those who have sensory loss are labeled as having HMSN2D.

The gene is expressed ubiquitously in neural and non-neural tissues and functions in attachment of tRNAs with appropriate glycyl amino acid. Earlier work in myositis suggested its potential role in pathogenesis of that muscle disease. Specifically, antibodies directed against this tRNA are identified in dermatomyositis [128]. The work provided emphasis of the potential role of GARS as an autoantigen. Why mutations in this gene lead to selective neuropathy or motor neuronopathy remains unclear [129–132].

Heat shock protein 27 (HMSN type 2F)

The initially described mutation S135F occurs in a conserved α-crystallin domain of the protein, heat shock protein 27 (HSP27) [133]. In vitro expression of this mutant resulted in poor viability of neuronal cells and impaired neurofilament assembly. Other families from Asia [134], among the Han Chinese, are identified with possible founder mutation [135].

Heat shock protein 22 (HMSN type 2L and dHMNII)

HSP22 chromosomally localizes to 12q24 [136], a region of many neuromuscular diseases [137]. Motor axonal symptoms are predominant with distal involvements hallmarked. Because motor symptoms are prominent, some classify this condition as distal hereditary motor neuropathy (dHMNII). The occurrence of variable sensory involvement in distal motor predominant processes is described previously and includes the genes GARS, RAB7, and HMSN2C localized to 12q23-24 [137].

Dynamin 2 (HMSN DI type B)

Dynamin 2, a ubiquitously expressed protein, seems important in membrane vesicle formation in clatherin-coated membranes. Mutations of this gene may lead to a variety of phenotypes, including centronuclear myopathy [138], and neutropenia with intermediate conduction slowing [139].

Tyrosyl-RNA transferase (HMSN DI type C)

A tRNA transferase for tyrosine, this protein, tyrosyl-RNA transferase (YARS), is expressed in spinal cord and brain. It is reported rarely in families and individuals who have a neuropathy with dominant inheritance. Unlike GARS (discussed previously), motor neuronopathy is not described but, rather, motor and sensory involvement [140].

Lamin A/C—axonal autosomal recessive neuropathy (HMSN type 2B1)

Inherited as an axonal form, lamin A/C has autosomal recessive inheritance. Lamin A/C is a nuclear envelope protein. As a group, the lamins are a large constituent of the nuclear lamina within the nuclear membrane. Their function is believed related directly to the proper handling of DNA chromatin with functions of replicational organization in addition to stabilizing the nucleus and its envelope protein [141]. Mutations of this gene have led to a variety of clinical phenotypes, including, rarely, an autosomal recessive axonal neuropathy among Algerian families [142]. The other clinical phenotypes include (1) skeletal muscle (Emery-Dreifuss muscular dystrophy [dominant or recessive] [143,144] and limb-girdle muscular dystrophy, autosomal dominant [LGMD1B] [145]); (2) cardiac conduction defects and cardiomyopathy (Emery-Dreifuss muscular dystrophy [143], LGMD1B, and dilated cardiomyopathy (CMD1A) [146]; (3) bone (mandibuloacral dysplasia) [147]; and (4) fat (partial lipodystrophy) [148].

HSAN

Like HMSN, this group (HSAN) is heterogenous (Table 3). The distinguishing features between different types of HSAN relate to age of onset, mode of inheritance, fiber type involvement and, increasingly, the molecular biologic cause. The clinical distinction between various forms often is possible only with specialized testing, including autonomic testing that looks at postganglionic small nerve fiber function and nerve pathology, with nerve morphometrics defining the specific sensory fiber involvements. It is important to understand that motor function need not be spared but is not the primary cause of disabilities; rather, sensory loss is foremost. Each condition should, however, include the following features: (1) having a genetic basis; (2) selective or predominant involvement of primary sensory with or without autonomic neurons (axons); and (3) small-diameter sensory and sudomotor function that often is impaired, affecting acral (distal limb) tissue injury.

Table 3
Hereditary sensory and autonomic neuropathy

			Neurons (axons)						
Disease	Onset	I	Aα	Aδ	C	Sudomotor	Locus	Gene	Putative functions
Type 1[a]	2+ decade	AD	+	++	++	LS+	9q22	*SPTLC1*	Ceramide regulation, apoptosis
							3q13	*RAB7*	Apoptosis
Type 2	C	AR	++	++	+	G	12p13	*HSN2*	—
Type 3[b]	C	AR	++	++	++	G	9q31	*IKBKAP*	—
Type 4	C	AR	N	±	++	G	1q21	*TrkA*	Nerve growth factor receptor
Type 5	C	AR	N	++	±	N	1q21	*TrkA*[c]	
							1p13	*NGFβ*	Nerve growth factor

Abbreviations: AD, autosomal dominant; AR, autosomal recessive; C, congenital; G, generalized; *HSN2*, putative protein; I, inheritance; LS+, lumbosacral plus; N, normal; *NGFβ*, nerve growth factor β; +, affected; ++, severely affected; ±, may be affected.

[a] Many autosomal dominant forms without known genetic cause.

[b] Typically Ashkenazi Jews.

[c] A single patient reported.

Gene defects in HSAN

SPTLC1 (HSAN1)

Within this specific genetic group, a great deal has been learned. Dominantly inherited symptoms typically begin in the second, third, or later decades of life. Plantar ulcers are common. Some kinships have severe lancinating pains of the feet and legs, whereas others have only loss of sensation, often with painless foot injuries. Peroneal atrophy with ankle dorsiflexion weakness is typical, with sensory loss major in disability. Families who have burning feet alone without sensory deficits likely represent a distinct entity and in at least one family linkage has been excluded to 9q22.1 [149], where the identified gene, serine palmitoyltransferase long-chain 1 (SPTLC1), resides [150,151]. SPTLC1 is believed to be the rate-limiting enzyme in the synthesis of sphingolipids, including ceramide and sphingomyelin [152,153]. Ceramide is important in regulation of programmed cell death in several tissue types, including differentiating neuronal cells [154].

HSN2 gene and theoretic protein (HS2 and HSN2)

The *HSN2* gene is unique by residing within another gene's (*PRKWNK*) intron. Mutations of *PRKWNK* cause autosomal dominant pseudohypoaldosteronism type II (PHAII), characterized by severe hypertension, hyperkalemia, and sensitivity to thiazide diuretics, which may result from a chloride shunt in the renal distal nephron [155]. The HSAN2 and PHAII phenotypes are discordant as are the mutations of either gene.

The five Canadian kindreds initially identified as having mutations in the *HSN2* gene [156] all originated from Newfoundland families and carried identical homozygous mutation, 594delA, causing a frameshift and truncation of the protein from 434 amino acids to 206 amino acids. A homozygous insertional mutation at 918-919insA, found in a Nova Scotian family, led to a truncation of the protein to 318 amino acids. The French Canadian kindreds had this conserved mutation but in heterozygote state and with an additional homozygous 943C to T nonsense mutation. Such mutations were not found in a large cohort of appropriate normals. Discordant mutations in the HSN2 gene have been identified in Japanese and Lebanese patients [157,158]. Despite convincing studies, Northern blot assays looking for the predicted *HSN2* transcript in multiple human tissues and more sensitive reverse transcription assays using polymerase chain reaction in various tissues, including dorsal root ganglion, fail to identify the predicted product conclusively. Further work is needed in expression studies of this predicted protein. It is likely, however, that the difficulties in isolation relate to the selective expression in nerve at low levels. A signaling peptide sequence is predicted from the known sequence of *HSN2*, and the investigators have speculated about the *HSN2* protein product as potentially important in nerve growth [156].

Inhibitor kappa light polypeptide gene enhancer in B-cells, kinase complex-associated protein (HSAN type 3, familial dysautonomia, and Riley-Day syndrome)

HSAN3 complex disorder has prominent autonomic involvement with (1) autosomal recessive inheritance; (2) congenital or infantile onset; (3) predominance in Ashkenazi Jews; (4) peripheral sensory (all classes), autonomic neurons (axons), lesser involvement of motor neurons (axons), and possibly other CNS neurons; (5) history of poor sucking, repeated episodes of fever; (6) blotchy skin; and (7) absence of fungiform papillae of the tongue [159,160]. Mutations in the inhibitor kappa light polypeptide gene enhancer in B-cells, kinase complex-associated protein (IKBKAP) gene, located at 9q31, cause HSAN3. Two mutations are identified and both disrupt phosphorylation (IKBKAP, IVS20DS, T-C, + 6; ARG696-PRO) [161]. Why such defects lead to a dysautonomia and sensory neuropathy is unknown. Genetic testing for the two mutations may allow for ease of carrier and affected assessment in the Ashkenazi Jew population, where a strong founder effect likely accounts for limited responsible mutation.

Tyrosine receptor kinase A (HSAN type IV)

This disorder includes (1) autosomal recessive inheritance; (2) congenital or infantile onset; (3) repeated high fevers, which may cause death; (4) decreased pain sensation and absence of sweating; (5) mental retardation in some patients; and (6) virtual absence of unmyelinated fibers in sural nerve. Rare patients who have HSAN V are described with (1) probable autosomal recessive inheritance, (2) congenital or infant onset, (3) selective loss of small myelinated fibers and normal unmyelinated fibers, and (4) normal motor sensory and sudomotor examinations [162].

Mutations in the neurotrophin receptor, TrkA, are causative of this disorder. Central and peripheral nerve tissues rely on neurotrophins and their receptors for proper formation. The gene, TrkA, is believed important for inducing neurite outgrowth and promotion of embryonic sensory and sympathetic neurons. Multiple mutations, including deletion, splice-site mutations, and missense mutations—all in the tryosine kinase domain of TrkA, are found causative [163,164].

Spinocerebellar ataxias with neuropathy

These system atrophies affect the spinocerebellar tracts and are inherited as autosomal dominant and recessive disorders. Currently, there are more than 20 dominant syndromes described and fewer known recessive forms. Peripheral nerve studies among spinocerebellar ataxias are limited, and primary axonal pathology is believed to predominate. Patients have progressive central ataxia with spinocerebellar degeneration and varied degrees of cognitive, ocular, autonomic, and hyperkinetic dysfunction. The most common disorder is inherited as autosomal recessive spinocerebellar ataxias (ie, Friedreich's ataxia, the most common spinocerebellar syndrome). Other recessive forms include spinocerebellar atrophy with peripheral axonal degeneration (SCAN1), vitamin E deficiency (resulting from α-tocopherol transfer protein deficiency or abetalipoproteinemia), ataxia telangiectasia, infantile-onset spinocerebellar ataxia, Marinesco-Sjögren syndrome, spastic ataxia of Charlevoix-Saguenay, Refsum disease, carbohydrate-deficiency ataxia, and Cayman Island ataxia, among others [165].

Friedreich's ataxia is caused by expansion of a GAA triplet repeat located within the first intron of the frataxin gene [166]. The gene is believed to be a - nuclear origin mitochondrial protein that plays a role in iron homeostasis. With deficiency of the gene product, there is an accumulation of iron in the mitochondria, poor mitochondrial enzymes function, enhanced sensitivity to oxidative stress, and eventually free radical–mediated cell death.

Hereditary spastic paraplegias with neuropathy

As with the spinocerebellar syndromes, the lower motor neuron involvement for these primary central spastic disorders typically is not clinically primary in deficit and, therefore, is not as well studied as desired. Of the more than 10 autosomal dominant genetically characterized spastic paraplegias, several are noted for variable extremity weakness and atrophy (SPGSPG9-10q23.3-q24.2, SPG17-11q12-q14, and SPG10-12q13). The conduction velocities of nerves typically are normal in the upper extremities, and in the lower extremity, normal or low normal, with reduction in CMAP amplitudes. On needle examination, fibrillations and fasciculations often are seen distally with increased size of motor unit potentials. Detailed descriptions of the electrophysiology and nerve biopsy reports are lacking in these and other forms, including SPG3A, where specific genetic cause is known [167].

There are no fewer than seven autosomal recessive forms of spastic paraplegia with identified chromosomal location and four are noted with either distal amyotrophy or neuropathy. Specific genes are identified in SPG7-16q-*paraplegian* and SPG20-13q-*spartin* (Table 4) [168].

Miscellaneous hereditary neuropathies

Historical classifications of some forms of HMSN are discussed later. Among those in which spastic paraplegias are predominant, characterization as "complicated" hereditary spastic paraplegias may be more appropriate. There also exists a group of disorders in which motor features are so prominent that motor neuronopathy is most appropriate, and specific genetic causes are found in some. When distal weakness is predominant, they may be referred to as dHMNII (Table 5).

Table 4
Hereditary spastic paraplegias with neuropathy

Disease	Locus	Gene	Functions	Clinical
Autosomal dominant				
SPG9	10q23	—	—	Motor neuronopathy, cataracts, GERD
SPG10	12q13	*KIF5A*	Axonal transport	±Distal atrophy
SPG17	11q12	—	—	Hand atrophy (Silver's syndrome)
Autosomal recessive				
SPG7	16q	*Paraplegin*	Mitochondrial function	±Neuropathy, dysarthria, dysphagia, optic disc pallor
SPG11	15q	—	—	Corpus callosum atrophy, mental retardation, extremity weakness, nystagmus
SPG15	14q	—		Motor neuronopathy, pigmented macula, mental retardation, dysarthria
SPG20	13q	*Spartin*	Microtubule formation	Distal wasting (Troyer syndrome)
X-linked				
SPG2	Xq21	*PLP*	Intrinsic myelin structure	±Varied CNS white matter disease, neuropathy
SPG16	Xq11	—		±Motor aphasia, mental retardation, gastrointestinal

Abbreviation: PLP, proteolipid protein.

Hereditary brachial plexus neuropathy

Attacks of brachial plexus neuropathy associated with inflammation [169] have undergone recent gene discovery. Specifically, Kuhlenbaumer and colleagues [170] reported, in six European families, mutation in a septin-like molecule SEPT9 at chromosome position 17q25. Mutations were not seen in four American kindreds with shared haplotypes but in two separate American families of European descent. Of 12 American kindreds, I identified only one that carries mutation within the gene at R88W, also of European descent without conserved haplotype. The described mutations in this gene were not identified in 56 cases of sporadic brachial plexus neuropathy (Parsonage-Turner syndrome) [171]. The gene is one of several GTP-binding scaffold proteins and is implicated in membrane dynamics, vesicle trafficking, apoptosis, and cytoskeletal remodeling.

Multisystem inherited neuropathies, "metabolic"

These inherited neuropathies have neural and non-neural tissues involvement (Table 6) [172]. Diverse presenting symptoms and signs exist. As

Table 5
Miscellaneous hereditary neuropathies: hereditary motor sensory neuropathy and others

Disease	Locus	Gene	Putative functions	Clinical
HMSN type 5 (Autosomal dominant)				
HMSN 5	—	—	—	Spastic paraplegia plus (see Table 4)
HMSN type 6 (autosomal recessive)				
HMSN 6	—	- *MFN2*	-Mitochondrial fusion	Optic atrophy
HMSN type 7 (unclear)				
HMSN 7	—	—	—	Retinitis pigmentosa
HNPP (autosomal dominant)				
HNPP	17p11.2-12	*PMP22*	Myelin function	Tomaculous neuropathy
Distal HMN				
Type 2 (AD)	12q24	*HSP22*	Axonal transport	? Allelic to scapuloperoneal amyotrophy and HMSN2C
Type 5 (AD)	7p15	—	—	Prominent hand, lower extremity spasticity
Jerash type (AR)	9p21	—	—	Pyramidal signs, childhood
SMARD1 (AR)	11q13	*IGHMBP2*	Not clear	Diaphragm; infantile death
Dynactin	2p13	*Dynactin*	Axonal transport	Vocal cord and face paralysis
Hereditary brachial plexus neuropathy				
HBPN	17q25	*SEPT9*	Possible cytoskeletal function	Attacks of brachial plexopathy

Abbreviation: IGHMBP2, immunoglobulin mu-binding protein 2.

a group, these diseases are rare when neurofibromatosis type 1 is excluded. Neurofibromatosis type 1 rivals in frequency the HMSNs (approximately 1 in 2000 affected). Specific pathologic features on nerve biopsies are common, but metabolic or genetic testing may preclude the need for nerve or other tissue biopsies. Because treatments are available in some, their recognition becomes important. Detailed description of these disorders is beyond the scope of this review and is reviewed elsewhere (see Table 6).

Current genetic testing considerations

Ethical and practical issues have arisen with the availability of the new genetic testing [173]. Previously, identification of affected and unaffected persons was limited to neurologic examination and electrophysiologic testing of the kinship [4]. It is now more complex: multiple genetic tests are available, testing is costly, and results frequently have low sensitivity and often are of uncertain significance. These issues make it difficult to decide who and which genes should be tested. If a test is ordered, the physician needs to be in a position to provide proper interpretation and counsel to a patient. The pretest discussion needs to include (1) comment of the variable clinical severity or expression of the disease; (2) future potential for work; (3) insurance issues; (4) risk for emotional upset; and (5) specific implications for family planning. Sometimes, other unforeseen complications occur as a result of testing, such as a chance discovery of an individual's illegitimate or adopted status. Because preventative or reversible treatments for gene abnormalities are not readily available, the decision to undergo genetic testing must be made carefully. For the rare disorders in which medical interventions are available, testing of asymptomatic family members seems reasonable. For the other inherited disorders, asymptomatic people probably should not be tested. In contrast, clinically affected individuals suspected of having a defined variety of inherited neuropathy should be tested, because testing can confirm a diagnosis and provide for improved counsel. By taking a detailed family history and telephoning or examining relatives, the need for genetic testing may be diminished [4].

Knowing the sensitivity and specificity of each genetic test is important. Among many of the axonal forms of hereditary motor and sensory neuropathies, the sensitivity of available genetic testing may be low compared with their demyelinating counterparts. A recent report, however, suggests the benefit of genetic testing in individuals who have axonal phenotypes and who do not have family history [174]. Specifically, from 153 stored and unrelated neuropathy DNA samples, Boerkoel and colleagues performed aggressive testing of multiple known causative genes of CMT and found 100 individuals who had an identified mutation. One third of those identified as having the mutation were reported to have de novo "sporadic" mutation and many had axonal phenotypes. Their experience suggests the usefulness of genetic testing beyond our own Mayo peripheral nerve group experience. An algorithm approach considering clinical phenotype with electrophysiology is helpful (see Fig. 1).

To avoid erroneous results, choose accredited facilities for testing [1]. In these laboratories, false-positive results can occur and generally are the result of chance discovery of polymorphisms. Polymorphisms represent normal DNA sequences occurring at different frequencies in different populations or races. These polymorphic base pair changes may or may not change amino acid. When the base pair change does not alter amino acid sequences, the results should be viewed skeptically. Rare mutations not predicted to change the protein might do so by producing alternative splicing. Such mutations occur at exon-intron boundaries. With indeterminate results, tracking base change with affected status is emphasized. Kindred studies, transcription assays, transcription expression, and functional assays typically are research based, however, and referral to tertiary care centers is emphasized. If the DNA sequence is ambiguous, studying the protein can be helpful. Protein assays typically are available commercially only for disorders characterized as inborn errors of metabolism.

Practical council in inherited neuropathies

Practice-based gene replacement, gene product manipulation, or other molecular therapies currently are not available for most inherited neuropathies. Nevertheless, physicians can make meaningful treatment interventions. The mainstay of those interventions is supportive with special attention to:

1. Genetic counseling, including discussion of inheritance pattern and potential for predicted specific impairments depending on disease, relevant to vocational council and risk injury assessment
2. Care of acral appendage, especially in the varieties of HSAN in which mutilating injuries are preventable
3. Proper bracing and supportive devices where appropriate
4. Emphasis on routine health maintenance, including weight control, screening for early diabetes, thyroid disease, and alcoholism, all of which may make impairments worse
5. Council of increased risk for worsened neuropathy with certain chemotherapeutic agents, including platinum-based agents, vinca alkaloids, and, likely, paclitaxel, thalidomide, and bortezomib products
6. Reassurance that these disorders often are compatible with normal life expectancy and life enjoyment

Future molecular directions

The increasing appreciation of complex factors in disease modification will emphasize further the need for clinical phenotypic and expression

Table 6
Hereditary multisystem disorders with neuropathy (partial list)

Disease	Inheritance	Locus	Gene	Clinical	Possible treatments
Familial amyloid					
Transthyretin amyloidosis	AD	18q11	*Transthyretin*	Varied presentation	Liver transplant
Apo A-1	AD	11q23	*Apo A-1*	Prominent nephrosis	—
Gelsolin	AD	9q34	*Gelsolin*	Facial paresis, corneal lattice dystrophy	—
Leukodystrophy					
Metachromatic	AR	22q13	*Arylsulfatase*	Schwann cells with metachromatic granules	Bone marrow transplant
Krabbe	AR	14q31	*GALC*	Prismatic inclusions in endoneurial macrophages	Bone marrow transplant
Adrenoleukodystrophy	XR		*ABCD1*		Bone marrow transplant, Lorenzo's oil
Peroxisomal					
Refsum disease	AR	10p	*PAHX*	Varied onion bulbs	Low phytol-low phytanic acid diet
Fabry	XR	Xq22	*α-Galactosidase*	Varied osmophilic granules	α-Glactosidase A
Lipoprotein deficiency					
Tangiers	XR	9q22	*ABC1*	Myelin droplets	—
Cerebrotendinous Xanthomatosis	AR	2q33	*CYP27A1*	Minor Schwann cell lipids	Chenodeoxycholic acid
Abetalipoproteinemia					Vitamins E, A, and K

Porphyrias					
Acute intermittent	AD	11q	*Porphobilinogen deaminase*	Axonal greater than demyelinating	Avoidance of precipitant factors
Defective DNA maintenance					
Xeroderma pigmentosa	AR	3p25	*XPC*	Axonal degeneration	Avoidance of sun
Ataxia telangiectasia	AR	11q22	*ATM*	Sensory greater than motor	Early cancer screening
Mitochondrial (Mt) defects					
Kearns-Sayre	Varied	Mt	Varied mutations	Demyelinating radiculopathy	Possible superoxide scavengers
Miscellaneous					
Giant axonal neuropathy	AR	16q24	*Gigaxonin*	Giant axonal swellings, kinky hair	—
Neurofibromatosis type 1	AD	17q11	*NF1*	Nerve tumors	Symptomatic tumor resection
Neurofibromatosis type 2		22q12	*Merlin*	Acoustic schwannomas	Symptomatic tumor resection

Abbreviations: ABCD1, ATP-binding cassette-subfamily D1; AD, autosomal dominant; AR, autosomal recessive; *ATM*, ataxia telangiectasia mutated; *CYP27A1*, sterol 27-hydroxylase; *GALC*, galactosylceramidase; *PAHX*, phytanoyl-CoA hydroxylase; *XPC*, xeroderma pigmentosa complementation group C; XR, X-linked recessive.

characterization. Understanding of nerve molecular architecture and function is predicted to improve and lead to more specific targeted approaches in diagnosis and treatment. Current DNA testing platforms for inherited neuropathies remain expensive, insensitive for many, and largely are limited to neuropathies with mendelian patterns of inheritance. Using mass spectrometry in the rapid identification of mutations leading to alteration of protein structure holds promise for some disorders in which the protein abnormality is expressed within blood [175]. Identification of complex susceptibility factors and modifiers of genetically defined neuropathies are predicted in the current "proteomic era." These discoveries will have implications for inherited and acquired neuropathies.

Using the tools that have allowed for understanding and diagnosis of neuropathy, specific drug developments are possible. Specifically, implementation of computer software and protein modelling programs already allow for the development of small molecules that may facilitate treatment of toxic gain or loss of function diseases, including denervating neuromuscular junction diseases and other degenerative neurologic disorders [176–178].

References

[1] New GENE TESTS. Available at: http://www.geneclinics.org/. Accessed Winter 2006.
[2] New OMIM. Available at: http://www.ncbi.nlm.nih.gov/. Accessed Winter 2006.
[3] New IPNMDB. Available at: http://www.molgen.ua.ac.be/cmt/. Accessed Winter 2006.
[4] Dyck PJ, Oviatt KF, Lambert EH. Intensive evaluation of referred unclassified neuropathies yields improved diagnosis. Ann Neurol 1981;10:222–6.
[5] Kleopa KA, Scherer SS. Inherited neuropathies. Neurol Clin 2002;20:679–709.
[6] Scherer SS. Finding the causes of inherited neuropathies. Arch Neurol 2006;63:812–6.
[7] Michael E, Shy JRL, Phillip F, et al. Hereditary motor and sensory neuropathies: an overview of clinical, genetic, electrophysiologic, and pathologic features. In: Dyck PJ, Thomas PK, editors. Peripheral neuropathy. 4th ed. Philadelphia: Elsevier Saunders; 2005. p. 1623–58.
[8] Klein CJ, Dyck PJ. HMSNII (CMT2) and miscellaneous inherited system atrophies of nerve axon: clinical-molectular correlates. In: Dyck PJ, Thomas PK, editors. Peripheral neuropathy. 4th ed. Philadelphia: Elsevier Saunders; 2005. p. 1717–51.
[9] Dyck PJ, et al. Histologic and lipid studies of sural nerves in inherited hypertrophic neuropathy: preliminary report of a lipid abnormality in nerve and liver in Dejerine-Sottas disease. Mayo Clin Proc 1970;45:286–327.
[10] Dyck PJ, Karnes JL, Lambert EH. Longitudinal study of neuropathic deficits and nerve conduction abnormalities in hereditary motor and sensory neuropathy type 1. Neurology 1989;39:1302–8.
[11] Collins MPK. Neuropathies with systemic vasculitis. In: Dyck PJ, Thomas, PK, editors. Peripheral neuropathy. 4th ed. Philadelphia: Elsevier Saunders; 2005. p. 2335–404.
[12] Dyck PJE J, Dyck PJ. Microvasculitis. In: Dyck PJ, Thomas PK, editors. Peripheral neuropathy. Philadelphia: Elsevier Saunders; 2005. p. 2405–14.
[13] Susuki K, et al. Acute motor axonal neuropathy rabbit model: immune attack on nerve root axons. Ann Neurol 2003;54:383–8.
[14] Griffin JW, et al. Guillain-Barre syndrome in Northern China. The spectrum of neuropathological changes in clinical defined cases. Brain 1995;118:577–95.

[15] McKhann GM, et al. Acute motor axonal neuropathy: a frequent cause of acute flaccid paralysis in China. Ann Neurol 1993;33:333–42.
[16] Umapathi T, Chaudhry V. Toxic neuropathy. Curr Opin Neurol 2005;18:574–80.
[17] Virchow E. Ein Fall von progressiven Muskelatrophie. Arch Pathol Anat 1855;8:537.
[18] Eichorst U. Ueber Heredtat de Progresiven Muskelatrophie. Berl Klin Wochenschr 1873; 10(497).
[19] Charcot JM. P, Sur une forme particuliere d'atrophie musculaire progressive souvent familial debutant par les pieds et les jambes et atteignant plus tard les mains. Rev Med (Paris) 1886;6:97.
[20] Tooth H. The peroneal type of progressive muscular atrophy. London: Lewis; 1886.
[21] Davidenkow S. Uber die neurotische Muskelatrophie Charcot Marie: Klinisch-genetische Studien. Z Neurol 1927;107:259.
[22] Dyck PJ, Lambert EH. Lower motor and primary sensory neuron diseases with peroneal muscular atrophy. II. Neurologic, genetic, and electrophysiologic findings in various neuronal degenerations. Arch Neurol 1968;18:619–25.
[23] D'Urso D, Muller HW. Ins and outs of peripheral myelin protein-22: mapping transmembrane topology and intracellular sorting. J Neurosci Res 1997;49:551–62.
[24] Naef RS. U, Many facets of the peripheral myelin protein PMP22 in myelination and disease. Microscop Res Techniques 1998;41:359–71.
[25] Hanemann CO, Muller HW. Pathogenesis of Charcot-Marie-Tooth 1A (CMT1A) neuropathy. Trends Neurosci 1998;21:282–6.
[26] Windebank A. Inherited recurrent focal neuropathies. In: Dyck PJ, Low PA, Poduslo JF, editors. Peripheral neuropathy. Philadelphia: Saunders; 1993. p. 1137–60.
[27] Gabreels-Festen AA, et al. The status of HMSN type III. Neuromuscul Disord 1994;4: 63–9.
[28] Dejerine H, Sottas J. Sur la nevritte interstitielle hypertropphique et progressive de L'enfance. CR Soc Biol (Paris) 1893;45:63.
[29] Ionasescu VV, Ionasescu R, Searby C. Screening of dominantly inherited Charcot-Marie-Tooth neuropathies. Muscle Nerve 1993;16:1232–8.
[30] Wise CA, et al. Molecular analyses of unrelated Charcot-Marie-Tooth (CMT) disease patients suggest a high frequency of the CMTIA duplication. Am J Hum Genet 1993;53: 853–63.
[31] Chance PF, et al. DNA deletion associated with hereditary neuropathy with liability to pressure palsies. Cell 1993;72:143–51.
[32] Pentao L, et al. Charcot-Marie-Tooth type 1A duplication appears to arise from recombination at repeat sequences flanking the 1.5 Mb monomer unit. Nat Genet 1992;2: 292–300.
[33] Lopes J, et al. Sex-dependent rearrangements resulting in CMT1A and HNPP. Nat Genet 1997;17:136–7.
[34] Bissar-Tadmouri N, et al. Mutational analysis and genotype/phenotype correlation in Turkish Charcot-Marie-Tooth Type 1 and HNPP patients. Clin Genet 2000;58:396–402.
[35] Nicholson GA, et al. A frame shift mutation in the PMP22 gene in hereditary neuropathy with liability to pressure palsies. Nat Genet 1994;6:263–6.
[36] Gabreels-Festen AA, et al. Charcot-Marie-Tooth disease type 1A: morphological phenotype of the 17p duplication versus PMP22 point mutations. Acta Neuropathol (Berl) 1995;90:645–9.
[37] Roa BB, et al. Charcot-Marie-Tooth disease type 1A. Association with a spontaneous point mutation in the PMP22 gene. N Engl J Med 1993;329:96–101.
[38] Valentijn LJ, et al. Identical point mutations of PMP-22 in Trembler-J mouse and Charcot-Marie-Tooth disease type 1A. Nat Genet 1992;2:288–91.
[39] Marrosu MG, et al. A novel point mutation in the peripheral myelin protein 22 (PMP22) gene associated with Charcot-Marie-Tooth disease type 1A. Neurology 1997; 48:489–93.

[40] Roa BB, et al. Evidence for a recessive PMP 22 point mutation in Charcot-Marie-Tooth disease type 1A. Nat Genet 1993.
[41] Numakura C, et al. Hemizygous mutation of the peripheral myelin protein 22 gene associated with Charcot-Marie-Tooth disease type 1. Ann Neurol 2000;47:101–3.
[42] Parman Y, et al. Recessive inheritance of a new point mutation of the PMP22 gene in Dejerine-Sottas disease. Ann Neurol 1999;45:518–22.
[43] Roa BB, et al. Dejerine-Sottas syndrome associated with point mutation in the peripheral myelin protein 22 (PMP22) gene. Nat Genet 1993;5:269–73.
[44] Ionasescu VV, et al. Dejerine-Sottas disease with de novo dominant point mutation of the PMP22 gene. Neurology 1995;45:1766–7.
[45] Ionasescu VV, Searby C, Greenberg SA. Dejerine-Sottas disease with sensorineural hearing loss, nystagmus, and peripheral facial nerve weakness: de novo dominant point mutation of the PMP22 gene. J Med Genet 1996;33:1048–9.
[46] Ionasescu VV, et al. Dejerine-Sottas neuropathy in mother and son with same point mutation of PMP22 gene. Muscle Nerve 1997;20:97–9.
[47] Dyck J, Lambert EH. Lower motor and primary sensory neruon diseases with peroneal muscular atrophy. I. Neurologic, genetic, and electrophysiologic findings in hereditary polyneuropathies. II. Neurologic, genetic, and electrophysiologic findings in various neuronal degenerations. Arch Neurol 1968;18:603, 619.
[48] Yoshikawa H, et al. Elevated expression of messenger RNA for peripheral myelin protein 22 in biopsied peripheral nerves of patients with Charcot-Marie-Tooth disease type 1A. Ann Neurol 1994;35:445–50.
[49] Schenone A, et al. Underexpression of messenger RNA for peripheral myelin protein 22 in hereditary neuropathy with liability to pressure palsies. Neurology 1997;48:445–9.
[50] Lupski JR, et al. DNA duplication associated with Charcot-Marie-Tooth disease type 1A. Cell 1991;66:219–32.
[51] LeGuern E, et al. Patients homozygous for the 17p11.2 duplication in Charcot-Marie-Tooth type 1A disease. Ann Neurol 1997;41:104–8.
[52] Sahenk Z, et al. NT-3 promotes nerve regeneration and sensory improvement in CMT1A mouse models and in patients. Neurology 2005;65:681–9.
[53] Sereda MW, et al. Therapeutic administration of progesterone antagonist in a model of Charcot-Marie-Tooth disease (CMT-1A). Nat Med 2003;9:1533–7.
[54] Passage E, et al. Ascorbic acid treatment corrects the phenotype of a mouse model of Charcot-Marie-Tooth disease. Nat Med 2004;10:396–401.
[55] Greenfield S, et al. Protein composition of myelin of the peripheral nervous system. J Neurochem 1973;20:1207–16.
[56] Shapiro L, et al. Crystal structure of the extracellular domain from P0, the major structural protein of peripheral nerve myelin. Neuron 1996;17:435–49.
[57] Lai C, et al. Two forms of 1B236/myelin-associated glycoprotein, a cell adhesion molecule for postnatal neural development, are produced by alternative splicing. Proc Natl Acad Sci U S A 1987;84:4337–41.
[58] Lemke G, Axel R. Isolation and sequence of a cDNA encoding the major structural protein of peripheral myelin. Cell 1985;40:501–8.
[59] Yan WX, et al. P0 protein is a target antigen in chronic inflammatory demyelinating polyradiculoneuropathy. Ann Neurol 2001;50:286–92.
[60] Donaghy M, et al. Steroid responsive polyneuropathy in a family with a novel myelin protein zero mutation. J Neurol Neurosurg Psychiatry 2000;69:799–805.
[61] Shy ME. Hereditary motor and sensory neuropathies related to MPZ (Po) muations. In: Dyck PJ, Thomas PK, editors. Peripheral neuropathy. 4th edition. Philadelphia: Elsevier Saunders; 2005. p. 1681–706.
[62] Burns TM, et al. Novel myelin protein zero mutation (Arg36Trp) in a patient with acute onset painful neuropathy. Neuromuscul Disord 2006;16:308–10.

[63] Kilfoyle DH, et al. Myelin protein zero mutation His39Pro: hereditary motor and sensory neuropathy with variable onset, hearing loss, restless legs and multiple sclerosis. J Neurol Neurosurg Psychiatry 2006;77:963–6.
[64] Almsaddi M, Bertorini TE, Seltzer WK. Demyelinating neuropathy in a patient with multiple sclerosis and genotypical HMSN-1. Neuromuscul Disord 1998;8:87–9.
[65] Maurer M, et al. Bone marrow transfer from wild-type mice reverts the beneficial effect of genetically mediated immune deficiency in myelin mutants. Mol Cell Neurosci 2001;17:1094–101.
[66] Street VA, et al. Mapping of Charcot-Marie-Tooth disease type 1C to chromosome 16p identifies a novel locus for demyelinating neuropathies. Am J Hum Genet 2002;70:244–50.
[67] Street VA, et al. Mutation of a putative protein degradation gene LITAF/SIMPLE in Charcot-Marie-Tooth disease 1C. Neurology 2003;60:22–6.
[68] Saifi GM, et al. SIMPLE mutations in Charcot-Marie-Tooth disease and the potential role of its protein product in protein degradation. Hum Mutat 2005;25:372–83.
[69] Chung KW, et al. Two missense mutations of EGR2 R359W and GJB1 V136A in a Charcot-Marie-Tooth disease family. Neurogenetics 2005;6:159–63.
[70] Boerkoel CF, et al. EGR2 mutation R359W causes a spectrum of Dejerine-Sottas neuropathy. Neurogenetics 2001;3:153–7.
[71] Warner LE, et al. Functional consequences of mutations in the early growth response 2 gene (EGR2) correlate with severity of human myelinopathies. Hum Mol Genet 1999;8:1245–51.
[72] Warner LE, et al. Mutations in the early growth response 2 (EGR2) gene are associated with hereditary myelinopathies. Nat Genet 1998;18:382–4.
[73] Joseph LJ, et al. Molecular cloning, sequencing, and mapping of EGR2, a human early growth response gene encoding a protein with "zinc-binding finger" structure. Proc Natl Acad Sci U S A 1988;85:7164–8.
[74] Zorick TS, et al. The transcription factors SCIP and Krox-20 mark distinct stages and cell fates in Schwann cell differentiation. Mol Cell Neurosci 1996;8:129–45.
[75] Topilko P, et al. Krox-20 controls myelination in the peripheral nervous system. Nature 1994;371:796–9.
[76] Jordanova A, et al. Mutations in the neurofilament light chain gene (NEFL) cause early onset severe Charcot-Marie-Tooth disease. Brain 2003;126(Pt 3):590–7.
[77] Georgiou DM, et al. A novel NF-L mutation Pro22Ser is associated with CMT2 in a large Slovenian family. Neurogenetics 2002;4:93–6.
[78] Mersiyanova IV, et al. A new variant of Charcot-Marie-Tooth disease type 2 is probably the result of a mutation in the neurofilament-light gene. Am J Hum Genet 2000;67:37–46.
[79] De Jonghe P, et al. Further evidence that neurofilament light chain gene mutations can cause Charcot-Marie-Tooth disease type 2E. Ann Neurol 2001;49:245–9.
[80] Yamamoto M, et al. Glu528del in NEFL is a polymorphic variant rather than a disease-causing mutation for Charcot-Marie-Tooth disease in Japan. Neurogenetics 2004;5:75–7.
[81] Brownlees J, et al. Charcot-Marie-Tooth disease neurofilament mutations disrupt neurofilament assembly and axonal transport. Hum Mol Genet 2002;11:2837–44.
[82] Rozental R, Giaume C, Spray DC. Gap junctions in the nervous system. Brain Res Brain Res Rev 2000;32:11–5.
[83] Ressot C, Bruzzone R. Connexin channels in Schwann cells and the development of the X-linked form of Charcot-Marie-Tooth disease. Brain Res Brain Res Rev 2000;32:192–202.
[84] Ionasescu VV, et al. X-linked recessive Charcot-Marie-Tooth neuropathy: clinical and genetic study. Muscle Nerve 1992;15:368–73.
[85] Nicholson GA, Yeung L, Corbett A. Efficient neurophysiologic selection of X-linked Charcot-Marie-Tooth families: ten novel mutations. Neurology 1998;51:1412–6.
[86] Birouk N, et al. X-linked Charcot-Marie-Tooth disease with connexin 32 mutations: clinical and electrophysiologic study. Neurology 1998;50:1074–82.

[87] Lewis RA, Shy ME. Electrodiagnostic findings in CMTX: a disorder of the Schwann cell and peripheral nerve myelin. Ann N Y Acad Sci 1999;883:504–7.
[88] Hahn AF, et al. Genotype/phenotype correlations in X-linked dominant Charcot-Marie-Tooth disease. Ann N Y Acad Sci 1999;883:366–82.
[89] Tabaraud F, et al. Demyelinating X-linked Charcot-Marie-Tooth disease: unusual electrophysiological findings. Muscle Nerve 1999;22:1442–7.
[90] Gutierrez A, et al. Unusual electrophysiological findings in X-linked dominant Charcot-Marie-Tooth disease. Muscle Nerve 2000;23:182–8.
[91] Panas M, et al. Episodes of generalized weakness in two sibs with the C164T mutation of the connexin 32 gene. Neurology 2001;57:1906–8.
[92] Marques W Jr, et al. Central nervous system involvement in a novel connexin 32 mutation affecting identical twins. J Neurol Neurosurg Psychiatry 1999;66:803–4.
[93] Sahenk Z, Chen L. Abnormalities in the axonal cytoskeleton induced by a connexin32 mutation in nerve xenografts. J Neurosci Res 1998;51:174–84.
[94] Ionasescu V, Ionasescu R, Searby C. Correlation between connexin 32 gene mutations and clinical phenotype in X-linked dominant Charcot-Marie-Tooth neuropathy. Am J Med Genet 1996;63:486–91.
[95] Nelis E, Haites N, Van Broeckhoven C. Mutations in the peripheral myelin genes and associated genes in inherited peripheral neuropathies. Hum Mutat 1999;13:11–28.
[96] Nakagawa M, et al. Clinical phenotype in X-linked Charcot-Marie-Tooth disease with an entire deletion of the connexin 32 coding sequence. J Neurol Sci 2001;185:31–7.
[97] Abrams CK, et al. Mutations in connexin 32: the molecular and biophysical bases for the X- linked form of Charcot-Marie-Tooth disease. Brain Res Brain Res Rev 2000;32: 203–14.
[98] Cuesta AP, Sevilla L, Garcia-Planells T, et al. The gene encoding ganglioside-induced differentiation-associate protein 1 is mutated in axonal Charcot-Marie-Tooth type 4A disease. Nat Genet 2002;30:22–4.
[99] Claramunt R, et al. Genetics of Charcot-Marie-Tooth disease type 4A: mutations, inheritance, phenotypic variability, and founder effect. J Med Genet 2005;42:358–65.
[100] Birouk N, et al. Phenotypical features of a Moroccan family with autosomal recessive Charcot-Marie-Tooth disease associated with the S194X mutation in the GDAP1 gene. Arch Neurol 2003;60:598–604.
[101] Baxter RV, et al. Ganglioside-induced differentiation-associated protein-1 is mutant in Charcot-Marie-Tooth disease type 4A/8q21. Nat Genet 2002;30:21–2.
[102] Nelis E, et al. Mutations in GDAP1: autosomal recessive CMT with demyelination and axonopathy. Neurology 2002;59:1865–72.
[103] Boerkoel CF, et al. CMT4A: identification of a Hispanic GDAP1 founder mutation. Ann Neurol 2003;53:400–5.
[104] Berger P, et al. Loss of phosphatase activity in myotubularin-related protein 2 is associated with Charcot-Marie-Tooth disease type 4B1. Hum Mol Genet 2002;11:1569–79.
[105] Bolino A, et al. Charcot-Marie-Tooth type 4B is caused by mutations in the gene encoding myotubularin-related protein-2. Nat Genet 2000;25:17–9.
[106] Bolino A, et al. Molecular characterization and expression analysis of Mtmr2, mouse homologue of MTMR2, the Myotubularin-related 2 gene, mutated in CMT4B. Gene 2002;283:17–26.
[107] Kalaydjieva L, et al. N-myc downstream-regulated gene 1 is mutated in hereditary motor and sensory neuropathy-Lom. Am J Hum Genet 2000;67:47–58.
[108] Morar B, et al. Mutation history of the roma/gypsies. Am J Hum Genet 2004;75: 596–609.
[109] Hunter M, et al. Mutation screening of the N-myc downstream-regulated gene 1 (NDRG1) in patients with Charcot-Marie-Tooth Disease. Hum Mutat 2003;22:129–35.
[110] Scherer SS, Arroyo EJ. Recent progress on the molecular organization of myelinated axons. J Peripher Nerv Syst 2002;7:1–12.

[111] Dytrych L, et al. Two PDZ domain proteins encoded by the murine periaxin gene are the result of alternative intron retention and are differentially targeted in Schwann cells. J Biol Chem 1998;273:5794–800.
[112] Scherer SS, et al. Periaxin expression in myelinating Schwann cells: modulation by axon-glial interactions and polarized localization during development. Development 1995;121: 4265–73.
[113] Kijima K, et al. Periaxin mutation causes early-onset but slow-progressive Charcot-Marie-Tooth disease. J Hum Genet 2004;49:376–9.
[114] Takashima H, et al. Periaxin mutations cause a broad spectrum of demyelinating neuropathies. Ann Neurol 2002;51:709–15.
[115] Boerkoel CF, et al. Periaxin mutations cause recessive Dejerine-Sottas neuropathy. Am J Hum Genet 2001;68:325–33.
[116] Delague V, et al. Mapping of a new locus for autosomal recessive demyelinating Charcot-Marie-Tooth disease to 19q13.1–13.3 in a large consanguineous Lebanese family: exclusion of MAG as a candidate gene. Am J Hum Genet 2000;67:236–43.
[117] Zhao C, et al. Charcot-Marie-Tooth disease type 2A caused by mutation in a microtubule motor KIF1Bbeta. Cell 2001;105:587–97.
[118] Bomont P, et al. The gene encoding gigaxonin, a new member of the cytoskeletal BTB/kelch repeat family, is mutated in giant axonal neuropathy. Nat Genet 2000;26:370–4.
[119] Saito M, et al. Linkage mapping of the gene for Charcot-Marie-Tooth disease type 2 to chromosome 1p (CMT2A) and the clinical features of CMT2A. Neurology 1997;49: 1630–5.
[120] Pericak-Vance MA, et al. Confirmation of a second locus for CMT2 and evidence for additional genetic heterogeneity. Neurogenetics 1997;1:89–93.
[121] Kijima K, et al. Mitochondrial GTPase mitofusin 2 mutation in Charcot-Marie-Tooth neuropathy type 2A. Hum Genet 2005;116:23–7.
[122] Zuchner S, et al. Axonal neuropathy with optic atrophy is caused by mutations in mitofusin 2. Ann Neurol 2006;59:276–81.
[123] Zhu D, et al. Charcot-Marie-Tooth with pyramidal signs is genetically heterogeneous: families with and without MFN2 mutations. Neurology 2005;65:496–7.
[124] Jordens I, et al. The Rab7 effector protein RILP controls lysosomal transport by inducing the recruitment of dynein-dynactin motors. Curr Biol 2001;11:1680–5.
[125] Cantalupo G, et al. Rab-interacting lysosomal protein (RILP): the Rab7 effector required for transport to lysosomes. EMBO J 2001;20:683–93.
[126] Harrison RE, et al. Phagosomes fuse with late endosomes and/or lysosomes by extension of membrane protrusions along microtubules: role of Rab7 and RILP. Mol Cell Biol 2003;23: 6494–506.
[127] Puls I, et al. Mutant dynactin in motor neuron disease. Nat Genet 2003;33:455–6.
[128] Ge Q, Trieu EP, Targoff IN. Primary structure and functional expression of human Glycyl-tRNA synthetase, an autoantigen in myositis. J Biol Chem 1994;269:28790–7.
[129] Ionasescu V, et al. Autosomal dominant Charcot-Marie-Tooth axonal neuropathy mapped on chromosome 7p (CMT 2D). Hum Mol Genet 1996;5:1373–5.
[130] Christodoulou K, et al. Mapping of a distal form of spinal muscular atrophy with upper limb predominance to chromosome 7p. Hum Mol Genet 1995;4:1629–32.
[131] Sambuughin N, et al. Autosomal dominant distal spinal muscular atrophy type V (dSMA-V) and Charcot-Marie-Tooth disease type 2D (CMT2D) segregate within a single large kindred and map to a refined region on chromosome 7p15. J Neurol Sci 1998; 161:23–8.
[132] Antonellis A, et al. Glycyl tRNA synthetase mutations in Charcot-Marie-Tooth disease type 2D and distal spinal muscular atrophy type V. Am J Hum Genet 2003; 72:1293–9.
[133] Evgrafov OV, et al. Mutant small heat-shock protein 27 causes axonal Charcot-Marie-Tooth disease and distal hereditary motor neuropathy. Nat Genet 2004;36:602–6.

[134] Kijima K, et al. Small heat shock protein 27 mutation in a Japanese patient with distal hereditary motor neuropathy. J Hum Genet 2005;50:473–6.
[135] Tang B, et al. Mutation analysis of the small heat shock protein 27 gene in Chinese patients with Charcot-Marie-Tooth disease. Arch Neurol 2005;62:1201–7.
[136] Tang BS, et al. Small heat-shock protein 22 mutated in autosomal dominant Charcot-Marie-Tooth disease type 2L. Hum Genet 2005;116:222–4.
[137] Klein CJ, et al. The gene for HMSN2C maps to 12q23–24: a region of neuromuscular disorders. Neurology 2003;60:1151–6.
[138] Bitoun M, et al. Mutations in dynamin 2 cause dominant centronuclear myopathy. Nat Genet 2005;37:1207–9.
[139] Zuchner S, et al. Mutations in the pleckstrin homology domain of dynamin 2 cause dominant intermediate Charcot-Marie-Tooth disease. Nat Genet 2005;37:289–94.
[140] Jordanova A, et al. Disrupted function and axonal distribution of mutant tyrosyl-tRNA synthetase in dominant intermediate Charcot-Marie-Tooth neuropathy. Nat Genet 2006; 38:197–202.
[141] Stuurman N, Heins S, Aebi U. Nuclear lamins: their structure, assembly, and interactions. J Struct Biol 1998;122:42–66.
[142] De Sandre-Giovannoli A, et al. Homozygous defects in LMNA, encoding lamin A/C nuclear-envelope proteins, cause autosomal recessive axonal neuropathy in human (Charcot-Marie-Tooth disorder type 2) and mouse [erratum: Am J Hum Genet 2002;70:1075]. Am J Hum Genet 2002;70:726–36.
[143] Bonne G, et al. Mutations in the gene encoding lamin A/C cause autosomal dominant Emery-Dreifuss muscular dystrophy. Nat Genet 1999;21:285–8.
[144] Raffaeledi Barletta M, et al. Different mutations in the LMNA gene casue atuosomal dominant and autosomal recessive Emery-Dreifuss muscular dystrophy. Am J Hum Genet 2000;66:1407–12.
[145] Muchir A, et al. Identification of mutations in the gene encoding lamins A/C in autosomal dominant limb girdle muscular dystrophy with atrioventricular conduction disturbances (LGMD1B). Hum Mol Genet 2000;9:1453–9.
[146] Fatkin D, et al. Missense mutations in the rod domain of the lamin A/C gene as causes of dilated cardiomyopathy and conduction-system disease. Am J Cardiol 1999;83:13H–8H [comment].
[147] Novelli G, et al. Mandibuloacral dysplasia is caused by a mutation in LMNA-encoding lamin A/C. Am J Hum Genet 2002;71:426–31.
[148] Shackleton S. LMNA, encoding lamin A/C, is mutated in partial lipodystrophy. 2000 [comment].
[149] Stogbauer F, et al. Autosomal dominant burning feet syndrome. J Neurol Neurosurg Psychiatry 1999;67:78–81.
[150] Dawkins JL, et al. Mutations in SPTLC1, encoding serine palmitoyltransferase, long chain base subunit-1, cause hereditary sensory neuropathy type I. Nat Genet 2001;27: 309–12.
[151] Bejaoui K, et al. SPTLC1 is mutated in hereditary sensory neuropathy, type 1. Nat Genet 2001;27:261–2.
[152] Snell EE, Dimari SJ, Brady RN. Biosynthesis of sphingosine and dihydrosphingosine by cell-free systems from Hansenula ciferri. Chem Phys Lipids 1970;5:116–38.
[153] Medlock KA, Merrill AH Jr. Inhibition of serine palmitoyltransferase in vitro and long-chain base biosynthesis in intact Chinese hamster ovary cells by beta- chloroalanine. Biochemistry 1988;27:7079–84.
[154] Herget T, et al. Production of ceramides causes apoptosis during early neural differentiation in vitro. J Biol Chem 2000;275:30344–54.
[155] Schambelan M, Sebastian A, Rector FC Jr. Mineralocorticoid-resistant renal hyperkalemia without salt wasting (type II pseudohypoaldosteronism): role of increased renal chloride reabsorption. Kidney Int 1981;19:716–27.

[156] Lafreniere RG, et al. Identification of a novel gene (HSN2) causing hereditary sensory and autonomic neuropathy type ii through the study of Canadian genetic isolates. Am J Hum Genet 2004;74:1064–73.
[157] Takagi M, et al. New HSN2 mutation in Japanese patient with hereditary sensory and autonomic neuropathy type 2. Neurology 2006;66:1251–2.
[158] Riviere JB, et al. A mutation in the HSN2 gene causes sensory neuropathy type II in a Lebanese family. Ann Neurol 2004;56:572–5.
[159] Dyck PJ, Klein CJ. Hereditary sensory and autonomic neuropathies. In: Noseworthy JH, editor. Neurological therapeutics principles and practice. London: Martin Dunitz; 2003. p. 2188–93.
[160] Axelrod FB, et al. Progressive sensory loss in familial dysautonomia. Pediatrics 1981;67: 517.
[161] Anderson SL, et al. Familial dysautonomia is caused by mutations of the IKAP gene. Am J Hum Genet 2001;68:753–8.
[162] Low PA, Burke WJ, McLeod JG. Congenital sensory neuropathy with selective loss of small myelinated fibers. Ann Neurol 1978;3:179.
[163] Mardy S, et al. Congenital insensitivity to pain with anhidrosis: novel mutations in the TRKA (NTRK1) gene encoding a high-affinity receptor for nerve growth factor. Am J Hum Genet 1999;64:1570–9.
[164] Indo Y, et al. Mutations in the TRKA/NGF receptor gene in patients with congenital insensitivity to pain with anhidrosis. Nat Genet 1996;13:485–8.
[165] McKusick V. Mendelian inheritance in man. Available at: http://www3.ncbi.nlm.nih.gov/Omim. 12th ed. Baltimore: Johns Hopkins University Press; 1998.
[166] Alper G, Narayanan V. Friedreich's ataxia. Pediatr Neurol 2003;28:335–41.
[167] Klein CJD, PJ. HMSN II (CMT2) and miscellaneous inherited system atrophies of nerve axon: clinical-molecular genetic correlations. In: Dyck PJ, Thomas PK, editors. Peripheral neuropathy. Philadelphia: Elsevier Saunders; 2005. p. 1717–51.
[168] Fink JK. The hereditary spastic paraplegias: nine genes and counting. Arch Neurol 2003; 60:1045–9.
[169] Klein CJ, et al. Inflammation and neuropathic attacks in hereditary brachial plexus neuropathy. J Neurol Neurosurg Psychiatry 2002;73:45–50.
[170] Kuhlenbaumer G, et al. Mutations in SEPT9 cause hereditary neuralgic amyotrophy. Nat Genet 2005;37:1044–6.
[171] Klein CJW, Cunningham JM, Klein DM, et al. Mutation of SEPT9 is rare in American kindreds with hereditary brachial plexus neuropathy and not found in sporadic brachial plexus neuropathy (Parsonage-Turner). Neurology 2006;66(5 Supp):A86.
[172] Thomas P. Other inherited neuropathies. In: Dyck P, editor. Peripheral neuropathies. Piladelphia: Saunders; 1993. p. 1194–218.
[173] Klein CJDPJ. Genetic testing in the peripheral neuropathies. J Peripher Nerv Syst 2005;10: 77–84.
[174] Boerkoel CF, et al. Charcot-Marie-Tooth disease and related neuropathies: mutation distribution and genotype-phenotype correlation. Ann Neurol 2002;51:190–201.
[175] Bergen HR 3rd, et al. Identification of transthyretin variants by sequential proteomic and genomic analysis. Clin Chem 2004;50:1544–52.
[176] Rodriguez-Lebron E, Paulson HL. Allele-specific RNA interference for neurological disease. Gene Ther 2006;13:576–81.
[177] Park JG, et al. Serotype-selective, small-molecule inhibitors of the zinc endopeptidase of botulinum neurotoxin serotype A. Bioorg Med Chem 2006;14:395–408.
[178] Lightstone FC, et al. Identification of novel small molecule ligands that bind to tetanus toxin. Chem Res Toxicol 2000;13:356–62.

ELSEVIER
SAUNDERS

Neurol Clin 25 (2007) 209–255

NEUROLOGIC
CLINICS

Nutritional Neuropathies

Neeraj Kumar, MD[a,b,*]

[a]Department of Neurology, Mayo Clinic, Rochester, MN 55905, USA
[b]Mayo Clinic College of Medicine, Rochester, MN 55905, USA

Optimal functioning of the central and peripheral nervous system is dependent on a constant supply of appropriate nutrients. Estimates provided by the United Nations Food and Agricultural Organization suggest that in 2004 approximately 852 million people in the world were malnourished [1]. Neurologic signs occur late in malnutrition. Neurologic consequences of nutritional deficiencies are not restricted to underdeveloped countries. Individuals at risk in developed countries include the poor and homeless; the elderly; patients on prolonged inadequate parenteral nutrition; those who have food fads or eating disorders, such as anorexia nervosa and bulimia; those suffering from malnutrition secondary to chronic alcoholism; and patients who have malabsorption syndromes, such as sprue, celiac disease, inflammatory bowel disease, and pernicious anemia (PA). Not infrequently, multiple nutritional deficiencies coexist. Of particular concern in the developed world is the epidemic of obesity. The rising rates of bariatric surgery are accompanied by neurologic complications related to nutrient deficiencies. The preventable and potentially treatable nature of these disorders makes this an important subject. Prognosis depends on prompt recognition and institution of appropriate therapy.

Particularly important for optimal functioning of the nervous system are the B-group vitamins (vitamin B_{12} [B_{12}], thiamine, niacin, and pyridoxine), vitamin E, copper, and possibly folic acid. Most of this review is limited to the discussion of peripheral nervous system manifestations related to the deficiency of these key nutrients. The second sections deals with the neurologic complications associated with bariatric surgery. In the final section, conditions discussed include those that have a geographic predilection or historical significance and those patients in whom either a precise nutrient

* 200 First Street, SW, Rochester, MN 55905.
E-mail address: kumar.neeraj@mayo.edu

0733-8619/07/$ - see front matter
doi:10.1016/j.ncl.2006.11.001

deficiency has not been identified definitively or disorders attributed to multiple coexisting deficiencies.

Nutrient deficiencies

Vitamin B_{12}

Even though B_{12} refers specifically to cyanocobalamin (cyanoCbl), for this review the terms cobalamin (Cbl) and B_{12} are used interchangeably. CyanoCbl is a stable synthetic pharmaceutical that has to be converted to other cobalamins to become metabolically active.

Function

The two active forms of Cbl are methylCbl and adenosylCbl (Fig. 1) [2]. MethylCbl is a cofactor for a cytosolic enzyme, methionine synthase, in a methyl transfer reaction that converts homocysteine (Hcy) to methionine. Methionine is adenosylated to S-adenosylmethionine (SAM), a methyl group donor required for biologic methylation reactions involving proteins, neurotransmitters, and phospholipids. Decreased SAM production leads to reduced myelin basic protein methylation and white matter vacuolization in Cbl deficiency [3]. Methionine also facilitates the formation of formyltetrahydrofolate (formylTHF), which is involved in purine synthesis. During the process of methionine formation, methylTHF donates the methyl group and is converted into THF, a precursor for purine and pyrimidine synthesis. Impaired DNA synthesis could interfere with oligodendrocyte growth and myelin production. AdenosylCbl is a cofactor for L-methylmalonyl–coenzyme A (CoA) mutase, which catalyzes the conversion of L-methylmalonyl–CoA to succinyl-CoA in an isomerization reaction. Accumulation of methylmalonate and propionate may provide abnormal substrates for fatty acid synthesis. The branched-chain and abnormal odd-number carbon fatty acids may be incorporated into the myelin sheath [4]. Definite evidence supporting this hypothesis is lacking. Data from animal models of the Cbl neuropathy suggest impairment of the methylCbl-dependent methionine synthetase reaction is the more important defect [5]. In the Cbl-deficient fruit bat with neurologic manifestations, no defect in the methylation of myelin lipid or basic protein has been shown. It is suggested that overproduction of the myelinolytic tumor necrosis factor-α and the reduced synthesis of epidermal growth factor and interleukin-6 may play a role in the pathogenesis of the neurologic manifestations of Cbl deficiency [6].

Requirements and sources

The recommended dietary allowance (RDA) of Cbl for adults is 2.4 μg per day and the median intake from food in the United States is 3.5 μg per day for women and 5 μg per day for men (Table 1) [7]. No adverse effects are associated with excess Cbl intake. Foods of animal orgin, such as meats,

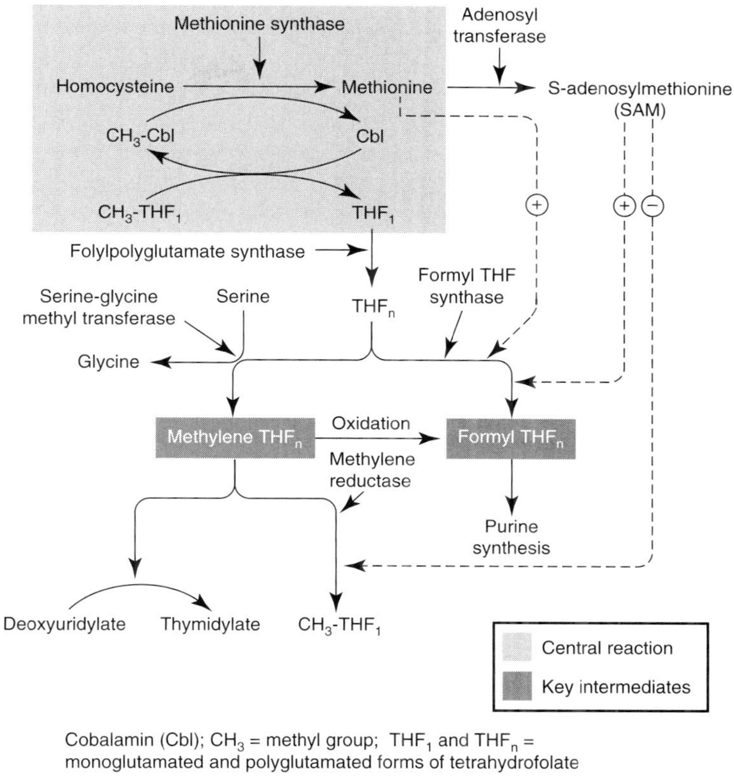

Fig. 1. Biochemistry of Cbl and folate deficiency. See text for details. CH_3, methyl group; THF_1 and THF_n, monoglutamated and polyglutamated forms of tetrahydrofolate. (*Adapted from* Tefferi A, Pruthi RK. The biochemical basis of cobalamin deficiency. Mayo Clin Proc 1994;69:181–6; with permission.)

eggs, and milk, are the major dietary sources. The richest sources of Cbl include shellfish; organ meats, such as liver; some game meat; and certain fish. In the United States, milk and Cbl-fortified cereals are particularly efficient sources. Even though vegetables lack Cbl, strict vegetarians generally do not develop overt clinical deficiency, because an adequate amount is present in legumes.

Physiology

In the stomach, Cbl bound to food is dissociated from proteins in the presence of acid and pepsin [7,8]. The released Cbl binds to R proteins secreted by salivary glands and gastric mucosa. In the small intestine, pancreatic proteases partially degrade the R proteins-Cbl complex at neutral pH and release Cbl, which then binds with intrinsic factor (IF). IF is a Cbl-binding protein secreted by gastric parietal cells. The IF-Cbl complex binds to specific receptors in the ileal mucosa and is internalized. In addition to the IF-mediated

Table 1
Summary of sources, causes of deficiency, neurologic significance, laboratory tests, and treatment for deficiency states related to cobalamin, folate, copper, and vitamin E

Nutrient	Sources	Major causes of deficiency	Neurologic significance associated with deficiency	Laboratory tests	Treatment
Cobalamin	Meats, egg, milk, fortified cereals	PA, food-Cbl malabsorption (elderly), gastric surgery, acid reduction therapy, gastrointestinal disease, N_2O toxicity	Myelopathy or myeloneuropathy, peripheral neuropathy, neuropsychiatric manifestations, optic neuropathy	Serum Cbl, serum MMA, plasma total Hcy, anemia, macrocytosis, neutrophil hypersegmentation, Schilling test, serum gastrin, IF, and parietal cell antibodies	Intramuscular B_{12} 1000 μg twice weekly for 2 weeks, followed by weekly for 2 months and monthly thereafter
Folate	In virtually all foods	Alcoholism, gastrointestinal disease, folate antagonists	Neurological manifestations are rare and indistiguishable from those due to Cbl deficiency	Serum folate, RBC folate, plasma total Hcy	Oral folate 1 mg 3 times/d followed by a maintenance dosage of 1 mg/d
Copper	Organ meats, seafood, nuts, whole grain products	Gastric surgery, zinc toxicity, gastrointestinal disease	Myelopathy or myeloneuropathy	Serum copper and ceruloplasmin	Oral elemental copper: 6 mg/d for a week followed by 4 mg/d for a week and 2 mg/d thereafter

Vitamin E	Vegetable oils, leafy vegetables, fruits, meats, nuts	Chronic cholestasis, pancreatic insufficiency, AVED, homozygous hypobetalipoproteinemia, abetalipoproteinemia, chylomicron retention disease	Spinocerebellar syndrome with peripheral neuropathy, ophthalmoplegia, pigmentary retinopathy	Serum vitamin E Ratio of serum α-tocopherol to sum of serum cholesterol and triglycerides	Variable dose and route (see text)
Thiamine	Enriched, fortified, or whole grain products	Recurrent vomiting, gastric surgery, alcoholism, dieting, increased demand with marginal nutritional status	Beriberi (dry, wet, infantile), WE, KS	Urinary thiamine, serum thiamine, erythrocyte transketolase activation assay, RBC TDP	50 to 100 mg (intravenous, intramuscular, oral)
Niacin	Meat, fish, poultry, enriched bread, fortified cereals	Corn as primary carbohydrate source, alcoholism, malabsorption, carcinoid and Hartnup syndrome	Encephalopathy (peripheral neuropathy)	Urinary excretion of methylated niacin metabolites	25 to 50 mg of nicotinic acid (intramuscular, oral)
Pyridoxine	Meat, fish, eggs, soybeans, nuts, dairy products	B_6 antagonists, alcoholism, gastrointestinal disease	Infantile seizures, peripheral neuropathy (pure sensory neuropathy with toxicity)	Plasma PLP	50 to 100 mg of pyridoxine daily (oral)

Abbreviations: AVED, ataxia with vitamin e deficiency; Cbl, cobalamin; Hcy, homocysteine; IF, intrinsic factor; KS, Korsakoff's syndrome; MMA, methylmalonioc acid; N_2O, nitrous oxide; PA, pernicious anemia; PLP, pyridoxal phosphate; RBC, red blood cells; TDP, thiamine diphosphate; WE, Wernicke's encephalopathy.

absorption of ingested Cbl, there is a nonspecific absorption of Cbl that occurs by passive diffusion at all mucosal sites. This is a relatively inefficient process by which 1% to 2% of the ingested amount is absorbed [9]. Cbl is transferred across the intestinal mucosa into portal blood where it binds to transCbl II (TC II). The liver takes up approximately 50% of the Cbl and the rest is transported to other tissues. TC II is the form that delivers Cbl to the tissues through receptors for TC II [10]. TC II–bound Cbl is taken up by cells through receptor-mediated endocytosis. Intracellular lysosomal degradation releases Cbl for conversion to methylCbl or adenosylCbl. Most of the Cbl secreted in the bile is reabsorbed. If circulating Cbl exceeds the Cbl binding capacity of blood, the excess is excreted in the urine. The estimated daily loss of Cbl is 1 μg. This is minute compared with body stores of 2500 μg. Hence, even in the presence of severe malabsorption, 2 to 5 years may pass before Cbl deficiency develops [11]. Similarly, a clinical relapse in PA after interrupting Cbl therapy takes approximately 5 years before it is recognized.

Causes of deficiency

The majority of patients who have Cbl deficiency have PA [8,12]. Cbl deficiency is particularly common in the elderly [13]. In a study, the prevalence of metabolic Cbl deficiency in the 65- to 99-year-old age group was 14.5% [14]. This most likely is the result of the high incidence of atrophic gastritis and achlorhydria-induced food-Cbl malabsorption rather than reduced intake [13,15]. Cbl deficiency commonly is seen after gastric surgery [16]. Acid reduction therapy, as with H_2-blockers, also can cause Cbl deficiency [17]. Other causes of Cbl deficiency include conditions associated with malabsorption, such as ileal disease or resection, bacterial overgrowth, and tropical sprue. Competition for Cbl secondary to parasitic infestation by the fish tapeworm, *Diphyllobothrium latum*, may cause Cbl deficiency. Certain hereditary enzymatic defects also can manifest as disorders of Cbl metabolism [18]. Increased prevalence of B_{12} deficiency is recognized in HIV-infected patients who have neurologic symptoms but the precise significance of this is unclear [19,20]. In AIDS-associated myelopathy, the Cbl- and folate-dependent transmethylation pathway is depressed and CSF and serum levels of SAM are reduced [21].

Nitrous oxide (N_2O) is a commonly used inhalational anesthetic that is abused because of its euphoriant properties. N_2O irreversibly oxidizes the cobalt core of Cbl and renders methylCbl inactive [22]. Clinical manifestations of Cbl deficiency appear relatively rapidly with N_2O toxicity because the metabolism is blocked at the cellular level. They may, however, be delayed up to 8 weeks [23]. Postoperative neurologic dysfunction can be seen with N_2O exposure during routine anesthesia if subclinical Cbl deficiency is present [23,24]. The other setting associated with N_2O (laughing gas) toxicity is inhalant abuse [25]. Earlier reports were among dentists and other medical personnel. More recently it is reported among university students [26]. Rarely, it may be seen in medical personnel working in poorly ventilated surgeries [25]. A generalized toxic polyneuropathy is reported after excessive intentional inhalation of compressed N_2O delivery from cartridges through a whipped-cream dispenser [27].

B_{12} deficiency only rarely is the consequence of diminished dietary intake. Strict vegetarians may develop Cbl deficiency after years. The consequences often are mild and often only subclinical. Clinical consequences are more likely when poor intake begins in childhood wherein limited stores and growth requirements act as additional confounders. Not infrequently the cause of Cbl deficiency is unknown.

Clinical significance

Neurologic manifestations may be the earliest and often the only manifestation of Cbl deficiency [12,28,29]. The severity of the hematologic and neurologic manifestations may be inversely related in a particular patient [29,30]. Relapses generally are associated with the same neurologic phenotype [31]. The recognized neurologic manifestations may include a myelopathy with or without an associated neuropathy, cognitive impairment, optic neuropathy, and paresthesias without abnormal signs [29].

The best characterized neurologic manifestation of Cbl deficiency is a myelopathy commonly referred to as subacute combined degeneration [32,33]. This term refers to the pathologic process seen in B_{12} deficiency myelopathy. The most severely involved regions are the cervical and upper thoracic posterior columns. Changes also are seen in the lateral columns. Involvement of the anterior columns is rare. Spongiform changes and foci of myelin and axon destruction are seen in the spinal cord white matter. There is myelin loss followed by axonal degeneration and gliosis [33]. The neurologic features typically include a spastic paraparesis, extensor plantar response, and impaired perception of position and vibration. Symptoms start in the feet and are symmetric. Neuropsychaitric manifestations include decreased memory, personality change, psychosis, and, rarely, delirium [12,29]. MRI abnormalities include a signal change in the subcortical white matter and posterior and lateral columns [34,35]. Contrast enhancement involving the dorsal or lateral columns may be present [36]. The dorsal column may show a decreased signal on T1-weighted images [36]. Other reported findings include cord atrophy and anterior column involvement [37,38]. Treatment may be accompanied by reversal of cord swelling, contrast enhancement, and signal change [34–36,38]. Similar MRI findings are seen with N_2O toxicity [26].

Clinical, electrophysiologic, and pathologic involvement of the peripheral nervous system is described. Earlier studies failed to provide pathologic evidence of peripheral neuropathy [33]. More recently, detailed pathologic studies of distal sensory or motor nerves and electrophysiologic studies demonstrate axonal degeneration with or without associated demyelination [39–41]. In a recent study, Cbl deficiency was detected in 27 of 324 patients who had a polyneuropathy [42]. Clues to possible B_{12} deficiency in a patient who had polyneuropathy included a relatively sudden onset of symptoms, findings suggestive of an associated myelopathy, onset of symptoms in the hands, macrocytic red blood cells (RBCs), and the presence of a risk factor for Cbl deficiency. Autonomic dysfunction with orthostatic hypotension is described [40,43,44]. Electrophysiologic abnormalities include nerve conduction studies suggestive of a sensorimotor axonopathy and abnormalities on somatosensory evoked potentials, visual evoked potentials, and motor evoked potentials [35,45].

Cbl can be normal in some patients who have Cbl deficiency and serum methylmalonic acid (MMA) and total Hcy levels are useful in diagnosing patients who have Cbl deficiency [11,46–49]. The sensitivity of the available metabolic tests has facilitated the development of the concept of subclinical Cbl deficiency [50]. This refers to biochemical evidence of Cbl deficiency in the absence of hematologic or neurologic manifestations. These biochemical findings should respond to Cbl therapy. The frequency of subclinical Cbl deficiency is estimated to be at least 10 times that of clinical Cbl deficiency [50]. Subclinical Cbl deficiency increases with age [51,52]. These individuals may have subtle neurologic and neurophysiologic abnormalities of uncertain significance that respond to Cbl therapy [53]. It is equally important to recognize that the presence of a low Cbl in the association with neurologic manifestations does not imply cause and effect or indicate the presence of metabolic Cbl deficiency. The incidence of cryptogenic polyneuropathy and Cbl deficiency increases with age and the latter may be a chance occurrence rather than a cause of the neuropathy [54]. The clinical impact of subclinical Cbl deficiency and its appropriate management are uncertain. If it is unclear whether or not elevated MMA or Hcy is the result of Cbl deficiency, the response to empiric parenteral B_{12} replacement can be seen. A trend to normalize with replacement favors Cbl deficiency as the likely cause [55].

Investigations

Serum Cbl determination is the mainstay for evaluating Cbl status [11,56]. The older microbiologic and radioisotopic assays have been replaced by immunologically based chemiluminescence assays. Although a widely used screening test, serum Cbl measurement has technical and interpretive problems and lacks sensitivity and specificity for the diagnosis of Cbl deficiency [47,48,55]. A low Cbl level may be seen in pregnancy, with oral contraceptive or anticonvulsant use, with transCbl I (TC I) deficiency, with folate deficiency, in association with HIV infection, and in multiple myeloma [50]. The Cbl radioassay may give falsely low readings if performed soon after radionuclide isotope studies, such as bone scans [57]. Patients who have mild TC I deficiency may be responsible for 15% of all unexplained low Cbl levels and many of these patients may be heterozygotes for hereditary TC I deficiency [58]. Falsely elevated Cbl levels may be seen with renal failure, liver disease, and myeloproliferative disorders [59].

Levels of serum MMA and plasma total Hcy are useful as ancillary diagnostic tests in the diagnosis of Cbl deficiency [48,55]. MMA is a byproduct of methylmalonyl-CoA and it accumulates in Cbl deficiency. Its specificity is superior to that of plasma Hcy [60]. Elevated MMA levels may be seen with renal insufficiency, in infancy, with methylmalonyl-CoA mutase deficiency, and possibly with volume contraction [50,56]. Urinary MMA levels may be useful to exclude falsely elevated serum levels resulting from renal insufficiency. Although plasma total Hcy is a sensitive indicator of Cbl deficiency, its major limitation is its poor specificity [47,48,51]. Causes of an elevated Hcy level include renal insufficiency, folate deficiency, alcohol abuse, hypothyroidism, increased age, hypovolemia, psoriasis, inherited metabolic disorders, and certain inborn errors of Hcy metabolism [50,56]. Elevated Hcy levels also are noted in associated with isoniazid (INH) use, renal transplantation, leukemia, and enzyme polymorphisms (eg, methylenetetrahydrofolate reductase [MTHFR]) [50].

A rise in mean corpuscular volume may precede development of anemia [61]. The presence of neutrophil hypersegmentation may be a sensitive marker for Cbl deficiency and may be seen in the absence of anemia or macrocytosis. The Cbl-TC II complex is believed to be the metabolically active fraction of circulating Cbl [62]. It is suggested that measuring the Cbl attached to TC II might lead to greater sensitivity and specificity [63]. The clinical usefulness seems limited [64].

In order to determine the cause of Cbl deficiency, tests directed at determining the cause of suspected malabsorption are undertaken. Concerns regarding cost, accuracy, and radiation exposure have led to a significant decrease in the availability of the Schilling test. An elevated serum gastrin and decreased pepsinogen I is seen in 80% to 90% of patients who have PA, but the specificity of these tests is limited [65]. Elevated gastrin levels are a marker for hypochlorhydria or achlorhydria, which invariably are seen with PA. Elevated gastrin levels may be seen in up to 30% of the elderly [15]. Elevated serum gastrin levels are approximately 70% specific and sensitive for PA [66]. Anti-IF factor antibodies are specific but lack sensitivity and are found in approximately 50% to 70% of patients who have PA [67–69]. Recent studies suggest that antiparietal cell antibodies may not be seen as commonly as believed earlier and, therefore, have limited usefulness [69]. Further, false-positive results for the gastric parietal cell antibody are common. They may be seen in 10% of people over age 70 and also are present in other autoimmune endocrinopathies.

Management

The goals of treatment are to reverse the signs and symptoms of deficiency, replete body stores, ascertain the cause of deficiency, and monitor response to therapy. With normal Cbl absorption, oral administration (3 to 5 μg) may suffice. In patients who have food-bound Cbl malabsorption resulting from achlorhydria, cyanoCbl (50 to 100 μg) given orally often is adequate [70]. Patients who have Cbl deficiency resulting from achlorhydria-induced food-bound Cbl malabsorption show normal absorption of crystalline B_{12} but are unable to digest and absorb Cbl in food because of achlorhydria. The more common situation is one of impaired absorption where parenteral therapy is required. A short course of daily or weekly therapy often is followed by monthly maintenance therapy. A common regimen is intramuscular injection, 100 μg daily for 2 weeks or 1000 μg twice weekly for 2 weeks followed by weekly injections of 1000 μg for 2 months. Lifelong therapy with monthly intramuscular injection (1000 μg) often is required. If the oral dose is large enough, even patients who have an absorption defect may respond to oral Cbl [71].

Patients who have B_{12} deficiency are prone to develop neurologic deterioration after N_2O anesthesia. It is preventable by prophylactic B_{12} given weeks before surgery in individuals who have a borderline B_{12} level who are expected to receive N_2O anesthesia. Intramuscular B_{12} should be given to patients who have acute N_2O poisoning. Methionine supplementation also is proposed as a first-line therapy [72]. With chronic exposure, immediate cessation of exposure should be ensured. In AIDS-associated myelopathy, possible benefit of administration of the SAM precursor, L-methionine, is suggested by a pilot study [73] but not confirmed in a subsequent double-blind study [74].

Response to treatment may relate to extent of involvement and delay in starting treatment [29]. Remission correlates inversely with the time lapsed between symptom onset and therapy initiation. Most of the symptomatic improvement occurs during the first 6 months [75]. Response of the hematologic derangements is prompt and complete. Reticulocyte count begins to rise within 3 days and peaks at approximately 7 days. RBC count begins to rise by 7 days and is followed by a decline in mean corpuscular volume with normalization by 8 weeks. MMA and Hcy levels normalize by 10 days. Cbl levels rise after injection regardless of the benefit. Hence, MMA and Hcy are more reliable ways to monitor response to therapy. In patients who have severe B_{12} deficiency, replacement therapy may be accompanied by hypokalemia resulting from proliferation of bone marrow cells that use potassium. Response of the neurologic manifestations is more variable and may be incomplete.

HydroxoCbl has superior retention and may permit injections every 2 to 3 months [76]. Compared with hydroxoCbl, cyanoCbl binds to serum proteins less well and is excreted more rapidly [77]. Intranasal administration of hydroxoCbl is associated with fast absorption and normalization of Cbl levels [78]. Advantages of delivering Cbl by the nasal or sublingual route are unproven. Oral preparations of IF are available but not reliable. Antibodies to IF may nullify its effectiveness in the intestinal lumen.

Neurologically affected patients may have high folate levels [79]. Folate therapy may delay recognition of the Cbl deficiency and cause neurologic deterioration. Anemia resulting from Cbl deficiency often responds to folate therapy but the response is incomplete and transient. It is unclear if routine folate supplementation may compromise the early diagnosis of the hematologic manifestations or worsen the neurologic consequences. Not infrequently, iron deficiency also is seen in patients who have PA [80].

Folic acid

Function

Folate functions as a coenzyme or cosubstrate by modifying, accepting, or transferring one-carbon moieties in single-carbon reactions involved in the metabolism of nucleic and amino acids [81,82]. The biologically active folates are in the THF form. MethylTHF is the predominant folate and is required for the Cbl-dependent remethylation of Hcy to methionine. Methylation of deoxyuridylate to thymidylate is mediated by methyleneTHF (see Fig. 1). Impairment of this reaction results in accumulation of uracil, which replaces the decreased thymine in nucleoprotein synthesis and initiates the process that leads to megaloblastic anemia.

Requirements and sources

The RDA for men and women is 400 μg per day of dietary folate equivalents [81]. Dietary folate equivalents adjust for the lower bioavailability of food folate compared with that of folic acid. The tolerable upper intake level (UL) for adults is set at 1000 μg per day of folate from fortified food or as a supplement, exclusive of food folate. Folate is found in virtually all foods (see Table 1). Spinach, yeast, peanuts, liver, beans (such as kidney beans and lima beans), and broccoli are particularly rich sources. Folate in food usually is reduced, often is methylated, may be protein bound, and is in the polyglutamate form. Folate in foods may have a bioavailability of less than 50%. Folic acid supplements are in the monoglutamate form and have a bioavailability approaching 100%. Fortification of cereals and grain products with folic acid (140 μg/100 g) has been mandated in the United States since 1998 to prevent neural tube defects. There is a concern that excess fortification may be associated with an adverse outcome in individuals who have Cbl deficiency. The reduced folates in food are labile and readily lost under certain cooking conditions, such as boiling.

Physiology

Folate is absorbed by saturable and unsaturable mechanisms [82]. The saturable process is specific and occurs in the proximal small intestines. The specific absorption is mediated by the reduced folate carrier, which has a high affinity for reduced folates and is located in the cellular brush border membranes [83]. In the enterocyte, folate is converted into methylTHF and a carrier-mediated mechanism exports it into the bloodstream. Nonspecific, unsaturable absorption predominates in the ileum. The absorbed folate is cleared from the bloodstream and enters various compartments. The reduced folate carrier also is involved in cellular uptake of reduced folates in tissues. Cellular folate uptake also occurs nonspecifically via passive diffusion. Once internalized, folate undergoes polyglutamation that permits its attachment to enzymes. Polyglutamated folates have greater metabolic activity and are retained better by cells compared with monoglutamated folates [84]. Daily folate losses may approximate 1% to 2% of body stores. The ratio of body stores to daily requirement is 100:1 [82]. Therefore, a few months of poor nutrition can result in folate deficiency. Clinically significant depletion of normal folate stores may be seen within 3 months, more rapidly with low stores or coexisting alcoholism. Serum folate falls within 3 weeks of decrease in folate intake or absorption; RBC folate declines weeks to months later [85].

Causes of deficiency

Folate deficiency rarely exists in the pure state [82]. It often is associated with conditions that affect other nutrients. Hence, attribution of neurologic manifestations resulting from folate deficiency requires exclusion of other potential causes.

Marginal intake in association with conditions that compromise folate status, such as alcoholism, result in folate deficiency, particularly when hard liquor is consumed. Beer contains folate. Alcohol abuse affects enterohepatic recycling of Cbl, affects folate metabolism, forms aldehyde adducts with folates, and accelerates folate breakdown [86]. Other populations at increased risk of folate deficiency include premature infants and adolescents. Increased folate requirements also are seen in pregnancy, lactation, and chronic hemolytic anemia. Folate deficiency also may result from restricted diets, such as those used to manage phenylketonuria. Folate deficiency is seen with small bowel disorders associated with malabsorption, such as tropical sprue, celiac disease, and inflammatory bowel disease. Folate absorption may be decreased in conditions associated with reduced gastric secretions, such as gastric surgery (partial gastrectomy), atrophic gastritis, acid-suppressive therapy, and acid neutralization by treatment of pancreatic insufficiency [87–89].

Several drugs, such as aminopterin, methotrexate (amethopterin), pyrimethamine, trimethoprim, and triamterene, act as folate antagonists and produce folate deficiency by inhibiting dihydrofolate reductase [90]. The mechanism by which anticonvulsants, antituberculosis drugs, and oral contraceptives result in folate deficiency is uncertain.

Clinical significance

In adults who have acquired folate deficiency, neurologic manifestations are rare and mild. The reason for this is not clear, because methionine synthase requires folate as cosubstrate. The megaloblastic anemia resulting from folate deficiency is indistinguishable from that seen in Cbl deficiency.

The occurrence and frequency of neurologic manifestations of folate deficiency is a matter of debate [91]. It likely is less common compared with the myeloneuropathy and cognitive symptoms associated with Cbl deficiency. The myeloneuropathy or neuropathy seen in association with folate deficiency is indistinguishable from Cbl deficiency [92–96]. Folate deficiency is associated with affective disorders [97]. A low folate level may be seen in elderly asymptomatic individuals and more commonly with psychiatric disease and Alzheimer's dementia [98]. In recent years, there has been evidence that suggests that chronic folate deficiency may increase stroke risk and cause cognitive impairment [99]. The precise significance of these observations awaits further studies.

Congenital errors of folate metabolism can be related either to defective transport of folate through various cells or to defective intracellular use of folate resulting from some enzyme deficiencies. These often are associated with severe central neurologic dysfunction [100].

Metabolic folate deficiency, suggested by elevated plasma total Hcy levels that improve with folate therapy, can be seen in asymptomatic individuals [91]. The increased Hcy seen with folate deficiency is associated with an increased risk of cardiovascular and cerebrovascular disease [91]. In a recent study, moderate reduction of Hcy levels with folate, Cbl, and vitamin B_6 (B_6) had no effect on vascular outcomes in patients who had stroke at 2 years follow-up [101].

Investigations

Microbiologic assays for folate measurement largely have been replaced by radioisotopic assays. More recently, automated immunologic methods using chemiluminescence or other nonisotopic detection are used. Folate results are dependent on the method used and laboratory where they were performed [102]. Generally, serum folate, 2.5 µg/L, is taken as the cut-off for folate deficiency. Plasma Hcy levels are slightly elevated and respond to folate supplementation in persons who have folate levels as high as 5 µg/L [103]. This has led to the suggestion that serum folate levels between 2.5 and 5 µg/L may be indicative of a mildly compromised folate status. Serum folate fluctuates daily and does not correlate with tissue stores [104]. Erythrocyte folate is more reliable than plasma folate because its levels are less affected by short-term fluctuations in intake [105]. RBC folate assay, however, is subject to greater variation depending on the method and laboratory [102]. Reticulocytes have a higher folate content than mature RBCs. Their presence can affect RBC folate levels as can blood transfusions. Plasma Hcy levels are shown to be elevated in 86% of patients who have clinically significant folate deficiency [48].

Management

In women of childbearing age who have epilepsy, a daily folate supplement, 0.4 mg, is recommended for prophylaxis against neural tube defects.

With documented folate deficiency, an oral dosage, 1 mg 3 times a day, may be followed by a maintenance dosage, 1 mg a day. Acutely ill patients may need parenteral administration, 1 to 5 mg. Despite malabsorption, patients respond to oral folic acid because it is absorbed readily by nonspecific mechanisms. Even in high doses, toxicity resulting from folic acid is rare [106]. Doses higher than 1 mg need a prescription because of concerns regarding masking Cbl deficiency. Coexisting Cbl deficiency, therefore, should be ruled out before instituting folate therapy. Reduced folates, such as folinic acid (N5-formylTHF), is required only when folate metabolism is impaired by drugs, such as methotrexate, or by an inborn error of metabolism. In a patient therapy with subacute combined degeneration resulting from folate deficiency, methyl folate use was associated with a significant response [95]. Therapy with folic or folinic acid could be considered in patients who have folate deficiency who have neuropsychiatric symptoms, neuropathy or myelopathy, and normal B_{12} levels [90]. Plasma Hcy likely is the best biochemical tool for monitoring response to therapy; it decreases within a few days of instituting folate therapy but does not respond to inappropriate Cbl therapy [107]. Because folate deficiency generally is seen in association with a broader dietary inadequacy, the associated comorbidities need to be addressed.

Copper

Copper deficiency–associated myelopathy is described in various animal species [108]. Often seen in ruminants, it is referred to as swayback or enzootic ataxia. Menkes' disease is the copper deficiency–related disease in humans and is the result of congenital copper deficiency. Comparative pathologic studies show similarity between Menkes' disease and swayback [108]. Only in recent years have the neurologic manifestations of acquired copper deficiency in humans been recognized. The most common manifestation is that of a myelopathy or myeloneuropathy that resembles the subacute combined degeneration seen with Cbl deficiency [109,110].

Functions

Copper functions as a prosthetic group in several metalloenzymes, which act as oxidases [111,112]. Many of these have a critical role in maintaining the structure and function of the nervous system. Some of these include copper/zinc superoxide dismutase (antioxidant defense), cytochrome *c. oxidase* (ATP synthesis), dopamine β-monooxygenase (norepinephrine biosynthesis), tyrosinase (dopamine and melanin synthesis), peptidylglycine α-amidating monooxygenase (neuropeptide processing), ferroxidase I (ie, ceruloplasmin) and ferroxidase II (iron metabolism), hephaestatin (ferroxidase activity), and lysyl oxidase (cross-linkages of elastin and collagen for development of connective tissues).

Requirements and sources

The RDA of copper for adult men and women is 900 μg per day; the median intake of from food in the United States is 1.0 to 1.6 mg per day; and the UL is 10,000 μg per day [111]. Copper is distributed widely in foods. Foods rich in copper include organ meats, seafood, nuts, seeds, wheat bran cereals, whole grain products, and cocoa products (see Table 1). Foods with a low copper content include tea, potatoes, milk, and chicken.

Physiology

Copper absorption occurs primarily in the small intestine [112]. Some absorption may occur in the stomach where the acidic environment facilitates solubilization of copper by dissociating it from copper-containing dietary macromolecules. As dietary copper increases, the fraction absorbed declines and the amount absorbed increases. Absorption occurs by a saturable active transport process at lower levels of dietary copper and by passive diffusion at high levels of dietary copper. The Menkes P-type ATPase (ATP7A) is responsible for copper trafficking to the secretory pathway for efflux from enterocytes and other cells [113]. Absorbed copper is bound to albumin and transported via the portal vein to the liver for uptake by liver parenchymal cells. Copper then is released into the plasma. Ninety-five percent of the copper is bound to ceruloplasmin. The Wilson P-type ATPase (ATP7B) is responsible for copper trafficking to the secretory pathway for ceruloplasmin biosynthesis and for endosome formation before biliary secretion [113]. Biliary copper is adjusted to maintain balance. Urinary excretion normally is low, less than 0.1 mg per day. Excretion of copper into the gastrointestinal tract is the major pathway that regulates copper homeostasis and prevents deficiency or toxicity.

Causes of deficiency

Although rare, acquired copper deficiency is well documented in humans [112,114,115]. Because of copper's ubiquitous distribution and low daily requirement, acquired dietary copper deficiency is rare. Dietary factors may affect copper bioavailability. These include antacids, iron deficiency, ascorbic acid, and amount of copper, molybdenum, or zinc in the diet. Excessive zinc ingestion is a well-recognized cause of copper deficiency [116,117]. The zinc-induced inhibition of copper absorption could be the result of competition for a common transporter or a consequence of induction of metallothionein in enterocytes. Metallothionein has a higher binding affinity for copper than for zinc [118]. Copper is retained within the enterocytes and lost as the intestinal cells are sloughed off. It may occur in malnourished infants [119], nephrotic syndrome [120], and enteropathies associated with malabsorption [121]. Copper deficiency may be a complication of prolonged total parenteral nutrition [122], particularly when copper supplementation in total parenteral nutrition is withheld because of cholestasis [123]. Enteral feeding with inadequate copper also is known to result in copper deficiency [124]. Copper deficiency after gastric surgery (for peptic ulcer disease or bariatric surgery) increasingly is recognized [125–127]. Not infrequently, the cause of copper deficiency is unknown. Emerging knowledge about copper transport may help clarify the etiology of idiopathic hypocupremia [128].

Clinical significance

The most common neurologic manifestation is that of a myelopathy presenting with a spastic gait and prominent sensory ataxia resulting from dorsal column dysfunction [109,110,117,121,126,127,129,134]. The onset may be subacute. Also reported are central nervous system demyelination [135,136] and optic neuritis [137]. Hyperzincemia may be present even in the absence of exogenous zinc ingestion [109,110,130,131,136]. The precise significance of this is unclear. Copper and Cbl deficiency may coexist [109]. Continued neurologic deterioration in patients who have a history of Cbl deficiency–related myelopathy who have a normal B_{12} level on B_{12} replacement should be evaluated for copper deficiency. Clinical or electrophysiologic evidence of an associated peripheral neuropathy is common. Neurophysiologic studies show varying degrees of axonal peripheral neuropathy [138]. Abnormalities in somatosensory evoked potential studies indicating central conduction delay is a common finding [138]. Other reported electrophysiologic abnormalities noted in patients who have copper deficiency and neurologic manifestations include prolonged visual evoked potentials [135] and impaired central conduction on transcranial magnetic stimulation [129]. Spinal cord MRI in patients who have copper deficiency myelopathy may show increased signal on T2-weighted images, most commonly in the paramedian cervical cord (Fig. 2A, B) [133]. Follow-up imaging may show resolution of the dorsal column signal change with improvement in serum copper [133].

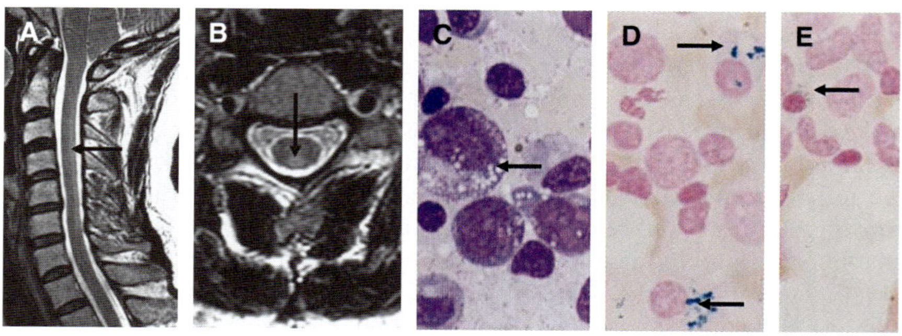

Fig. 2. Sagittal (*A*) and axial (*B*) T2-weighted MRI in a patient who had copper deficiency showing increased signal in the paramedian aspect of the dorsal cervical cord. (*From* Kumar N, Ahlskog JE, Klein CJ, et al. Imaging features of copper deficiency myelopathy: a study of 25 cases. Neuroradiology 2006;48:78–83; with permission [panels A–B]). Bone marrow study (*C–E*) in a patient who had copper deficiency myelopathy showing vacuolated myeloid precursors (*C*). Also shown is iron staining (*D* and *E*) showing iron-containing plasma cells (*D*) and ringed sideroblasts (*E*). (*Reprinted from* Kumar N. Copper deficiency myelopathy (human swayback). Mayo Clin Proc 2006;81(10):1371–84; with permission [panels C–D].)

The hematologic manifestations of acquired copper deficiency include anemia, neutropenia, and a left shift in granulocytic and erythroid maturation with vacuolated precursors, iron-containing plasma cells, and ringed sideroblasts in the bone marrow (see Fig. 2C–E) [116]. Patients may be given a diagnosis of sideroblastic anemia or myelodysplastic syndrome [116,132,137]. Thrombocytopenia and resulting pancytopenia are relatively rare [139]. The neurologic syndrome resulting from acquired copper deficiency may be present without the hematologic manifestations [109,117,140].

Investigations

Laboratory indicators of copper deficiency include serum copper or ceruloplasmin and urinary copper excretion but these parameters are not sensitive to marginal copper status. Changes in serum copper usually parallel the ceruloplasmin concentration. Ceruloplasmin is an acute-phase reactant and the rise in ceruloplasmin probably is responsible for the increase in serum copper seen in a variety of conditions, such as pregnancy, oral contraceptive use, liver disease, malignancy, hematologic disease, myocardial infections, smoking, diabetes, uremia, and various inflammatory and infections diseases [141]. Copper deficiency could be masked under these conditions. Urinary copper declines only when dietary copper is low [112]. It is suggested that serum copper may be inadequate for assessing total body copper stores and activity of copper enzymes, such as erythrocyte superoxide dismutase and platelet or leukocyte cytochrome c oxidase, may be a better indicator of metabolically active copper stores [142,143]. Red cell superoxide dismutase does not increase with other conditions that increase serum copper.

Treatment

With severe copper deficiency, serum copper and ceruloplasmin fall, often to low levels, and respond promptly to copper supplementation [115]. In patients who have zinc-induced copper deficiency, discontinuing the zinc may suffice and no additional copper supplementation may be required [144]. Despite a suspected absorption defect, oral copper supplementation generally is the preferred route of supplementation. Studies in yeast show that the copper transport pathways are high-affinity pathways, active in conditions of low copper concentration, and increasing the concentration of copper may result in the pathways being bypassed [128]. This may explain why in a majority of patients, normal serum copper levels can be achieved by increasing the amount of copper ingested. In most patients, oral administration, 2 mg of elemental copper a day, seems to suffice. A comparable dose of elemental copper may be given intravenously. At times, prolonged oral therapy may not result in improvement and parenteral therapy may be required. Some have used initial parenteral administration followed by oral therapy [134]. Commonly used copper salts include copper gluconate and copper chloride. A commonly used regimen is administration of elemental copper, 6 mg a day orally for a week, 4 mg a day for the second week, and 2 mg a day thereafter [110]. Alternatively, elemental copper, 2 mg, may be administered intravenously for 5 days and periodically thereafter. Periodic assessment of serum copper is essential to determine adequacy of replacement and to decide on the appropriate long-term maintenance.

Response of the hematologic parameters (including bone marrow findings) is prompt and often complete [109,110,116,124,131,132,137]. Hematologic recovery may be accompanied by reticulocytosis. Recovery of neurologic signs and symptoms seen in association with copper deficiency is variable. Improvement in neurologic symptoms generally is absent, although progression typically is halted [109,110,131,136]. Improvement when present is slight, often subjective, and preferentially involves sensory symptoms. Early recognition and prompt treatment may prevent significant neurologic morbidity.

Vitamin E

In humans, α-tocopherol is the active form of vitamin E. The terms, vitamin E and α-tocopherol, are used interchangeably. Vitamin E is the collective name for molecules with the antioxidant activity of α-tocopherol. The chemically synthesized α-tocopherol is not identical to the naturally occurring form. Vitamin E supplements contain esters of α-tocopherol, such as α-tocopheryl acetate, succinate, or nicotinate. The esters prevent vitamin E oxidation and prolong its shelf life. These esters are hydrolyzed readily in the gut and absorbed in the unesterified form [145]. The exception to this is in patients who have malabsorption.

Function

Vitamin E serves as an antioxidant and free radical scavenger. It prevents the formation of toxic free radical products, seems to protect cellular membranes from oxidative stress, and inhibits the peroxidation of polyunsaturated fatty acids of membrane phospholipids.

Requirements and sources

The RDA for men and women is 15 mg (35 μmol) per day of α-tocopheral [146]. The UL for adults is set at 1000 mg (2325 μmol) per day. Rich sources of vitamin E include vegetable oils, leafy vegetables, fruits, meats, nuts, and unprocessed cereal grains (see Table 1). The bioavailability of vitamin E is dependent on the fat content of food [147]. Vitamin E bioavailability from fortified breakfast cereal is greater than that from encapsulated supplements [148].

Physiology

The overall efficiency of vitamin E absorption is less than 50%. Vitamin E is absorbed from the gastrointestinal tract by a nonenergy-requiring diffusion mechanism. Vitamin E absorption requires bile acids, fatty acids, and monoglycerides for micelle formation. After uptake by enterocytes, all forms of dietary vitamin E are incorporated into chylomicrons. During chylomicron catabolism in plasma, vitamin E is transferred to circulating lipoproteins, which deliver it to tissues. The chylomicron remnants are taken up by the liver, which selects the α-tocopherol form for secretion in very low-density lipoproteins (VLDLs). In the liver, the α-tocopherol transfer protein (TTP) incorporates α-tocopherol into VLDLs, which are secreted into plasma. Lipolysis of VLDL results in enrichment of circulating lipoproteins with RRR-α-tocopherol, which is delivered to peripheral tissue. Most ingested vitamin E is eliminated by the fecal route. The majority of vitamin E in the human body is localized in the adipose tissue. Analysis of adipose tissue α-tocopherol content provides a useful estimate of long-term vitamin E intake. More than 2 years is required for adipose tissue α-/γ-tocopherol ratios to reach new steady-state levels in response to changes in dietary intake [149].

Causes of deficiency

Because of the ubiquitous distribution of tocopherols in foods, vitamin E deficiency virtually is never the consequence of a dietary inadequacy [150]. Vitamin E absorption requires biliary and pancreatic secretions. Hence, vitamin E deficiency is seen with chronic cholestasis and pancreatic insufficiency. Vitamin E deficiency also is seen with other conditions associated with malabsorption, such as celiac disease, Crohn's disease, cystic fibrosis, blind loop syndrome, and extensive small bowel resection. It is suggested that the vitamin E supplementation in total parenteral nutrition may be inadequate to maintain vitamin E stores [151].

Vitamin E deficiency may be seen resulting from genetic defects in α-TTP (ataxia with vitamin E deficiency [AVED]), in apolipoprotein B (homozygous hypobetalipoproteinemia), or in the microsomal triglyceride transfer protein (abetalipoproteinemia). An additional cause is defect in chylomicron synthesis and secretion (chylomicron retention disease). AVED is an autosomal recessive disorder in which isolated vitamin E deficiency occurs without generalized fat malabsorption or gastrointestinal disease. Mutations in the α-TTP gene on chromosome 8q13 are responsible [152,153]. The defect lies in impaired incorporation of vitamin E into hepatic lipoproteins for tissue delivery [154]. Patients who have hypobetalipoproteinemia or abetalipoproteinemia have an inability to secrete chylomicrons or other apolipoprotein B-containing lipoproteins, specifically VLDLs and low-density lipoproteins (LDLs) [150]. Homozygous hypobetalipoproteinemia patients have a defect in the apoB gene. ApoB-containing lipoproteins secreted into the circulation turn over rapidly. Abetalipoproteinemia patients have a genetic defect in microsomal triglyceride transfer protein, which prevents normal lipidation of apoB, and the secretion of apoB-containing lipoproteins is nonexistent. In chylomicron retention disease, there is impaired assembly and secretion of chylomicrons and chylomicron retention in the intestinal mucosa is present [155].

Clinical significance

The neurologic manifestations of vitamin E deficiency include a spinocerebellar syndrome with variable peripheral nerve involvement [156–158]. The phenotype is similar to that of Friedreich's ataxia. The clinical features include ataxia, hyporeflexia, and proprioceptive and vibratory loss. Cutaneous sensations may be affected to a lesser degree. Findings suggestive of cerebellar involvement include dysarthria, tremor, and nystagmus. Ophthalmoplegia, ptosis, and pigmentary retinopathy are reported. An associated myopathy may be present [159,160]. It is rare for vitamin E deficiency to present as an isolated neuropathy [161]. Somatosensory evoked potential studies may show evidence of central delay and nerve conduction studies may show evidence of an axonal neuropathy [162,163]. Spinal MRI in patients who have vitamin E deficiency–related myeloneuropathy may show increased signal in the cervical cord dorsal column [164]. In children who have cholestatic liver disease, neurologic abnormalities appear as early as the second year of life. In AVED, hypolipoproteinemia, and abetalipoproteinemia, neurologic manifestations start by the first or second decade. Development of neurologic symptoms in adults who have acquired fat malabsorption syndromes takes decades.

The neuropathy associated with vitamin E deficiency preferentially involves centrally directed fibers of large myelinated neurons. Loss of myelinated nerve fibers may be seen on sural nerve biopsy before onset of neurologic signs and symptoms [165]. Reduction of peripheral nerve tocopherol may precede the axonal degeneration [166]. Swollen dystrophic axons (spheroids) are seen in the gracile and cuneate nuclei of the brainstem. Lipofuscin may accumulate in the dorsal sensory neurons and peripheral Schwann's cell cytoplasm. The peripheral nerves, posterior columns, and sensory roots show degeneration of large myelinated fibers.

Investigations

Serum vitamin E levels are dependent on the concentrations of serum lipids, cholesterol, and VLDL. Hyperlipidemia or hypolipidemia independently can increase or decrease serum vitamin E without reflecting similar alterations in tissue levels of the vitamin [167]. Effective serum α-tocopherol concentrations are calculated by dividing the serum α-tocopherol by the sum of serum cholesterol and triglycerides [168,169]. Serum α-tocopherol concentrations may be in the normal range in patients who have α-tocopherol deficiency resulting from cholestatic liver disease, a disorder that also is associated with high lipid levels [170]. In patients who have neurologic manifestations resulting from vitamin E deficiency, the serum vitamin E levels frequently are undetectable. Additional markers of fat malabsorption, such as increased stool fat and decreased serum carotene levels, may be present.

Management

In patients who have vitamin E deficiency resulting from cholestasis and malabsorption, large oral dosages (up to 200 IU/kg per day) [54] or intramuscular administration of dl-α-tocopherol (0.8 to 2.0 IU/kg per day) are used [171]. In patients who have cystic fibrosis and who are receiving oral pancreatic enzyme therapy, dosages of 5 to 10 IU/kg per day are sufficient [54]. With cholestatic liver disease, treatment with fat-soluble vitamin E may be ineffective because of fat malabsorption. A water-miscible product, d-α-tocopherol glycol 1000 succinate, is shown to raise plasma and tissue levels of α-tocopherol to normal [172]. The target should be a normal ratio of α-tocopherol to total lipids. Because of limited absorption, patients who have abetalipoproteinemia may need high doses [173]. Plasma α-tocopherol levels are not affected significantly but measurement of adipose tissue levels show the increased concentration [174]. In AVED, supplementation with vitamin E (600 IU twice daily) raises plasma concentration to normal and is accompanied by beneficial effects on neurologic function. An empiric approach is to start with a lower dose, increase it gradually, and, based on the clinical and laboratory responses, consider a higher dose or parenteral formulation. Supplements of bile salts may be of value in some patients.

Thiamine

Beriberi has the distinction of being the first-identified human nutritional deficiency disorder. During the industrial revolution of the nineteenth century, introduction of milled rice was accompanied by epidemics of beriberi [54]. A connection between the consumption of polished rice and beriberi was shown in the latter part of the nineteenth century. In the 1950s, universal enrichment of rice, grains, and flour products with thiamine was successful in achieving significant worldwide control. The terms vitamin B_1 (B_1) and thiamine are used interchangeably.

Function

Thiamine functions as a coenzyme in the metabolism of carbohydrates and branched-chain amino acids [175]. After cellular uptake, thiamine is phosphorylated into thiamine diphosphate (TDP), the metabolically active form that is involved in several enzyme systems. TDP is a cofactor for the pyruvate dehydrogenase complex, α-ketoglutarate dehydrogenase (α-KGDH), and transketolase (TK). Pyruvate dehydrogenase and α-KGDH are involved in the oxidative decarboxylation of α-ketoacids, such as pyruvate and α-ketoglutarate, to acetyl-CoA and succinate, respectively. TK transfers activated aldehydes in the hexose monophosphate shunt in the generation of nicotinamide adenine dinucleotide phosphate for reductive biosynthesis. Thiamine deficiency results in reduced synthesis of high-energy phosphates and lactate accumulation. It is suggested that decreased α-KGDH, rather than decreased pyruvate dehydrogenase complex, constitutes the "biochemical lesion" in thiamine deficiency encephalopathy [176]. α-KGDH is the rate-limiting enzyme in the tricarboxylic acid cycle. Decreased activity of α-KGDH results in decreased synthesis of amino acid neurotransmitters, such as glutamate and γ-aminobutyric acid [177]. TDP may be phosphorylated further to thiamine triphosphate, which may activate high-conductance chloride channels and have a role in regulating cholinergic neurotransmission because of its regulatory properties on proteins involved in the clustering of acetylcholine receptors [178].

Requirements and sources

The RDA for adults is 1.2 mg per day for men and 1.1 mg per day for women [175,179]. The median intake of thiamine from food in the United States is approximately 2 mg per day. The highest concentrations of thiamine are found in yeast and in the pericarp of grain. Most cereals and breads are fortified with thiamine. Organ meats are a good source of thiamine. Dairy products, seafood, and fruits are poor sources. Thiamine does not occur in fats and oils. Prolonged cooking of food, baking of bread, and pasteurization of milk all are potential causes of thiamine loss.

Physiology

At low concentrations, thiamine is absorbed in jejunum and ileum by active transport [175]. At higher concentration absorption takes place by passive diffusion. After gastrointestinal uptake, thiamine is transported by portal blood to the liver. The areas most vulnerable to thiamine deficiency are those with the highest turnover rates, such as the caudal brain and cerebellum [180]. The half-life of thiamine is only 10 to 14 days [54]. Because of the rapid turnover rates and absence of significant storage amounts, a continuous dietary supply of thiamine is necessary. A thiamine-deficient diet may result in manifestations of thiamine deficiency in just 18 days [181].

Causes of deficiency

Causes of thiamine deficiency include decreased intake, decreased absorption, defective transport, increased losses, and enhanced requirements [162,175,179,182]. Thiamine deficiency may be seen with persistent vomiting, anorexia nervosa, dieting, malnutrition, severe gastrointestinal or liver disease, gastrointestinal surgery (including bariatric surgery), and AIDS. Thiamine deficiency in alcoholism results from inadequate dietary intake, reduced gastrointestinal absorption, and reduced liver thiamine stores. Additionally, alcohol inhibits transport of thiamine in the gastrointestinal system and blocks phosphorylation of thiamine to TDP [183]. Thiamine requirement is dependent on the body's metabolic rate with the requirement being the greatest during periods of high metabolic demand or high glucose intake. Symptoms of thiamine deficiency may be seen in high-risk patients during periods of vigorous exercise and high carbohydrate intake as with intravenous glucose administration and refeeding. In patients who have a marginal nutritional status, increased metabolic demand, as is seen in hyperthyroidism, malignancy, and systemic infections, may precipitate symptoms. Pregnant and lactating women have increased thiamine requirements and infant beriberi may be seen in infants who are breastfed by thiamine-deficient asymptomatic mothers. Maternal thiamine deficiency may result from eating a staple diet of polished rice with foods containing thiaminase or antithiamine compounds.

Clinical significance

The best-characterized human neurologic disorders related to thiamine deficiency are beriberi, Wernicke encephalopathy (WE), and Korsakoff's syndrome (KS). The three forms of beriberi are dry beriberi, wet beriberi, and infantile beriberi [175]. Dry beriberi is characterized by a sensorimotor, distal, axonal peripheral neuropathy often associated with calf cramps, muscle tenderness, and burning feet [184,185]. Autonomic neuropathy may be present. A rapid progression of the neuropathy may mimic Guillain-Barré syndrome (GBS) [185]. Classic descriptions report hoarseness and tongue and facial weakness [54]. Pathologic studies of beriberi in nonalcoholics are limited [163,184,186]. Axonal degeneration is noted in distal nerves. Chromatolysis of dorsal root ganglion (DRG) neurons and anterior horn cell (AHC) neurons may be seen resulting from axonal degeneration. Segmental demyelination is rare and likely secondary to axonal degeneration. Severe cases may have involvement of the vagus and phrenic nerves. Degeneration of the posterior columns may be present. Pedal edema may be seen resulting from coexisting wet beriberi. Wet beriberi is associated with a high-output congestive heart failure with peripheral neuropathy. This distinction is of limited significance, because the wet form may be converted to the dry form after diuresis. Shoshin beriberi is the name given to a fulminant form that presents with tachycardia and circulatory collapse. Acute quadriplegia resulting from central-pontine myelinolysis is reported in Shoshin beriberi [187]. Although called infantile beriberi, it bears little resemblance to the adult form. Infantile beriberi is seen between 2 and 6 months of age and may present with the cardiac, aphonic, or pseudomeningitic forms [175].

The clinical features of WE include a subacute onset of ocular palsies, nystagmus, gait ataxia, and confusion [162,188]. Involvement of the hypothalamic and brainstem autonomic pathways may be associated with hypothermia and orthostatic hypotension. Skin changes, tongue redness, features of liver disease, and truncal ataxia may be present. More than 80% of patients may have an associated peripheral neuropathy. Reliance on the described triad of ophthalmoplegia, ataxia, and confusion and not recognizing thiamine deficiency in nonalcoholics may result in missing the diagnosis [182]. Typical MRI findings include increased T2 or proton density or diffusion-weighted imaging signal around the third ventricle, periaqueductal midbrain, dorsomedial thalami, and mamillary bodies [189]. Rarely, symmetric cortical involvement with contrast enhancement may occur [190]. The signal abnormalities resolve with treatment but shrunken mamillary bodies may persist as sequelae. The frequency of WE in various autopsy studies ranges from 0.8% to 2.8%, far in excess from what is expected from clinical studies [182,191,192]. In one series, only 20% of the cases were diagnosed during life [192]. Sudden death may occur and is related to hemorrhagic brainstem lesions [193]. In some autopsy-confirmed cases of WE, the only clinical manifestation was that of psychomotor retardation [194]. KS is an amnestic-confabulatory syndrome that follows WE and emerges as ocular manifestations and encephalopathy subside. Rarely, KS may be present without WE or may be present at the time of diagnosis of WE. Neuropathologic findings in WE include symmetric lesions of the periventricular regions of the thalamus and hypothalamus, nuclei at the level of the third and fourth ventricle, and superior cerebellar vermis [195,196]. Involvement of the mammillary bodies is characteristic. Histology shows necrosis, neuronal loss, edema, prominent capillaries with endothelial proliferation, and hemorrhagic foci. In the late stages, there is cell loss with astrocytic and microglial proliferation. Patients who have KS also have involvement of the dorsal median nucleus of the thalamus.

Investigations

Urinary thiamine excretion and serum thiamine levels may be decreased but do not reflect tissue concentrations accurately and are not reliable indicators of thiamine status. The preferred tests are the erythrocyte transketolase activation assay or measurement of TDP in RBC hemolysates using high-performance liquid chromatography [197,198]. The erythrocyte transketolase activation assay is an assay of functional status and is based on measurement of transketolase activity in hemolysates of RBCs in the absence of (and in the presence of) added excess cofactor (TDP). Because these laboratory abnormalities normalize quickly, a blood sample should be drawn before initiation of treatment.

Management

Intravenous glucose infusion in patients who have thiamine deficiency may consume the available thiamine and precipitate an acute WE. At-risk patients should receive parenteral thiamine before administration of glucose or parenteral nutrition. Patients suspected of having beriberi or WE should receive parenteral thiamine promptly. The recommended dose of thiamine in beriberi is 100 mg intravenously followed by 100 mg intramuscularly daily for 5 days and permanent oral maintenance [196]. At times, high-dosage thiamine (100 mg intravenously every 8 hours) may be required [190]. The parenteral form is used when there is doubt about adequate gastrointestinal absorption. Oral maintenance, 50- to 100-mg thiamine, is used. A lipophilic form of thiamine (benfotiamine) is used in chronic alcoholism-related neuropathy, 320 mg per day for 4 weeks followed by 120 mg per day for an additional 3 weeks [199].

In wet beriberi, a rapid improvement is seen with clearing of symptoms within 24 hours to 1 week [184]. Improvement in motor and sensory symptoms takes weeks or months [184,185]. Response in WE is variable. Apathy and lethargy improve over days or weeks. Even with thiamine treatment, the mortality is 10% to 20%. As the global confusional state recedes, some patients are left with KS: a disorder of impaired memory and learning. Ophthalmoplegia improves rapidly (ie, ocular signs improve in a few hours) [200]. A fine horizontal nystagmus may persist in 60% of patients. Improvement in gait ataxia and memory is variable and often delayed [201].

Niacin

Function

Niacin in humans is an end product of tryptophan metabolism. It is converted into nicotinamide adenine dinucleotide and nicotinamide adenine dinucleotide phosphate. Both are coenzymes important in carbohydrate metabolism.

Requirements and sources

Dietary requirements of niacin consider the tryptophan and niacin content [202]. The RDA for adults is 16 mg per day of niacin equivalent for men and 14 mg per day of niacin equivalent for women. One mg of niacin equivalent equals 51 mg of niacin or 60 mg of tryptophan. The median intake of preformed niacin is approximately 28 mg for men and 18 mg for women. The UL for niacin in adults is 35 mg per day and is based on flushing as the critical side effect. In most developed countries, niacin commonly is added as an enrichment to bread. Most niacin intake comes from meat, fish, poultry, enriched and whole grain bread and bread products, and fortified ready-to-eat cereals (see Table 1).

Physiology

Niacin and its amide are absorbed through the intestinal mucosa by simple diffusion [203]. Fifteen percent to 30% of niacin is protein bound. Complexed and free niacin are taken up by tissue. Niacin is retained by metabolic trapping to nicotinamide adenine dinucleotide. Niacin and nicotinamide are metabolized by separate pathways. The major metabolite of niacin is nicotinuric acid and the major metabolite of nicotinamide is N^1-methylnicotinamide and its oxidized products, 2- and 4-pyridones.

Causes of deficiency

Pellagra is rare in developed countries [203]. Niacin deficiency is seen predominantly in populations dependent on corn as the primary carbohydrate source. Corn lacks niacin and tryptophan. Nonendemic pellagra rarely is seen with alcoholism and malabsorption. Pellagra may be seen in the carcinoid syndrome, because tryptophan is converted to serotonin instead of being used in niacin synthesis. Biotransformation of tryptophan to nicotinic acid requires several vitamins and minerals, such as B_2, B_6, iron, and copper. Because tryptophan is necessary for niacin synthesis, B_6 deficiency can result in secondary niacin deficiency. Diets deficient in these nutrients can predispose to pellagra. INH depletes B_6 and can trigger pellagra. Excess of neutral amino acids in the diet, such as leucine, can compete with tryptophan for uptake and predispose to niacin deficiency by impairing its synthesis from tryptophan. Hartnup syndrome is an autosomal recessive disorder characterized by impaired synthesis of niacin from tryptophan and results in pellagra-like symptoms.

Clinical significance

Pellagra affects the gastrointestinal tract, skin, and nervous system [202,203]. The classical hallmarks of pellagra are alluded to by mnemonic dermatitis, diarrhea, and dementia. Skin changes include a reddish-brown hyperkeratotic rash, which has a predilection for the face, chest, and dorsum of the hands and feet. Gastrointestinal manifestations include anorexia, abdominal pain, diarrhea, and stomatitis. The neurologic syndrome resulting from niacin deficiency is not well characterized. Reported cases are confounded by the presence of coexisting nutrient deficiencies, as is common in alcoholics. Reported manifestations include a confusional state which may progress to coma, spasticity, and myoclonus. Unexplained progressive encephalopathy in alcoholics that is not responsive to thiamine should raise the possibility of pellagra. The peripheral neuropathy seen in pellagra is indistinguishable from the peripheral neuropathy seen with thiamine deficiency and may be the result of deficiencies of other vitamins, likely B-group, because it does not respond to niacin supplementation alone [54,202,204,205].

Investigations

The most reliable and sensitive measures of niacin status are urinary excretion of the methylated metabolites, N^1-methylnicotinamide and its 2-pyridone derivative (N^1-methyl-2-pyridone-5-carboxamide) [202]. There are no sensitive and specific blood measures of niacin status. It is suggested that measures of erythrocyte nicotinamide adenine dinucleotide and plasma metabolites may serve as markers of niacin status.

Management

Oral nicotinic acid (50 mg 3 times a day) or parenteral doses (25 mg 3 times a day) are used for treatment of symptomatic patients [162]. Nicotinamide has comparable therapeutic efficacy in pellagra. Advanced stages of pellagra can be cured with intramuscular nicotinamide (50 to 100 mg 3 times a day for 3 to 4 days followed by similar quantities orally) [203].

Vitamin B_6

The term pyridoxine generally is used interchangeably with B_6. Pyridoxal and pyridoxamine are two other naturally occurring compounds that have comparable biologic activity. All three compounds are converted readily to pyridoxal phosphate (PLP).

Function

B_6 is essential for cellular functions and growth because of its involvement in important metabolic reactions [206]. PLP serves as a coenzyme in many reactions involved in the metabolism of amino acids, lipids, nucleic acid, and one-carbon units, in the pathways of gluconeogenesis, and in neurotransmitter and heme biosynthesis. The interconversion and metabolism of B_6 is dependent on riboflavin, niacin, and zinc. Niacin, carnitine, and folate require B_6 for their metabolism.

Requirements and sources

The RDA for young adults is 1.3 mg; the median intake of B_6 from food in the United States is approximately 2 mg per day for men and 1.4 mg per day for women; and the UL for adults is 100 mg per day [207]. Meat, fish, eggs, soybeans, nuts, and dairy products are rich in B_6. Starchy vegetables, noncitrus foods, and whole grain cereal products are additional sources. Milling of grain, cooking, and thermal processing can result in significant losses (see Table 1).

Physiology

Humans and other mammals cannot synthesize B_6 and, thus, must obtain this micronutrient from exogenous sources via intestinal absorption [206]. B_6 uptake by intestinal epithelial cells occurs by a carrier-mediated, pH-dependent mechanism that has saturable and nonsaturable components [208]. B_6 (mostly in the form of pyridoxal) enters the portal circulation and is transported bound to albumin in plasma and hemoglobin in RBCs. Absorbed dietary pyridoxine, pyridoxal, and pyridoxamine are phosphorylated for metabolic trapping. Tissue uptake of B_6 from circulation requires dephosphorylation. PLP and pyridoxal are the main circulating forms of B_6.

Causes of deficiency

Most diets are adequate in B_6 [206]. Its deficiency is seen with B_6 antagonists, such as INH, cycloserine, hydralazine, and penicillamine [209]. Alcohol intake antagonizes B_6 status through production of acetaldehyde, which competes with PLP for binding sites of PLP-dependent enzymes [210]. Individuals at risk of developing B_6 deficiency include pregnant and lactating women and elderly individuals. Plasma PLP levels are reduced in celiac disease, inflammatory bowel disease, and renal disease.

Clinical significance

Dietary deficiency of pyridoxine or congenital dependency on pyridoxine may manifest as infantile seizures. Adults are more tolerant of pyridoxine deficiency. Even with low levels, symptoms are rare. Chronic B_6 deficiency results in a microcytic hypochromic anemia. A form of sideroblastic anemia can be treated with pyridoxine supplementation [211]. Neuropathic symptoms in association with pellagra-like dermatitis are described in association with use of the B_6 antagonist desoxypyridoxine [212]. INH use is associated with painful distal paresthesias that can progress rapidly to limb weakness and sensory ataxia [213]. INH-associated neuropathy is dose related. Up to 50% of slow activators may develop a peripheral neuropathy when treated with INH [162]. Axonal degeneration and regeneration affect myelinated and unmyelinated fibers [214]. Excess consumption of B_6 is associated with a pure sensory peripheral neuropathy or ganglionopathy [215,216]. It is characterized by sensory ataxia, areflexia, impaired cutaneous and deep sensations, and positive Romberg's sign. The site of lesion most likely is the dorsal root ganglia. The presence of Lhermitte's sign in some patients suggests involvement of the spinal cord also [54]. The risk of developing this decreases at dosages less than 100 mg per day [207].

Investigations

Microbiologic assays measure total B_6 [207]. High-performance liquid chromatography methods allow estimation of the various forms of B_6. B_6 status can be assessed by measuring its levels in the blood or urine. The most commonly used measure is plasma PLP. A plasma PLP concentration of over 30 nmol/L is considered to indicate adequate status [217]. A concentration greater than 20 nmol/L is considered a more conservative cut-off value [207]. Functional indicators of B_6 status are based on PLP-dependent reactions. The methionine load test is used as a functional indicator of B_6 status. B_6 deficiency results in a higher postmethionine-load Hcy concentration resulting from impairment of the transsulfuration pathway. B_6 deficiency has little effect on fasting plasma Hcy concentration.

Management

INH-induced neuropathy is reversible by drug discontinuation or B_6 supplementation [216]. B_6 may be supplemented, 50 to 100 mg per day, to prevent development of the neuropathy. In an isolated report, peripheral neuropathy symptoms associated with hemodialysis were ameliorated with supplemental pyridoxine (250 mg per day) [218]. The neuropathy resulting from B_6 toxicity may reverse once the supplementation is withdrawn. Patients who have congenital dependency on pyridoxine develop symptoms despite a normal dietary supplementation of pyridoxine. High doses of B_6 are required and even after years and seizures reappear within days of B_6 withdrawal.

Bartiatric surgery

Types of surgeries

The epidemic of obesity and limited efficacy of medical treatments have led to increasing use of bariatric surgical procedures for the treatment of medically complicated obesity. Several different surgical procedures are used [219–222]. The earliest surgical treatments for obesity were malabsorptive procedures, such as the jejunocolic shunt and jejunoileal bypass. These operations were abandoned because of severe metabolic derangements and associated malnutrition, which required revision surgeries in many patients. Gastric restriction procedures used have included gastric partitioning, gastroplasty, and vertical banded gastroplasty. These procedures separate the stomach into a small pouch that empties into the greater stomach through a narrow channel, thus restricting the quantity and rate of food ingested without affecting digestion or absorption. The weight loss after these procedures, however, has not been found to be sustained either because the surgical technique was not durable or because patients developed maladaptive eating behaviors that circumvented the restriction. Gastric bypass procedures result in weight loss by a more physiologic mechanism. They restrict the volume ingested, cause partial malabsorption of fat, and induce a dumping syndrome with a high-carbohydrate meal, thus leading to sustained weight loss. The Roux-en-Y gastric bypass often is the procedure of choice and often is done laparoscopically. Recently, a laparoscopically placed adjustable gastric band has gained popularity. This procedure differs from previously performed restrictive procedures in that there is adjustment of the band in response to rate of weight loss and absence of an enterotomy or permanent change to the anatomy. Additional procedures that result in greater degrees of maldigestion and malabsorption combined with partial gastric resection are advocated for the treatment of patients who have “super” obesity (body mass index over 50 kg/m^2). These include distal gastric bypass, biliopancreatic diversion with duodenal switch modification, partial biliopancreatic bypass, and very, very long limb Roux-en-Y gastric bypass.

Vitamin deficiencies

B_{12} deficiency is the most common nutritional deficiency noted after bariatric surgery [16,223–228]. A low B_{12} level has been noted in 70% of patients undergoing gastric bypass surgery and B_{12} deficiency in nearly 40% [227]. It may result from inadequate intake, impaired hydrolysis of B_{12} from dietary protein, or abnormal IF and B_{12} interaction [16,224–226]. B1 deficiency frequently is seen [223,229]. B_1 deficiency after bariatric surgery is the result ofintractable vomiting, rapid weight loss, and inadequate vitamin repletion and associated neurologic complications due to B_1 deficiency, such as WE, and peripheral neuropathy may be seen as early as 6 weeks after gastric surgery [230,231]. Also recognized are deficiencies in other vitamins, such as folate [16,223,227] and vitamin D [232–234].

Mineral deficiencies

The most commonly identified mineral that is deficient after bariatric surgery is iron, seen in nearly half of patients [16,225,227]. Aches and pains occurring after 1 year of bypass surgery has been called "bypass bone disease" and is believed the result of bone demineralization from impaired calcium absorption, often with concurrent vitamin D deficiency [225]. Other identified minerals that are deficient include copper [125–127] and potassium [16].

Abnormal fat and carbohydrate metabolism

Reports of neurologic disorders after bariatric surgery resulting from rapid fat metabolism are of uncertain significance [235,236]. Recurrent spells of encephalopathy with lactic acidosis after high-carbohydrate diets arereported after jejunoileostomy [237]. The elevated D-lactate is believed to result from fermentation of carbohydrates in the colon or bypasses segment of the small bowel.

Types and frequency of neurologic complications

Neurologic complications after gastrectomy for ulcer disease or bariatric surgery are well recognized but frequently the cause is not determined [229,235,236,238–242]. Neurologic complications may be noted in 5% to 16% of patients undergoing surgery for obesity [229,240]. Specific vitamin and mineral deficiencies are identified after bariatric surgery. Central and peripheral neurologic complications often are multifactorial in etiology.

A recent review of reported cases of neurologic complications of bariatric surgery identified 96 patients [243]. A peripheral neuropathy was identified in 60 and encephalopathy in 30. Among the patients who had peripheral neuropathy, 40 had a polyneuropathy and 18 had a mononeuropathy. Lumbar plexopathy or radiculopathy were rare and each seen in one case only. Forty of the polyneuropathy cases were attributed to thiamine deficiency. Wernicke-Korsakoff syndrome or WE was identified in 27 cases, optic nerve involvement was identified in eight, a myelopathy in two, and primary muscle disease in seven.

In a controlled retrospective study of peripheral neuropathy after bariatric surgery, peripheral neuropathy developed in 71 of 435 patients: sensory-predominant polyneuropathy in 27, mononeuropathy in 39, and radiculoplexopathy in five [240]. A rapid progression of the peripheral neuropathy may mimic GBS [244]. The neuropathy after bariatric surgery may mimic a sensory ganglionopathy [235].

Risk factors for neurologic complications after bariatric surgery

Risk factors for neurologic complications include rate and absolute amount of weight loss, prolonged gastrointestinal symptoms, not attending a nutritional clinic after bariatric surgery, less vitamin and mineral supplementation, reduced serum albumin and transferrin, postoperative surgical complications requiring hospitalization, and having jejunoileal bypass [240]. In a series of 23 patients who had neurologic complications associated with bariatric surgery, protracted vomiting was noted in all affected patients [229].

Management

Prevention, diagnosis, and treatment of these disorders are necessary parts of lifelong care after bariatric surgery [245]. Long-term follow-up with dietary counseling is important. All bariatric surgery patients should have 6-month follow-up laboratory studies that include complete blood count, serum iron, iron-binding capacity, B_{12}, calcium, and alkaline phosphatase [225,246]. It is unclear which patients may develop copper deficiency after gastric surgery and if routine screening and supplementation should be considered. Oral supplementation containing the RDA for micronutrients can prevent abnormal blood indicators of most vitamins and minerals but are insufficient to maintain normal plasma B_{12} levels in approximately 30% of gastric bypass patients [228]. Multivitamins with mineral supplements may not prevent development of iron deficiency or subsequent anemia [247]. Indefinite use of the following daily supplements is suggested [225]: a multivitamin-mineral combination containing B_{12}, folic acid, vitamin D, and iron; an additional iron tablet, preferably with vitamin C; an additional B_{12} tablet of 50 to 100 μg; and a calcium supplement equivalent to 1 g of elemental calcium.

Other considerations

Alcoholic neuropathy

The direct role of alcohol in the pathogenesis of neuropathy related to chronic alcoholism has been a matter of debate [248]. The peripheral neuropathy associated with alcoholism generally is considered nutritional in origin [249]. Even though a specific nutrient often is not implicated, deficiencies in B-group vitamins, in particular thiamine, are believed the main cause. Alcohol displaces food in the diet, increases the demand for B-group vitamins, causes decreased absorption of lipid soluble vitamins resulting from pancreatic dysfunction, and possibly has a role as a secondary neurotoxin [196]. A slowly progressive, distally predominant, painful, symmetric, sensorimotor, axonal neuropathy is the typical finding [250,251]. Midline cerebellar degeneration may be an additional cause of gait ataxia.

Some patients may have a subacute presentation that mimics GBS [252]. Trophic skin changes and a distal neuropathic arthropathy may be present. It is likely that in at least a subgroup of patients the direct toxic effects of alcohol are responsible [250,251,253,254]. These patients may have a painful sensory neuropathy with autonomic involvement [251,253]. The presence of a vagal neuropathy may be associated with a higher mortality [255].

Tropical neuropathies and myeloneuropathies

There are many descriptions of neuropathies and myeloneuropathies from the tropics for which a nutritional cause has been postulated [196]. "Burning feet" were described first in 1826 by a British medical officer in the Indian army. Conditions described in the late nineteenth century included Strachan's Jamaican neuropathy, Cuban retrobulbar optic neuropathy, and the Cuban "amblyopia of the blockade." Similar disorders were reported among prisoners of war in tropical and subtropical regions during World War II and in victims of the Spanish Civil War. The term "happy feet" was used to describe similar symptoms in prisoners of war in camps in the tropics in World War II. Restoration of a normal diet and vitamin supplementation improved symptoms but often some deficits remained. Lack of multiple dietary components, in particular B-group vitamins, likely was the cause.

More recently, from 1991 to 1994, an epidemic in Cuba affected more than 50,000 persons and caused optic neuropathy, sensorineural deafness, dorsolateral myelopathy, and axonal sensory neuropathy [256,257]. Identified risk factors included irregular diet, weight loss, smoking, alcohol, and excessive sugar consumption [257]. Patients responded to B-group vitamins and folic acid. Overt malnutrition was not present.

The term, tropical myeloneuropathies, had been used to describe two major groups of conditions: patients who have prominent sensory ataxia (tropical ataxic neuropathy) and those who have prominent spastic paraparesis (tropical spastic paraparesis [TSP]). Human T-lymphotropic virus (HTLV)-I myelitis had been called TSP in many equatorial regions and HTLV-I–associated myelopathy (HAM) in Japan. HAM and TSP now are believed to be identical syndromes [258]. HTLV-II also is recognized to cause a chronic myelopathy that resembles TSP [259] or tropical ataxic neuropathy [260].

Organophosphate toxicity

Triorthocresyl phosphate is an organophosphate compound that has been used as an adulterant. In 1930, thousands of Americans developed neurologic deficits after consuming a popular illicit alcoholic beverage (Jamaica ginger extract or "jake") that had been adulterated with triorthocresyl phosphate [261]. Jamaican ginger paralysis was associated with peripheral neuropathy and spastic paraparesis.

An outbreak of acute polyneuropathy occurred in a tea plantation in Sri Lanka during 1977 to 1978 affecting adolescent girls [262]. The cause was attributed to tricresyl phosphate, which was present as a contaminant in a type of cooking oil that, because of its presumed nutritive value, was given in large amounts to pubertal girls in the postmenarche period. Contamination likely occurred when the oil was transported in containers previously used to store mineral oils. Sensory abnormalities were minimal. A distal axonopathy and pyramidal tract dysfunction were present. Significant improvement was noted over a 3-year period [263].

Organophosphate-induced delayed neurotoxicity (OPIDN) is a well-recognized complication of organophosphorus compounds [264]. OPIDN occurs 1 to 3 weeks after acute exposure and after a more uncertain duration after chronic exposure. The symptoms include distal paresthesias, progressive leg weakness, and cramping muscle pain. Distal weakness and wasting is seen. There may be evidence of upper limb involvement and central nervous system dysfunction. Sensory loss when present is mild. The RBC cholinesterase activity is depressed less rapidly than the serum cholinesterase activity and is a measure of chronic exposure to organophosphates [265]. Most modern organophosphate pesticides do not cause the delayed neurotoxic syndrome. OPIDN is the result of phosphorylation and subsequent aging of a protein neurotoxic esterase in the nervous system [266]. The signs and symptoms of acute organophosphate toxicity are the result of acetylcholinesterase inhibition and resulting muscarinic and nicotinic dysfunction. In some patients, after resolution of the cholinergic crisis, an intermediate syndrome develops [267]. This is characterized by weakness of neck flexors and proximal limb and respiratory muscles. This weakness may relate to depolarization blockade at the neuromuscular junction.

Prevention of organophosphate insecticide toxicity requires good occupational practices, including use of gloves and protective clothing. Pralidoxime is a reactivator of inhibited acetylcholinesterase and is the specific antidote for organophosphate poisoning. It is used in conjunction with atropine in the acute stages.

Lathyrism

Lathyrus sativus (grass pea or chickling pea) is an environmentally tolerant legume that resists drought conditions. Lathyrism is a self-limiting neurotoxic disorder that presents as a spastic paraparesis and afflicts individuals who consume *L sativus* as a staple. It is endemic in parts of Bangladesh, India, and Ethiopia. The spastic paraparesis is associated with greatly increased tone in thigh extensors, thigh adductors, and gastrocnemius, leading to a lurching scissoring gait characterized by patients walking on the balls of their feet [268]. Sensory symptoms may be reported at onset in the legs. In individuals who are affected severely, pyramidal signs also may be present in the upper limbs. The onset may be abrupt, subacute, or insidious. An early improvement in limb strength is seen and may be substantial. In the early stages, there may be diffuse and transitory central nervous system excitation of somatic motor and autonomic function, including the presence of bladder symptoms [268]. The degree of neurologic deficit has been classified as the "no-stick stage," "one-stick stage," "two-stick stage," and "crawler stage." Some patients stabilize in a subclinical, asymptomatic stage with minimal deficits. Electrophysiologic studies suggest subclinical anterior horn cell involvement [269]. Neuropathologic studies show loss of axons and myelin in the pyramidal tract in the lumbar cord and mild degeneration of the anterior horn cells at the same level [270]. Studies suggest that beta-N-oxalyl-amino-L-alanine, an excitotoxic amino acid in *L sativus*, is the responsible toxin [271]. It is a potent agonist of the excitatory neurotransmitter, glutamate. It is suggested that neurolathyrism may be prevented by mixing grass pea preparations with cereals [272] or detoxification of grass peas through aqueous leaching [273].

Cyanide toxicity

Weeks of high dietary cyanide exposure resulting from consumption of insufficiently processed cassava in parts of Africa, such as Zaire and Tanzania, results in konzo, a distinct tropical myelopathy characterized by the abrupt onset of symmetric, nonprogressive, spastic paraparesis [274,275]. Upper limb involvement and central visual field defects may be present. There is absence of sensory or autonomic disturbance. Improvement after onset is seen. Permanent deficits remain. Brain and spinal cord MRI are normal. Motor evoked potentials on magnetic brain stimulation may be absent [276]. Decreased sulfur intake with impaired conversion of cyanide to thiocyanate may be responsible [275]. Drought increases the natural occurrence of cyanogenic glucosides in the cassava roots [274]. Because of food shortages, the processing procedure normally used to remove cyanide before consumption is shortened. Minor improvement in food processing may be preventive [275]. The distribution of konzo is similar to that of HAM/TSP. The abrupt onset and nonprogressive course differentiates konzo from HAM/TSP. Lathyrism bears clinical similarities to konzo but has a different geographic distribution, is the result of a different diet, may have autonomic dysfunction, and does not have visual involvement. In parts of Africa, such as Nigeria, a syndrome characterized by slowly progressive ataxia, peripheral neuropathy, and optic atrophy is described [277]. Years of low dietary cyanide exposure resulting from cassava consumption likely is the cause.

Subacute myelo-opticoneuropathy

Subacute myelo-opticoneuropathy (SMON) is a myeloneuropathy with optic nerve involvement that affected approximately 10,000 individuals in Japan between 1955 and 1970 [278]. A similar syndrome also has been reported rarely outside Japan [279]. Epidemiologic studies suggest that SMON was the result of toxicity from the antiparasitic drug, clioquinol. SMON was characterized by subacute onset of lower limb paresthesias and spastic paraparesis with optic atrophy [280]. Tendon hyperreflexia and extensor plantar responses were seen, although at times the ankle jerk was absent. Electrophysiologic studies show delayed central conduction and normal conduction in peripheral sensory axons [281]. Autopsy studies show symmetric axonal degeneration in the corticospinal tracts in the lumbar spine, gracile columns at the cervicomedullary junction, and optic tracts [282]. Morphometric studies show only slight reduction of large myelinated fibers in the sural nerve [283].

Protein-calorie malnutrition

Protein and calorie deficiency in infants and children in underdeveloped countries results in two related disorders: marasmus and kwashiorkor [162]. Marasmus is the result of caloric insufficiency and results in growth failure and emaciation in early infancy. Kwashiorkor presents with edema, ascites, and hepatomegaly and is the result of protein deficiency. Generalized muscle wasting and weakness with hypotonia and hyporeflexia are seen. Cognitive deficits may be permanent. Autopsy studies show cerebral atrophy and immature neuronal development. During the initial stages of dietary treatment, an encephalopathy may be seen.

References

[1] Food and Agricultural Organization. The state of food insecurity in the world 2004. Rome: Food and Agriculture Organization of the United Nations; 2004. Available at: www.fao.org.

[2] Tefferi A, Pruthi RK. The biochemical basis of cobalamin deficiency. Mayo Clin Proc 1994;69:181–6.

[3] Scott JM, Dinn JJ, Wilson P, et al. Pathogenesis of subacute combined degeneration: a result of methyl group deficiency. Lancet 1981;2:334–7.

[4] Cardinale GJ, Carty TJ, Abeles RH. Effect of methylmalonyl coenzyme A, a metabolite which accumulates in vitamin B 12 deficiency, on fatty acid synthesis. J Biol Chem 1970;245:3771–5.

[5] Metz J. Cobalamin deficiency and the pathogenesis of nervous system disease. Annu Rev Nutr 1992;12:59–79.

[6] Scalabrino G. Cobalamin (vitamin B(12)) in subacute combined degeneration and beyond: traditional interpretations and novel theories [erratum appears in Exp Neurol 2005;194:561]. Exp Neurol 2005;192:463–79.

[7] Institute of Medicine. Vitamin B12. In: Food and Nutrition Board, editor. Dietary reference intakes: thiamin, riboflavin, niacin, vitamin B6, folate, vitamin B12, pantothenic acid, biotin, and choline. Washington, DC: National Academy Press; 1998. p. 306–56.

[8] Carmel R. Cobalamin (vitamin B12). In: Shils ME, Shike M, Ross AC, et al, editors. Modern nutrition in health and disease. 10th ed. Baltimore: Lippincott Williams and Wilkins; 2006. p. 482–97.

[9] Berlin H, Berlin R, Brante G. Oral treatment of pernicious anemia with high doses of vitamin B12 without intrinsic factor. Acta Med Scand 1968;184:247–58.

[10] Seetharam B, Alpers DH. Absorption and transport of cobalamin (vitamin B12). Annu Rev Nutr 1982;2:343–69.
[11] Green R, Kinsella LJ. Current concepts in the diagnosis of cobalamin deficiency. Neurology 1995;45:1435–40.
[12] Lindenbaum J, Healton EB, Savage DG, et al. Neuropsychiatric disorders caused by cobalamin deficiency in the absence of anemia or macrocytosis. N Engl J Med 1988;318: 1720–8.
[13] Carmel R. Cobalamin, the stomach, and aging. Am J Clin Nutr 1997;66:750–9.
[14] Pennypacker LC, Allen RH, Kelly JP, et al. High prevalence of cobalamin deficiency in elderly outpatients. J Am Geriatr Soc 1992;40:1197–204.
[15] Hurwitz A, Brady DA, Schaal SE, et al. Gastric acidity in older adults. JAMA 1997;278: 659–62.
[16] Halverson JD. Micronutrient deficiencies after gastric bypass for morbid obesity. Am Surg 1986;52:594–8.
[17] Marcuard SP, Albernaz L, Khazanie PG. Omeprazole therapy causes malabsorption of cyanocobalamin (vitamin B12). Ann Intern Med 1994;120:211–5.
[18] Rosenblatt DS, Cooper BA. Inherited disorders of vitamin B12 utilization. Bioessays 1990; 12:331–4.
[19] Kieburtz KD, Giang DW, Schiffer RB, et al. Abnormal vitamin B12 metabolism in human immunodeficiency virus infection. Association with neurological dysfunction. Arch Neurol 1991;48:312–4.
[20] Robertson KR, Stern RA, Hall CD, et al. Vitamin B12 deficiency and nervous system disease in HIV infection. Arch Neurol 1993;50:807–11.
[21] Di Rocco A, Bottiglieri T, Werner P, et al. Abnormal cobalamin-dependent transmethylation in AIDS-associated myelopathy. Neurology 2002;58:730–5.
[22] Deacon R, Lumb M, Perry J, et al. Selective inactivation of vitamin B12 in rats by nitrous oxide. Lancet 1978;2:1023–4.
[23] Schilling RF. Is nitrous oxide a dangerous anesthetic for vitamin B12-deficient subjects? JAMA 1986;255:1605–6.
[24] Kinsella LJ, Green R. 'Anesthesia paresthetica': nitrous oxide-induced cobalamin deficiency. Neurology 1995;45:1608–10.
[25] Layzer RB. Myeloneuropathy after prolonged exposure to nitrous oxide. Lancet 1978;2: 1227–30.
[26] Ng J, Frith R. Nanging. Lancet 2002;360:384.
[27] Sahenk Z, Mendell JR, Couri D, et al. Polyneuropathy from inhalation of N2O cartridges through a whipped-cream dispenser. Neurology 1978;28:485–7.
[28] Carmel R. Pernicious anemia. The expected findings of very low serum cobalamin levels, anemia, and macrocytosis are often lacking. Arch Intern Med 1988;148:1712–4.
[29] Healton EB, Savage DG, Brust JC, et al. Neurologic aspects of cobalamin deficiency. Medicine (Baltimore) 1991;70:229–45.
[30] Savage D, Gangaidzo I, Lindenbaum J, et al. Vitamin B12 deficiency is the primary cause of megaloblastic anaemia in Zimbabwe. Br J Haematol 1994;86:844–50.
[31] Savage D, Lindenbaum J. Relapses after interruption of cyanocobalamin therapy in patients with pernicious anemia. Am J Med 1983;74:765–72.
[32] Russell JSR, Batten FE, Collier J. Subacute combined degeneration of the spinal cord. Brain 1900;23:39–110.
[33] Pant SS, Asbury AK, Richardson EP Jr. The myelopathy of pernicious anemia. A neuropathological reappraisal. Acta Neurol Scand 1968;44(Suppl 5):1–36.
[34] Timms SR, Cure JK, Kurent JE. Subacute combined degeneration of the spinal cord: MR findings. AJNR Am J Neuroradiol 1993;14:1224–7.
[35] Hemmer B, Glocker FX, Schumacher M, et al. Subacute combined degeneration: clinical, electrophysiological, and magnetic resonance imaging findings. J Neurol Neurosurg Psychiatry 1998;65:822–7.

[36] Locatelli ER, Laureno R, Ballard P, et al. MRI in vitamin B12 deficiency myelopathy. Can J Neurol Sci 1999;26:60–3.
[37] Bassi SS, Bulundwe KK, Greeff GP, et al. MRI of the spinal cord in myelopathy complicating vitamin B12 deficiency: two additional cases and a review of the literature. Neuroradiology 1999;41:271–4.
[38] Karantanas AH, Markonis A, Bisbiyiannis G. Subacute combined degeneration of the spinal cord with involvement of the anterior columns: a new MRI finding. Neuroradiology 2000;42:115–7.
[39] Fine EJ, Hallett M. Neurophysiological study of subacute combined degeneration. J Neurol Sci 1980;45:331–6.
[40] McCombe PA, McLeod JG. The peripheral neuropathy of vitamin B12 deficiency. J Neurol Sci 1984;66:117–26.
[41] Heyer EJ, Simpson DM, Bodis-Wollner I, et al. Nitrous oxide: clinical and electrophysiologic investigation of neurologic complications. Neurology 1986;36:1618–22.
[42] Saperstein DS, Wolfe GI, Gronseth GS, et al. Challenges in the identification of cobalamin-deficiency polyneuropathy. Arch Neurol 2003;60:1296–301.
[43] White WB, Reik L Jr, Cutlip DE. Pernicious anemia seen initially as orthostatic hypotension. Arch Intern Med 1981;141:1543–4.
[44] Eisenhofer G, Lambie DG, Johnson RH, et al. Deficient catecholamine release as the basis of orthostatic hypotension in pernicious anaemia. J Neurol Neurosurg Psychiatry 1982;45: 1053–5.
[45] Fine EJ, Soria E, Paroski MW, et al. The neurophysiological profile of vitamin B12 deficiency. Muscle Nerve 1990;13:158–64.
[46] Allen RH, Stabler SP, Savage DG, et al. Diagnosis of cobalamin deficiency I: usefulness of serum methylmalonic acid and total homocysteine concentrations. Am J Hematol 1990;34: 90–8.
[47] Lindenbaum J, Savage DG, Stabler SP, et al. Diagnosis of cobalamin deficiency: II. Relative sensitivities of serum cobalamin, methylmalonic acid, and total homocysteine concentrations. Am J Hematol 1990;34:99–107.
[48] Savage DG, Lindenbaum J, Stabler SP, et al. Sensitivity of serum methylmalonic acid and total homocysteine determinations for diagnosing cobalamin and folate deficiencies. Am J Med 1994;96:239–46.
[49] Stabler SP. Screening the older population for cobalamin (vitamin B12) deficiency. J Am Geriatr Soc 1995;43:1290–7.
[50] Carmel R, Green R, Rosenblatt DS, et al. Update on cobalamin, folate, and homocysteine. Hematology 2003;1:62–81.
[51] Lindenbaum J, Rosenberg IH, Wilson PW, et al. Prevalence of cobalamin deficiency in the Framingham elderly population. Am J Clin Nutr 1994;60:2–11.
[52] Metz J, Bell AH, Flicker L, et al. The significance of subnormal serum vitamin B12 concentration in older people: a case control study. J Am Geriatr Soc 1996;44:1355–61.
[53] Karnaze DS, Carmel R. Neurologic and evoked potential abnormalities in subtle cobalamin deficiency states, including deficiency without anemia and with normal absorption of free cobalamin. Arch Neurol 1990;47:1008–12.
[54] Saperstein DS, Bahron RJ. Neuropathy associated with nutritional and vitamin deficiencies. In: Dyck PJ, Thomas PK, editors. Peripheral neuropathy. 10th ed. Philadelphia: Elsevier Saunders; 2005. p. 470–81.
[55] Stabler SP, Allen RH, Savage DG, et al. Clinical spectrum and diagnosis of cobalamin deficiency. Blood 1990;76:871–81.
[56] Snow CF. Laboratory diagnosis of vitamin B12 and folate deficiency: a guide for the primary care physician. Arch Intern Med 1999;159:1289–98.
[57] Kinsella LJ. Megaloblastic anemias—vitamin B12, Folate. In: Noseworthy JN, editor. Neurological therapeutics principles and practice. Abingdon, United Kingdom: Informa Healthcare; 2006. p. 1478–84.

[58] Carmel R. Mild transcobalamin I (haptocorrin) deficiency and low serum cobalamin concentrations. Clin Chem 2003;49:1367–74.
[59] Carmel R, Vasireddy H, Aurangzeb I, et al. High serum cobalamin levels in the clinical setting—clinical associations and holo-transcobalamin changes. Clin Lab Haematol 2001;23:365–71.
[60] Bolann BJ, Solli JD, Schneede J, et al. Evaluation of indicators of cobalamin deficiency defined as cobalamin-induced reduction in increased serum methylmalonic acid. Clin Chem 2000;46:1744–50.
[61] Carmel R. Macrocytosis, mild anemia, and delay in the diagnosis of pernicious anemia. Arch Intern Med 1979;139:47–50.
[62] Seetharam B. Receptor-mediated endocytosis of cobalamin (vitamin B12). Annu Rev Nutr 1999;19:173–95.
[63] Lindemans J, Schoester M, van Kapel J. Application of a simple immunoadsorption assay for the measurement of saturated and unsaturated transcobalamin II and R-binders. Clin Chim Acta 1983;132:53–61.
[64] Carmel R. Measuring and interpreting holo-transcobalamin (holo-transcobalamin II). Clin Chem 2002;48:407–9.
[65] Carmel R. Pepsinogens and other serum markers in pernicious anemia. Am J Clin Pathol 1988;90:442–5.
[66] Miller A, Slingerland DW, Cardarelli J, et al. Further studies on the use of serum gastrin levels in assessing the significance of low serum B12 levels. Am J Hematol 1989;31:194–8.
[67] Rothenberg SP, Kantha KR, Ficarra A. Autoantibodies to intrinsic factor: their determination and clinical usefulness. J Lab Clin Med 1971;77:476–84.
[68] Fairbanks VF, Lennon VA, Kokmen E, et al. Tests for pernicious anemia: serum intrinsic factor blocking antibody. Mayo Clin Proc 1983;58:203–4.
[69] Carmel R. Reassessment of the relative prevalences of antibodies to gastric parietal cell and to intrinsic factor in patients with pernicious anaemia: influence of patient age and race. Clin Exp Immunol 1992;89:74–7.
[70] Verhaeverbeke I, Mets T, Mulkens K, et al. Normalization of low vitamin B12 serum levels in older people by oral treatment. J Am Geriatr Soc 1997;45:124–5.
[71] Lederle FA. Oral cobalamin for pernicious anemia. Medicine's best kept secret? JAMA 1991;265:94–5.
[72] Stacy CB, Di Rocco A, Gould RJ. Methionine in the treatment of nitrous-oxide-induced neuropathy and myeloneuropathy. J Neurol 1992;239:401–3.
[73] Di Rocco A, Tagliati M, Danisi F, et al. A pilot study of L-methionine for the treatment of AIDS-associated myelopathy. Neurology 1998;51:266–8.
[74] Di Rocco A, Werner P, Bottiglieri T, et al. Treatment of AIDS-associated myelopathy with L-methionine: a placebo-controlled study. Neurology 2004;63:1270–5.
[75] Ungley CC. Subacute combined degeneration of the cord: I. Response to liver extracts. II. Trials with B12. Brain 1949;72:382–427.
[76] Skouby AP. Hydroxocobalamin for initial and long-term therapy for vitamin B12 deficiency. Acta Med Scand 1987;221:399–402.
[77] Tudhope GR, Swan HT, Spray GH. Patient variation in pernicious anaemia, as shown in a clinical trial of cyanocobalamin, hydroxocobalamin and cyanocobalamin–zinc tannate. Br J Haematol 1967;13:216–28.
[78] Slot WB, Merkus FW, Van Deventer SJ, et al. Normalization of plasma vitamin B12 concentration by intranasal hydroxocobalamin in vitamin B12-deficient patients. Gastroenterology 1997;113:430–3.
[79] Carmel R, Melnyk S, James SJ. Cobalamin deficiency with and without neurologic abnormalities: differences in homocysteine and methionine metabolism. Blood 2003;101: 3302–8.
[80] Carmel R, Weiner JM, Johnson CS. Iron deficiency occurs frequently in patients with pernicious anemia. JAMA 1987;257:1081–3.

[81] Institute of Medicine. Folate. In: Food and Nutrition Board, editor. Dietary reference intakes: thiamin, riboflavin, niacin, vitamin B6, folate, vitamin B12, pantothenic acid, biotin, and choline. Washington, DC: National Academy Press; 1998. p. 196–305.
[82] Carmel R. Folic acid. In: Shils ME, Shike M, Ross AC, et al, editors. Modern nutrition in health and disease. 10th ed. Baltimore: Lippincott Williams and Wilkins; 2006. p. 470–81.
[83] Sirotnak FM, Tolner B. Carrier-mediated membrane transport of folates in mammalian cells. Annu Rev Nutr 1999;19:91–122.
[84] Moran RG. Roles of folylpoly-gamma-glutamate synthetase in therapeutics with tetrahydrofolate antimetabolites: an overview. Semin Oncol 1999;26(2, Suppl 6):24–32.
[85] Eichner ER, Pierce HI, Hillman RS. Folate balance in dietary-induced megaloblastic anemia. N Engl J Med 1971;284:933–8.
[86] Halsted CH. Folate deficiency in alcoholism. Am J Clin Nutr 1980;33:2736–40.
[87] Elsborg L. Malabsorption of folic acid following partial gastrectomy. Scand J Gastroenterol 1974;9:271–4.
[88] Russell RM, Krasinski SD, Samloff IM, et al. Folic acid malabsorption in atrophic gastritis. Possible compensation by bacterial folate synthesis. Gastroenterology 1986;91: 1476–82.
[89] Russell RM, Golner BB, Krasinski SD, et al. Effect of antacid and H2 receptor antagonists on the intestinal absorption of folic acid. J Lab Clin Med 1988;112:458–63.
[90] Lambie DG, Johnson RH. Drugs and folate metabolism. Drugs 1985;30:145–55.
[91] Green R, Miller JW. Folate deficiency beyond megaloblastic anemia: hyperhomocysteinemia and other manifestations of dysfunctional folate status. Semin Hematol 1999;36:47–64.
[92] Grant HC, Hoffbrand AV, Wells DG. Folate deficiency and neurological disease. Lancet 1965;2:763–7.
[93] Reynolds EH, Rothfeld P, Pincus JH. Neurological disease associated with folate deficiency. BMJ 1973;2:398–400.
[94] Manzoor M, Runcie J. Folate-responsive neuropathy: report of 10 cases. BMJ 1976;1: 1176–8.
[95] Lever EG, Elwes RD, Williams A, et al. Subacute combined degeneration of the cord due to folate deficiency: response to methyl folate treatment. J Neurol Neurosurg Psychiatry 1986; 49:1203–7.
[96] Parry TE. Folate responsive neuropathy. Presse Med 1994;23:131–7.
[97] Shorvon SD, Carney MW, Chanarin I, et al. The neuropsychiatry of megaloblastic anaemia. BMJ 1980;281:1036–8.
[98] Reynolds EH. Benefits and risks of folic acid to the nervous system. J Neurol Neurosurg Psychiatry 2002;72:567–71.
[99] Diaz-Arrastia R. Homocysteine and neurologic disease. Arch Neurol 2000;57:1422–7.
[100] Zittoun J. Congenital errors of folate metabolism. Baillieres Clin Haematol 1995;8: 603–16.
[101] Toole JF, Malinow MR, Chambless LE, et al. Lowering homocysteine in patients with ischemic stroke to prevent recurrent stroke, myocardial infarction, and death: the Vitamin Intervention for Stroke Prevention (VISP) randomized controlled trial. JAMA 2004;291: 565–75.
[102] Gunter EW, Bowman BA, Caudill SP, et al. Results of an international round robin for serum and whole-blood folate. Clin Chem 1996;42:1689–94.
[103] Brouwer DA, Welten HT, Reijngoud DJ, et al. Plasma folic acid cutoff value, derived from its relationship with homocysteine. Clin Chem 1998;44:1545–50.
[104] Eichner ER, Hillman RS. Effect of alcohol on serum folate level. J Clin Invest 1973;52: 584–91.
[105] Lucock M, Yates Z. Measurement of red blood cell methylfolate. Lancet 2002;360:1021–2.
[106] Butterworth CE Jr, Tamura T. Folic acid safety and toxicity: a brief review. Am J Clin Nutr 1989;50:353–8.

[107] Stabler SP, Marcell PD, Podell ER, et al. Elevation of total homocysteine in the serum of patients with cobalamin or folate deficiency detected by capillary gas chromatography-mass spectrometry. J Clin Invest 1988;81:466–74.
[108] Tan N, Urich H. Menkes' disease and swayback. A comparative study of two copper deficiency syndromes. J Neurol Sci 1983;62:95–113.
[109] Kumar N, Gross JB Jr, Ahlskog JE. Copper deficiency myelopathy produces a clinical picture like subacute combined degeneration. Neurology 2004;63:33–9.
[110] Kumar N. Copper deficiency myelopathy (human swayback). Mayo Clin Proc 2006;81(10): 1371–84.
[111] Institute of Medicine. Copper. In: Food and NutritionBoard, editor. Dietary reference intakes for vitamin A, vitamin K, arsenic, boron, chromium, copper, iodine, iron, manganese, molybdenum, nickel, silicon, vanadium, and zinc. Washington, DC: National Academy Press; 2000. p. 224–57.
[112] Turnlund JR. Copper. In: Shils ME, Shike M, Ross AC, et al, editors. Modern nutrition in health and disease. 10th ed. Baltimore: Lippincott Williams and Wilkins; 2006. p. 286–99.
[113] Harris ZL, Gitlin JD. Genetic and molecular basis for copper toxicity. Am J Clin Nutr 1996; 63:836S–41S.
[114] Williams DM. Copper deficiency in humans. Semin Hematol 1983;20:118–28.
[115] Danks DM. Copper deficiency in humans. Annu Rev Nutr 1988;8:235–57.
[116] Fiske DN, McCoy HE 3rd, Kitchens CS. Zinc-induced sideroblastic anemia: report of a case, review of the literature, and description of the hematologic syndrome. Am J Hematol 1994;46:147–50.
[117] Kumar N, Gross JB Jr, Ahlskog JE. Myelopathy due to copper deficiency. Neurology 2003; 61:273–4.
[118] Yuzbasiyan-Gurkan V, Grider A, Nostrant T, et al. Treatment of Wilson's disease with zinc: X. Intestinal metallothionein induction. J Lab Clin Med 1992;120:380–6.
[119] Cordano A, Baertl JM, Graham GG. Copper deficiency in infancy. Pediatrics 1964;34: 324–36.
[120] Cartwright GE, Gubler CJ, Wintrobe MM. Studies on copper metabolism. XI. Copper and iron metabolism in the nephrotic syndrome. J Clin Invest 1954;33:685–98.
[121] Kumar N, Low PA. Myeloneuropathy and anemia due to copper malabsorption. J Neurol 2004;251:747–9.
[122] Karpel JT, Peden VH. Copper deficiency in long-term parenteral nutrition. J Pediatr 1972; 80:32–6.
[123] Spiegel JE, Willenbucher RF. Rapid development of severe copper deficiency in a patient with Crohn's disease receiving parenteral nutrition. JPEN J Parenter Enteral Nutr 1999;23:169–72.
[124] Tamura H, Hirose S, Watanabe O, et al. Anemia and neutropenia due to copper deficiency in enteral nutrition. JPEN J Parenter Enteral Nutr 1994;18:185–9.
[125] Hayton BA, Broome HE, Lilenbaum RC. Copper deficiency-induced anemia and neutropenia secondary to intestinal malabsorption. Am J Hematol 1995;48:45–7.
[126] Kumar N, McEvoy KM, Ahlskog JE. Myelopathy due to copper deficiency following gastrointestinal surgery. Arch Neurol 2003;60:1782–5.
[127] Kumar N, Ahlskog JE, Gross JB Jr. Acquired hypocupremia after gastric surgery. Clin Gastroenterol Hepatol 2004;2:1074–9.
[128] Valentine JS, Gralla EB. Delivering copper inside yeast and human cells. Science 1997;278: 817–8.
[129] Schleper B, Stuerenburg HJ. Copper deficiency-associated myelopathy in a 46-year-old woman. J Neurol 2001;248:705–6.
[130] Hedera P, Fink JK, Bockenstedt PL, et al. Myelopolyneuropathy and pancytopenia due to copper deficiency and high zinc levels of unknown origin: further support for existence of a new zinc overload syndrome. Arch Neurol 2003;60:1303–6.
[131] Greenberg SA, Briemberg HR. A neurological and hematological syndrome associated with zinc excess and copper deficiency. J Neurol 2004;251:111–4.

[132] Kumar N, Elliott MA, Hoyer JD, et al. "Myelodysplasia," myeloneuropathy, and copper deficiency. Mayo Clin Proc 2005;80:943–6.
[133] Kumar N, Ahlskog JE, Klein CJ, et al. Imaging features of copper deficiency myelopathy: a study of 25 cases. Neuroradiology 2005;48:78–83.
[134] Rowin J, Lewis SL. Copper deficiency myeloneuropathy and pancytopenia secondary to overuse of zinc supplementation. J Neurol Neurosurg Psychiatry 2005;76:750–1.
[135] Prodan CI, Holland NR. CNS demyelination from zinc toxicity? Neurology 2000;54:1705–6.
[136] Prodan CI, Holland NR, Wisdom PJ, et al. CNS demyelination associated with copper deficiency and hyperzincemia. Neurology 2002;59:1453–6.
[137] Gregg XT, Reddy V, Prchal JT. Copper deficiency masquerading as myelodysplastic syndrome. Blood 2002;100:1493–5.
[138] Crum BA, Kumar N. Electrophysiologic findings in copper deficiency myeloneuropathy. Neurology 2005;64(Suppl 1):A123.
[139] Wasa M, Satani M, Tanano H, et al. Copper deficiency with pancytopenia during total parenteral nutrition. JPEN J Parenter Enteral Nutr 1994;18:190–2.
[140] Kumar N, Gross JB, Ahlskog JE. Myelopathy due to copper deficiency [letter]. Neurology 2004;62:1656.
[141] Mason KE. A conspectus of research on copper metabolism and requirements of man. J Nutr 1979;109:1979–2066.
[142] Uauy R, Castillo-Duran C, Fisberg M, et al. Red cell superoxide dismutase activity as an index of human copper nutrition. J Nutr 1985;115:1650–5.
[143] Milne DB. Assessment of copper nutritional status. Clin Chem 1994;40:1479–84.
[144] Gyorffy EJ, Chan H. Copper deficiency and microcytic anemia resulting from prolonged ingestion of over-the-counter zinc. Am J Gastroenterol 1992;87:1054–5.
[145] Cheeseman KH, Holley AE, Kelly FJ, et al. Biokinetics in humans of RRR-alpha-tocopherol: the free phenol, acetate ester, and succinate ester forms of vitamin E. Free Radic Biol Med 1995;19:591–8.
[146] Institute of Medicine. Vitamin E. In: Food and Nutrition Board, editor. Dietary reference intakes for vitamin C, vitamin E, selenium, and carotenoids. Washington, DC: National Academy Press; 2000. p. 186–283.
[147] Hayes K, Pronczuk A, Perlman D. Vitamin E in fortified cow milk uniquely enriches human plasma lipoproteins. Am J Clin Nutr 2001;74:211–8.
[148] Leonard SW, Good CK, Gugger ET, et al. Vitamin E bioavailability from fortified breakfast cereal is greater than that from encapsulated supplements. Am J Clin Nutr 2004;79:86–92.
[149] Handelman GJ, Epstein WL, Peerson J, et al. Human adipose alpha-tocopherol and gamma-tocopherol kinetics during and after 1 y of alpha-tocopherol supplementation. Am J Clin Nutr 1994;59:1025–32.
[150] Traber MG. Vitamin E. In: Shils ME, Shike M, Ross AC, editors. Modern nutrition in health and disease. 10th ed. Baltimore: Lippincott Williams and Wilkins; 2006. p. 396–411.
[151] Steephen AC, Traber MG, Ito Y, et al. Vitamin E status of patients receiving long-term parenteral nutrition: is vitamin E supplementation adequate? JPEN J Parenter Enteral Nutr 1991;15:647–52.
[152] Ben Hamida C, Doerflinger N, Belal S, et al. Localization of Friedreich ataxia phenotype with selective vitamin E deficiency to chromosome 8q by homozygosity mapping. Nat Genet 1993;5:195–200.
[153] Cavalier L, Ouahchi K, Kayden HJ, et al. Ataxia with isolated vitamin E deficiency: heterogeneity of mutations and phenotypic variability in a large number of families. Am J Hum Genet 1998;62:301–10.
[154] Traber MG, Sokol RJ, Burton GW, et al. Impaired ability of patients with familial isolated vitamin E deficiency to incorporate alpha-tocopherol into lipoproteins secreted by the liver. J Clin Invest 1990;85:397–407.

[155] Aguglia U, Annesi G, Pasquinelli G, et al. Vitamin E deficiency due to chylomicron retention disease in Marinesco-Sjogren syndrome. Ann Neurol 2000;47:260–4.
[156] Harding AE. Vitamin E and the nervous system. Crit Rev Neurobiol 1987;3:89–103.
[157] Sokol RJ. Vitamin E deficiency and neurologic disease. Annu Rev Nutr 1988;8:351–73.
[158] Ben Hamida M, Belal S, Sirugo G, et al. Friedreich's ataxia phenotype not linked to chromosome 9 and associated with selective autosomal recessive vitamin E deficiency in two inbred Tunisian families. Neurology 1993;43:2179–83.
[159] Tomasi LG. Reversibility of human myopathy caused by vitamin E deficiency. Neurology 1979;29:1182–6.
[160] Burck U, Goebel HH, Kuhlendahl HD, et al. Neuromyopathy and vitamin E deficiency in man. Neuropediatrics 1981;12:267–78.
[161] Palmucci L, Doriguzzi C, Orsi L, et al. Neuropathy secondary to vitamin E deficiency in acquired intestinal malabsorption. Ital J Neurol Sci 1988;9:599–602.
[162] So YT, Simon RP. Deficiency diseases of the nervous system. In: Bradley WG, Daroff RB, Fenichel GM, et al, editors. Neurology in clinical practice, vol. II. 4th ed. Philadelphia: Butterworth Heinemann; 2004. p. 1693–708.
[163] Suarez GA. Peripheral neuropathy associated with alcoholism, malnutrition and vitamin deficiencies. In: Noseworthy JN, editor. Neurological therapeutics principles and practice, vol. 3. Abingdon, United Kingdom: Informa Healthcare; 2006. p. 2294–306.
[164] Vorgerd M, Tegenthoff M, Kuhne D, et al. Spinal MRI in progressive myeloneuropathy associated with vitamin E deficiency. Neuroradiology 1996;38(Suppl 1):S111–3.
[165] Sokol RJ, Bove KE, Heubi JE, et al. Vitamin E deficiency during chronic childhood cholestasis: presence of sural nerve lesion prior to 2 1/2 years of age. J Pediatr 1983;103:197–204.
[166] Traber MG, Sokol RJ, Ringel SP, et al. Lack of tocopherol in peripheral nerves of vitamin E-deficient patients with peripheral neuropathy. N Engl J Med 1987;317:262–5.
[167] Behrens WA, Thompson JN, Madere R. Distribution of alpha-tocopherol in human plasma lipoproteins. Am J Clin Nutr 1982;35:691–6.
[168] Horwitt MK, Harvey CC, Dahm CH Jr, et al. Relationship between tocopherol and serum lipid levels for determination of nutritional adequacy. Ann N Y Acad Sci 1972;203: 223–36.
[169] Traber MG, Jialal I. Measurement of lipid-soluble vitamins–further adjustment needed? Lancet 2000;355:2013–4.
[170] Sokol RJ, Heubi JE, Iannaccone ST, et al. Vitamin E deficiency with normal serum vitamin E concentrations in children with chronic cholestasis. N Engl J Med 1984;310:1209–12.
[171] Sokol RJ, Guggenheim MA, Iannaccone ST, et al. Improved neurologic function after long-term correction of vitamin E deficiency in children with chronic cholestasis. N Engl J Med 1985;313:1580–6.
[172] Sokol RJ, Butler-Simon N, Conner C, et al. Multicenter trial of d-alpha-tocopheryl polyethylene glycol 1000 succinate for treatment of vitamin E deficiency in children with chronic cholestasis. Gastroenterology 1993;104:1727–35.
[173] Azizi E, Zaidman JL, Eshchar J, et al. Abetalipoproteinemia treated with parenteral and oral vitamins A and E, and with medium chain triglycerides. Acta Paediatr Scand 1978; 67:796–801.
[174] Kayden HJ, Hatam LJ, Traber MG. The measurement of nanograms of tocopherol from needle aspiration biopsies of adipose tissue: normal and abetalipoproteinemic subjects. J Lipid Res 1983;24:652–6.
[175] Butterworth RF. Thiamin. In: Shils ME, Shike M, Ross AC, editors. Modern nutrition in health and disease. 10th ed. Baltimore: Lippincott Williams and Wilkins; 2006. p. 426–33.
[176] Butterworth RF. Effects of thiamine deficiency on brain metabolism: implications for the pathogenesis of the Wernicke-Korsakoff syndrome. Alcohol Alcohol 1989;24:271–9.
[177] Butterworth RF, Heroux M. Effect of pyrithiamine treatment and subsequent thiamine rehabilitation on regional cerebral amino acids and thiamine-dependent enzymes. J Neurochem 1989;52:1079–84.

[178] Bettendorff L. Thiamine in excitable tissues: reflections on a non-cofactor role. Metab Brain Dis 1994;9:183–209.
[179] Institute of Medicine. Vitamin B1. In: Food and Nutrition Board, editor. Dietary reference intakes: thiamin, riboflavin, niacin, vitamin B6, folate, vitamin B12, pantothenic acid, biotin, and choline. Washington, DC: National Academy Press; 1998. p. 58–86.
[180] Rindi G, Patrini C, Comincioli V, et al. Thiamine content and turnover rates of some rat nervous regions, using labeled thiamine as a tracer. Brain Res 1980;181:369–80.
[181] Singleton CK, Martin PR. Molecular mechanisms of thiamine utilization. Curr Mol Med 2001;1:197–207.
[182] Reuler JB, Girard DE, Cooney TG. Current concepts. Wernicke's encephalopathy. N Engl J Med 1985;312:1035–9.
[183] Rindi G, Imarisio L, Patrini C. Effects of acute and chronic ethanol administration on regional thiamin pyrophosphokinase activity of the rat brain. Biochem Pharmacol 1986;35: 3903–8.
[184] Ohnishi A, Tsuji S, Igisu H, et al. Beriberi neuropathy. Morphometric study of sural nerve. J Neurol Sci 1980;45:177–90.
[185] Koike H, Misu K, Hattori N, et al. Postgastrectomy polyneuropathy with thiamine deficiency. J Neurol Neurosurg Psychiatry 2001;71:357–62.
[186] Wright H. Changes in neuronal centers in beriberi neuritis. BMJ 1901;1:1610–6.
[187] Aguiar AC, Costa VM, Ragazzo PC, et al. Mielinolise pontina e extra-pontina associada a Shoshin beriberi em paciente etilista. Arq Neuropsiquiatr 2004;62:733–6.
[188] Caine D, Halliday GM, Kril JJ, et al. Operational criteria for the classification of chronic alcoholics: identification of Wernicke's encephalopathy. J Neurol Neurosurg Psychiatry 1997;62:51–60.
[189] Doherty MJ, Watson NF, Uchino K, et al. Diffusion abnormalities in patients with Wernicke encephalopathy. Neurology 2002;58:655–7.
[190] Foster D, Falah M, Kadom N, et al. Wernicke encephalopathy after bariatric surgery: losing more than just weight. Neurology 1987;2005:65.
[191] Torvik A, Lindboe CF, Rogde S. Brain lesions in alcoholics. A neuropathological study with clinical correlations. J Neurol Sci 1982;56:233–48.
[192] Harper C. The incidence of Wernicke's encephalopathy in Australia—a neuropathological study of 131 cases. J Neurol Neurosurg Psychiatry 1983;46:593–8.
[193] Harper C. Wernicke's encephalopathy: a more common disease than realised. A neuropathological study of 51 cases. J Neurol Neurosurg Psychiatry 1979;42:226–31.
[194] Butterworth RF, Gaudreau C, Vincelette J, et al. Thiamine deficiency and Wernicke's encephalopathy in AIDS. Metab Brain Dis 1991;6:207–12.
[195] Kril JJ. Neuropathology of thiamine deficiency disorders. Metab Brain Dis 1996;11: 9–17.
[196] Roman GC. Nutritional disorders of the nervous system. In: Shils ME, Shike M, Ross AC, editors. Modern nutrition in health and disease. 10th ed. Baltimore: Lippincott Williams and Wilkins; 2006. p. 1362–80.
[197] Dreyfus PM. Thiamine and the nervous system: an overview. J Nutr Sci Vitaminol (Tokyo) 1976;22(Suppl):13–6.
[198] Talwar D, Davidson H, Cooney J, et al. Vitamin B(1) status assessed by direct measurement of thiamin pyrophosphate in erythrocytes or whole blood by HPLC: comparison with erythrocyte transketolase activation assay. Clin Chem 2000;46:704–10.
[199] Woelk H, Lehrl S, Bitsch R, et al. Benfotiamine in treatment of alcoholic polyneuropathy: an 8-week randomized controlled study (BAP I Study). Alcohol and Alcoholism 1998;33:631–8.
[200] Cole M, Turner A, Frank O, et al. Extraocular palsy and thiamine therapy in Wernicke's encephalopathy. Am J Clin Nutr 1969;22:44–51.
[201] Salas-Salvado J, Garcia-Lorda P, Cuatrecasas G, et al. Wernicke's syndrome after bariatric surgery. Clin Nutr 2000;19:371–3.

[202] Institute of Medicine. Niacin. In: Food and Nutrition Board, editor. Dietary reference intakes: thiamin, riboflavin, niacin, vitamin B6, folate, vitamin B12, pantothenic acid, biotin, and choline. Washington, DC: National Academy Press; 1998. p. 123–49.

[203] Bourgeois C, Cervantes-Laurean D, Moss J. Niacin. In: Shils ME, Shike M, Ross AC, editors. Modern nutrition in health and disease. 10th ed. Baltimore: Lippincott Williams and Wilkins; 2006. p. 442–51.

[204] Spies TD, Aring CD. The effect of vitamin B1 on the peripheral neuritis of pellagra. JAMA 1938;110:1081–4.

[205] Spies TD, Vilter RW, Ashe WF. Pellagra, beriberi and riboflavin deficiency in human beings: diagnosis and treatment. JAMA 1939;113:931–7.

[206] Mackey AD, Davis SR, Gregory JFI. Vitamin B6. In: Shils ME, Shike M, Ross AC, et al, editors. Modern nutrition in health and disease. 10th ed. Baltimore: Lippincott Williams and Wilkins; 2006. p. 452–61.

[207] Institute of Medicine. Vitamin B6. In: Food and Nutrition Board, editor. Dietary reference intakes: thiamin, riboflavin, niacin, vitamin B6, folate, vitamin B12, pantothenic acid, biotin, and choline. Washington, DC: National Academy Press; 1998. p. 150–95.

[208] Said HM, Ortiz A, Ma TY. A carrier-mediated mechanism for pyridoxine uptake by human intestinal epithelial Caco-2 cells: regulation by a PKA-mediated pathway. Am J Physiol Cell Physiol 2003;285:C1219–25.

[209] Bhagavan HN, Brin M. Drug—vitamin B6 interaction. Curr Concepts Nutr 1983;12:1–12.

[210] Lumeng L. The role of acetaldehyde in mediating the deleterious effect of ethanol on pyridoxal 5′-phosphate metabolism. J Clin Invest 1978;62:286–93.

[211] Mason DY, Emerson PM. Primary acquired sideroblastic anaemia: response to treatment with pyridoxal-5-phosphate. BMJ 1973;1:389–90.

[212] Vilter RW, Mueller JF, Glazer HS, et al. The effect of vitamin B6 deficiency induced by desoxypyridoxine in human beings. J Lab Clin Med 1953;42:335–57.

[213] Goldman AL, Braman SS. Isoniazid: a review with emphasis on adverse effects. Chest 1972; 62:71–7.

[214] Victor M, Adams RD. The neuropathology of experimental vitamin B6 deficiency in monkeys. Am J Clin Nutr 1956;4:346–53.

[215] Schaumburg H, Kaplan J, Windebank A, et al. Sensory neuropathy from pyridoxine abuse. A new megavitamin syndrome. N Engl J Med 1983;309:445–8.

[216] Parry GJ, Bredesen DE. Sensory neuropathy with low-dose pyridoxine. Neurology 1985; 35:1466–8.

[217] Leklem JE. Vitamin B-6: a status report. J Nutr 1990;120(Suppl 11):1503–7.

[218] Okada H, Moriwaki K, Kanno Y, et al. Vitamin B6 supplementation can improve peripheral polyneuropathy in patients with chronic renal failure on high-flux haemadialysis and human recombinant erythropoietin. Nephrol Dial Transplant 2000;15:1410–3.

[219] Brolin RE. Bariatric surgery and long-term control of morbid obesity. JAMA 2002;288: 2793–6.

[220] Buchwald H, Buchwald JN. Evolution of operative procedures for the management of morbid obesity 1950–2000. Obes Surg 2002;12:705–17.

[221] Deitel M, Shikora SA. The development of the surgical treatment of morbid obesity. J Am Coll Nutr 2002;21:365–71.

[222] Livingston EH. Obesity and its surgical management. Am J Surg 2002;184:103–13.

[223] MacLean LD, Rhode BM, Shizgal HM. Nutrition following gastric operations for morbid obesity. Ann Surg 1983;198:347–55.

[224] Crowley LV, Olson RW. Megaloblastic anemia after gastric bypass for obesity. Am J Gastroenterol 1983;78:406–10.

[225] Crowley LV, Seay J, Mullin G. Late effects of gastric bypass for obesity. Am J Gastroenterol 1984;79:850–60.

[226] Schilling RF, Gohdes PN, Hardie GH. Vitamin B12 deficiency after gastric bypass surgery for obesity. Ann Intern Med 1984;101:501–2.

[227] Amaral JF, Thompson WR, Caldwell MD, et al. Prospective hematologic evaluation of gastric exclusion surgery for morbid obesity. Ann Surg 1985;201:186–93.
[228] Provenzale D, Reinhold RB, Golner B, et al. Evidence for diminished B12 absorption after gastric bypass: oral supplementation does not prevent low plasma B12 levels in bypass patients. J Am Coll Nutr 1992;11:29–35.
[229] Abarbanel JM, Berginer VM, Osimani A, et al. Neurologic complications after gastric restriction surgery for morbid obesity. Neurology 1987;37:196–200.
[230] Chaves LC, Faintuch J, Kahwage S, et al. A cluster of polyneuropathy and Wernicke-Korsakoff syndrome in a bariatric unit. Obes Surg 2002;12:328–34.
[231] Sola E, Morillas C, Garzon S, et al. Rapid onset of Wernicke's encephalopathy following gastric restrictive surgery. Obes Surg 2003;13:661–2.
[232] Banerji NK, Hurwitz LJ. Nervous system manifestations after gastric surgery. Acta Neurol Scand 1971;47:485–513.
[233] Marinella MA. Ophthalmoplegia: an unusual manifestation of hypocalcemia. Am J Emerg Med 1999;17:105–6.
[234] Alvarez-Leite JI. Nutrient deficiencies secondary to bariatric surgery. Curr Opin Clin Nutr Metab Care 2004;7:569–75.
[235] Feit H, Glasberg M, Ireton C, et al. Peripheral neuropathy and starvation after gastric partitioning for morbid obesity. Ann Intern Med 1982;96:453–5.
[236] Paulson GW, Martin EW, Mojzisik C, et al. Neurologic complications of gastric partitioning. Arch Neurol 1985;42:675–7.
[237] Dahlquist NR, Perrault J, Callaway CW, et al. D-Lactic acidosis and encephalopathy after jejunoileostomy: response to overfeeding and to fasting in humans. Mayo Clin Proc 1984;59:141–5.
[238] Banerji NK. Acute polyneuritis cranialis with total external ophthalmoplegia and areflexia. Ulster Med J 1971;40:14–6.
[239] Hoffman PM, Brody JA. Neurological disorders in patients following surgery for peptic ulcer. Neurology 1972;22:450.
[240] Thaisetthawatkul P, Collazo-Clavell ML, Sarr MG, et al. A controlled study of peripheral neuropathy after bariatric surgery. Neurology 2004;63:1462–70.
[241] Chang CG, Adams-Huet B, Provost DA. Acute post-gastric reduction surgery (APGARS) neuropathy. Obes Surg 2004;14:182–9.
[242] Berger JR. The neurological complications of bariatric surgery. Arch Neurol 2004;61:1185–9.
[243] Koffman BM, Greenfield LJ, Ali II, et al. Neurologic complications after surgery for obesity. Muscle Nerve 2006;33:166–76.
[244] Chang CG, Helling TS, Black WE, et al. Weakness after gastric bypass. Obes Surg 2002;12:592–7.
[245] Mason ME, Jalagani H, Vinik AI. Metabolic complications of bariatric surgery: diagnosis and management issues. Gastroenterol Clin North Am 2005;34:25–33
[246] Brolin RE. Gastric bypass. Surg Clin North Am 2001;81:1077–95.
[247] Brolin RE, Gorman RC, Milgrim LM, et al. Multivitamin prophylaxis in prevention of post-gastric bypass vitamin and mineral deficiencies. Int J Obes 1991;15:661–7.
[248] D'Amour ML, Butterworth RF. Pathogenesis of alcoholic peripheral neuropathy: direct effect of ethanol or nutritional deficit? Metab Brain Dis 1994;9:133–42.
[249] Victor M, Adams RD. On the etiology of alcoholic neurologic disease with special reference to the role of nutrition. Am J Clin Nutr 1961;9:379–97.
[250] Behse F, Buchthal F. Alcoholic neuropathy: clinical, electrophysiological, and biopsy findings. Ann Neurol 1977;2:95–110.
[251] Koike H, Mori K, Misu K, et al. Painful alcoholic polyneuropathy with predominant small-fiber loss and normal thiamine status. Neurology 2001;56:1727–32.
[252] Tabaraud F, Vallat JM, Hugon J, et al. Acute or subacute alcoholic neuropathy mimicking Guillain-Barre syndrome. J Neurol Sci 1990;97:195–205.

[253] Monforte R, Estruch R, Valls-Sole J, et al. Autonomic and peripheral neuropathies in patients with chronic alcoholism. A dose-related toxic effect of alcohol. Arch Neurol 1995;52: 45–51.
[254] Koike H, Iijima M, Sugiura M, et al. Alcoholic neuropathy is clinicopathologically distinct from thiamine-deficiency neuropathy. Ann Neurol 2003;54:19–29.
[255] Johnson RH, Robinson BJ. Mortality in alcoholics with autonomic neuropathy. J Neurol Neurosurg Psychiatry 1988;51:476–80.
[256] Roman GC. An epidemic in Cuba of optic neuropathy, sensorineural deafness, peripheral sensory neuropathy and dorsolateral myeloneuropathy. J Neurol Sci 1994;127:11–28.
[257] Cuban Neuropathy Field Investigation Team. Epidemic optic neuropathy in Cuba-Clinical characterization and risk factors. N Engl J Med 1995;333:1176–82.
[258] Roman GC, Osame M. Identity of HTLV-I-associated tropical spastic paraparesis and HTLV-I-associated myelopathy. Lancet 1988;1:651.
[259] Jacobson S, Lehky T, Nishimura M, et al. Isolation of HTLV-II from a patient with chronic, progressive neurological disease clinically indistinguishable from HTLV-I-associated myelopathy/tropical spastic paraparesis. Ann Neurol 1993;33:392–6.
[260] Harrington WJ Jr, Sheremata W, Hjelle B, et al. Spastic ataxia associated with human T-cell lymphotropic virus type II infection. Ann Neurol 1993;33:411–4.
[261] Morgan JP, Penovich P. Jamaica ginger paralysis. Forty-seven-year follow-up. Arch Neurol 1978;35:530–2.
[262] Senanayake N, Jeyaratnam J. Toxic polyneuropathy due to gingili oil contaminated with tri-cresyl phosphate affecting adolescent girls in Sri Lanka. Lancet 1981;1:88–9.
[263] Senanayake N. Tri-cresyl phosphate neuropathy in Sri Lanka: a clinical and neurophysiological study with a three year follow up. J Neurol Neurosurg Psychiatry 1981;44:775–80.
[264] Weiner ML, Jortner BS. Organophosphate-induced delayed neurotoxicity of triarylphosphates. Neurotoxicology 1999;20:653–73.
[265] Jaga K, Dharmani C. Sources of exposure to and public health implications of organophosphate pesticides. Pan American J Public Health 2003;14:171–85.
[266] Lotti M, Becker CE, Aminoff MJ. Organophosphate polyneuropathy: pathogenesis and prevention. Neurology 1984;34:658–62.
[267] Senanayake N, Karalliedde L. Neurotoxic effects of organophosphorus insecticides. An intermediate syndrome. N Engl J Med 1987;316:761–3.
[268] Ludolph AC, Hugon J, Dwivedi MP, et al. Studies on the aetiology and pathogenesis of motor neuron diseases. 1. Lathyrism: clinical findings in established cases. Brain 1987; 110(Pt 1):149–65.
[269] Drory VE, Rabey MJ, Cohn DF. Electrophysiologic features in patients with chronic neurolathyrism. Acta Neurol Scand 1992;85:401–3.
[270] Striefler M, Cohn DF, Hirano A, et al. The central nervous system in a case of neurolathyrism. Neurology 1977;27:1176–8.
[271] Spencer PS, Roy DN, Ludolph A, et al. Lathyrism: evidence for role of the neuroexcitatory aminoacid BOAA. Lancet 1986;2:1066–7.
[272] Getahun H, Lambein F, Vanhoorne M, et al. Food-aid cereals to reduce neurolathyrism related to grass-pea preparations during famine. Lancet 2003;362:1808–10.
[273] Spencer PS, Palmer VS. Lathyrism: aqueous leaching reduces grass-pea neurotoxicity. Lancet 2003;362:1775–6.
[274] Howlett WP, Brubaker GR, et al. Konzo, an epidemic upper motor neuron disease studied in Tanzania. Brain 1990;113(Pt 1):223–35.
[275] Tylleskar T, Banea M, Bikangi N, et al. Cassava cyanogens and konzo, an upper motoneuron disease found in Africa. Lancet 1992;339:208–11.
[276] Tylleskar T, Howlett WP, Rwiza HT, et al. Konzo: a distinct disease entity with selective upper motor neuron damage. J Neurol Neurosurg Psychiatry 1993;56:638–43.
[277] Osuntokun BO. Cassava diet, chronic cyanide intoxication and neuropathy in the Nigerian Africans. World Rev Nutr Diet 1981;36:141–73.

[278] Konagaya M, Matsumoto A, Takase S, et al. Clinical analysis of longstanding subacute myelo-optico-neuropathy: sequelae of clioquinol at 32 years after its ban. J Neurol Sci 2004;218:85–90.
[279] Baumgartner G, Gawel MJ, Kaeser HE, et al. Neurotoxicity of halogenated hydroxyquinolines: clinical analysis of cases reported outside Japan. J Neurol Neurosurg Psychiatry 1979; 42:1073–83.
[280] Sobue G, Ueno-Natsukari I, Okamoto H, et al. Phenotypic heterogeneity of an adult form of adrenoleukodystrophy in monozygotic twins. Ann Neurol 1994;36:912–5.
[281] Shibasaki H, Kakigi R, Ohnishi A, et al. Peripheral and central nerve conduction in subacute myelo-optico-neuropathy. Neurology 1982;32:1186–9.
[282] Konno H, Takase S, Fukui T. Neuropathology of longstanding subacute myelo-optico-neuropathy (SMON): an autopsy case of SMON with duration of 28 years. No To Shinkei 2001;53:875–80.
[283] Shiraki H. The neuropathology of subacute myelo-optico-neuropathy, "SMON", in the humans:—with special reference to the quinoform intoxication. Jpn J Med Sci Biol 1975; 28(Suppl):101–64.

ELSEVIER
SAUNDERS

Neurol Clin 25 (2007) 257–276

NEUROLOGIC
CLINICS

Toxic Neuropathies Associated with Pharmaceutic and Industrial Agents

Zachary London, MD, James W. Albers, MD, PhD*

Department of Neurology, University of Michigan, 1324 Taubman Center, Ann Arbor, MI 48109-0322, USA

The diagnosis of peripheral neuropathy can be established readily on the basis of clinical and electrodiagnostic criteria. Clinicians generally think of neuropathy, as a manifestation of an underlying systemic disorder, such as diabetes mellitus, or as a hereditary disorder of myelination. Investigations aimed at identifying the source of a neuropathy are fueled appropriately by the desire to find a reversible cause or at least to provide information about prognosis. The most common causes of peripheral neuropathy are genetic, inflammatory, or systemic, and many of these conditions can be diagnosed with simple blood tests.

In up to 20% of cases of neuropathy, however, the standard battery of laboratory tests is unrevealing. In these instances, it is natural for patients and physicians to wonder whether or not an unsuspected toxicant could be responsible. This suspicion can be heightened when patients have

Dr. Albers has received personal compensation from Eli Lily and Co. for consulting and for serving on a scientific advisory board, and he has a research grant from the National Institutes of Health and a research contract from the US Air Force. He previously received research grants from Dow AgroSciences, Dow Chemical Co., Prana Biotechnology, and CSX Transportation. Dr. Albers also has been retained as a consultant to firms or companies concerned with the manufacture or use of toxic substances, including medications, solvents, metals, and pesticides. Support of these activities has included personal and institutional remuneration.

Portions of this article rely on materials reproduced from: Albers JW, Teener JW. Toxic neuropathies. In: Kimura J, editor. Peripheral nerve diseases. Handbook of clinical neurophysiology. Vol. 7. Philadelphia: Elsevier; 2006. p. 677–702; Albers JW, Wald JJ. Industrial and environmental toxic neuropathies. In: Brown WF, editor. Neuromuscular function and disease: basic, clinical, and electrodiagnostic aspects. Philadelphia: WB Saunders; 2002. p. 1143–68; and Albers JW. Toxic neuropathies. Continuum: lifelong learning in neurology neurotoxicology 1999;5:27–50.

* Corresponding author.

E-mail address: jwalbers@med.umich.edu (J.W. Albers).

doi:10.1016/j.ncl.2006.10.001 ***neurologic.theclinics.com*** unexplained systemic manifestations or when other close contacts also have developed symptoms of neuropathy. In other cases, exposure to a specific agent is suspected as the cause of peripheral neuropathy. At times like this, it can be tempting to equate exposure (or opportunity for exposure) with causation. Patients may be anxious to know if they need to take steps to eliminate an ongoing industrial or environmental exposure, and in some cases litigation is involved. Perhaps an even more common situation is patients who have idiopathic neuropathy and who undergo exhaustive work-up and are found to have abnormal levels of an unsuspected toxicant. For example, routine screening for urine arsenic is a common practice, and elevated levels periodically are discovered in patients who do not have a known exposure. The physician then is left with the task of determining if these values represent true toxicity.

In all of these situations, it helpful to have an understanding of the clinical, laboratory, and electrodiagnostic features of specific toxic neuropathies. Whenever a toxic neuropathy is suspected, it also is essential to understand the scientific methodology necessary to verify or refute this suspicion. The purpose of this article is to discuss the clinical investigation of a suspected toxic neuropathy, to review some of the more common or representative toxicants, and to identify the methods for establishing causation.

The clinical evaluation of suspected toxic neuropathy

Perhaps the most compelling reason to be familiar with the various toxic neuropathies is that these conditions are, by nature, reversible with removal of the offending agent. Thus, even though these conditions are rare, there is an urgency to arrive at the correct diagnosis so measures can be taken to eliminate ongoing toxic exposure. Early diagnosis also can identify other individuals who may be at risk. Unfortunately, identifying a toxicant as the causative agent for a patient's neuropathy can be a difficult task, as there are no neurologic or electrodiagnostic features that distinguish toxic neuropathy from other causes of peripheral neuropathy reliably. Thus, toxic neuropathies always must be considered once a clinical diagnosis of neuropathy is established.

The first step in working up a suspected toxic neuropathy is to establish that a patient does, in fact, have clinical and electrodiagnostic evidence of peripheral neuropathy. The history should focus on sensory, motor, and autonomic complaints, including temporal profile, magnitude, and description of the symptoms. Most toxic neuropathies involve the longest and largest axons, causing numbness, paresthesias, or weakness in a stocking or stocking-glove distribution [1].

If a toxic neuropathy is suspected based on a patient's symptoms and signs and an apparent lack of a systemic or hereditary cause, the diagnostic yield can be increased by asking directed questions about potential pharmaceutic, industrial, recreational, or environmental exposures. It is useful particularly to become familiar with common pharmaceutic agents that can be associated with neuropathy. Examples include amitriptyline, cimetidine, cisplatin, colchicine, dapsone, disulfiram, ethambutol, gold, hydralazine, isoniazid, lithium, paclitaxel, phenytoin, nitrofurantoin, metronidazole, thalidomide, and vincristine. It also is important to ask about over-the-counter preparations and vitamins, because some agents, such as the essential vitamin, pyridoxine, can be potent neurotoxicants at high doses. It is also worthwhile to ask about potential occupational exposures, including specific chemicals, whenever possible. Industrial exposures have become increasingly uncommon compared with their reported frequency in the early twentieth century. This almost certainly is the result of increased awareness of the neurotoxic properties of the chemicals used in manufacturing and the institution of preventive measures to reduce exposure. Exposures to known neurotoxicants still occur, however, often in epidemic form, and new industrial chemicals that may cause neuropathy periodically are introduced into society.

It is important, also, to solicit information about recreational exposures, such as use of chemicals in hobbies. Recreational drugs, such as alcohol, nitrous oxide, and n-hexane (from sniffing glue) are well-established causes of neuropathy. These causes of neuropathy easily can be missed, because patients may hesitate to volunteer information about recreational drug use. Even a negative response to direct questioning does not exclude such agents from further consideration.

Finally, it is important to take a thorough review of systems and perform a thorough general examination, because many neurotoxicants also cause systemic toxicity (Table 1). For example, arsenic poisoning can cause abnormal skin pigmentation and nail abnormalities (Mees' lines), and thallium intoxication can cause alopecia. Often, patients complain of nonspecific systems suggestive of gastrointestinal, cardiovascular, hepatic, or renal toxicity. These features should raise clinical suspicion for a toxic neuropathy, even though they may not suggest a specific toxicant.

Physical examination should focus foremost on findings that are suggestive of peripheral neuropathy. Objective findings, such as motor weakness and loss of reflexes, are more significant than subjective findings, such as sensory loss, without supportive evidence of impaired sensation (eg, a positive Romberg's sign). Examination of the skin, hair, and nails may help identify features of systemic toxicity. Most patients found to have toxic neuropathy do not exhibit any of these cardinal features. Furthermore, features that are believed the most suggestive of a toxic exposure, such as Mees' lines, often appear long after patients develop symptoms of neuropathy, limiting their initial diagnostic usefulness.

Electromyography (EMG) and nerve conduction studies are an essential part of the investigation for neuropathy, because they can confirm the diagnosis of peripheral neuropathy and give valuable information about

Table 1
Selected systemic clues associated with specific neurotoxicants

Neurotoxicant	Systemic feature
Acrylamide	Irritant dermatitis, palmar erythema, desquamation, hyperhydrosis, axonal swellings
Arsenic	Gastrointestinal symptoms, hyperpigmentation, hyperkeratosis, Mees' lines, cardiomyopathy, hepatomegaly, renal failure, anemia, basophilic stippling of red blood cells
Colchicine	Myopathy (neuromyopathy)
Dapsone	After decades of use, possibly slow acetylators
Ethyl alcohol	Nutritional factors, Wernicke's syndrome (dementia, ophthalmoplegia, and ataxia), midline cerebellar degeneration, abnormal liver function, cirrhosis
n-hexane	Irritant dermatitis, axonal swellings
Lead	Gastrointestinal symptoms, musculoskeletal complaints, weight loss, gum lead line, bone lead line, Mees' lines, renal failure, anemia, basophilic stippling of red blood cells
Lithium	Postural tremor
Mercury, elemental	Anorexia, gingivitis, hypersalivation, papular rash, hyperkeratosis, lens opacities, postural tremor, nephrotic syndrome, respiratory tract irritation, metal fume fever
Nitrofurantoin	Elderly with impaired renal function
Nitrous oxide	Myelopathy
Organophosphate pesticides	Irritant dermatitis, acute cholinergic effects, corticospinal tract residua, noncardiogenic pulmonary edema
Phenytoin	Gingival hyperplasia, cerebellar ataxia
Thallium	Gastrointestinal symptoms, irritant dermatitis, alopecia, noncardiogenic pulmonary edema
Trichloroethylene	Vasodilation with ethanol ingestion, irritant dermatitis, elevated liver function tests, cirrhosis
Toluene	Respiratory tract irritation, irritant dermatitis
L-tryptophan	Peau d'orange, eosinophilia

Adapted from Ford D. Exposure assessment. Continuum: lifelong learning in neurology neurotoxicology; 1999. p. 9–25.

pathophysiology and severity [2]. Nerve conduction studies, in particular, provide a degree of information that cannot be determined on a clinical basis alone. First, nerve conduction studies can determine whether or not the neuropathy involves sensory axons, motor axons, or both. Second, they can determine whether or not there is conduction slowing. Any neuropathy that causes loss of large-caliber myelinated axons can cause mildly reduced conduction velocities, but conduction slowing out of proportion to axonal loss can help focus the differential diagnosis significantly. Third, nerve conduction studies can identify the pattern of neuropathy, such as a typical stocking-glove polyneuropathy or a mononeuritis multiplex. Needle EMG is of secondary importance in the evaluation of neuropathy. It is useful predominantly for identifying the degree of axonal involvement and ruling out polyradiculopathy, which can mimic peripheral neuropathy.

Many neurotoxicants cause similar clinical manifestations, but electrodiagnostic testing can be used to divide the neuropathies produced by neurotoxicants into broad categories. These categories are not exclusive, and some toxicants can cause more than one type of neuropathy, often depending on whether or not patients are subjected to a massive acute exposure or a low-dose chronic exposure. Nevertheless, this classification scheme is useful because it incorporates the suggested pathophysiology of the abnormality and can reduce an exhaustive list of potential neurotoxicants to a more manageable differential. These major categories include motor or motor greater than sensory neuropathy with or without conduction slowing, sensory neuropathy or neuronopathy, sensory greater than motor neuropathy with or without conduction slowing, and mononeuritis multiplex.

Discussion of every known toxic neuropathy is beyond the scope of this article. Rather, it focuses on selected examples that are the most common or most characteristic of each of the categories described.

Motor and motor greater than sensory neuropathy, with conduction slowing

Some neurotoxicants can mimic acute inflammatory demyelinating polyradiculoneuropathy (AIDP), with a motor or motor greater than sensory neuropathy with conduction slowing. Examples include arsenic (shortly after exposure), n-hexane, amiodarone, carbon disulfide, cytosine arabinoside, methyl n-butyl ketone, perhexiline, saxitoxin, and suramin.

Arsenic

Arsenic is a metalloid best known for its use as a poison in homicide and suicide. Industrial exposure may occur in lead and copper smelting, mining, and pesticide manufacturing [3]. Sources of environmental exposure include tainted well-water, wood preservatives, and arsenic-contaminated fossil fuels [4,5].

The neurotoxic effects of arsenic differ, depending on whether or not patients are subjected to an acute massive exposure or a chronic, low-level exposure. High-dose exposure can lead to a syndrome that can mimic AIDP [6]. Neuropathy begins 5 to 10 days after exposure and progresses over weeks. As with many toxic neuropathies, there may be a "coasting" effect, with continued progression of disease for a period of weeks after removal from exposure. Patients can develop flaccid areflexic quadriparesis, bifacial weakness, and even diaphragm paralysis, requiring ventilatory support [7,8].

Clinical manifestations can help distinguish arsenic toxicity from inflammatory demyelinating neuropathy, including a variety of systemic symptoms that may develop before the onset of neuropathy. Gastrointestinal disturbance with abdominal pain and vomiting, tachycardia, and hypotension are common, although these symptoms also may be seen in AIDP [9]. Nonspecific systemic manifestations may follow, including hepatomegaly, renal failure, anemia, and cardiomyopathy, which are atypical for AIDP. Other systemic features are more specific to arsenic toxicity, such as brownish desquamation of the hands and feet (arsenical dermatitis) and Mees' lines on fingernails and toenails. Unfortunately, the skin and nail changes may not appear until a month or more after isolated ingestion of arsenic, by which time the diagnosis rarely is still in question.

If an initial EMG is performed within days, decreased motor unit recruitment may be the only finding. Over the first few weeks, EMG may show motor greater than sensory neuropathy with reduced amplitudes, borderline–low conduction velocities, prolonged F waves, and even partial conduction block in several motor nerves. The nerve conduction studies even may fulfill criteria for the diagnosis of an acquired demyelinating neuropathy [10]. Cases even are reported in which the sural sensory response is normal, but the median sensory response is absent, a finding often found in AIDP [11]. Follow-up studies are more consistent with a typical dying-back axonopathy, with absent sensory and motor responses and denervation/reinnervation changes on needle EMG.

Chronic exposure to low levels of arsenic, such as can be seen in industrial settings, often results in dermatologic manifestations first, including hyperpigmentation, hyperkeratosis, and mucosal irritation [12]. Ongoing exposure may lead to a painful length-dependent neuropathy with proportionally fewer motor symptoms [3].

Laboratory testing can aid in the diagnosis of arsenic poisoning in acute and chronic settings. Urine arsenic levels greater than 25 μg in a 24-hour specimen generally are considered abnormal, although levels may be elevated falsely by the ingestion of seafood, in particular bottom-feeding finfish. Small amounts of arsenic bind to keratin in growing tissues, allowing diagnosis to be made by measuring levels in hair and nails. This is useful particularly in the setting of chronic or low-level exposure or for detecting a remote exposure that has since ceased. Blood arsenic levels are not helpful, because serum arsenic is cleared within 2 to 4 hours [13].

Chelation with penicillamine or dimercaprol should be started as soon as possible after exposure [14,15]. The usefulness of chelation in preventing progression of acute arsenical neuropathy is unknown, however.

Hexacarbons

N-hexane and methyl-n-butyl ketone are hexacarbons used in industrial solvents and household glues. Most of the industrial exposures producing neuropathy occurred in the cabinet- and shoe-making industries, where hexacarbon solvents were used extensively until the 1970s. More recently, cases of n-hexane neuropathy were reported in automotive technicians using degreasing solvents and cleansers. The most common source of n-hexane exposure today is the intentional inhalation of household glues for the purpose of intoxication [16,17].

Both n-hexane and methyl-n-butyl ketone are metabolized to 2,5-hexanedione in the liver, which probably is the neurotoxic agent [18]. Substantial n-hexane toxicity causes central nervous system depression and narcosis, but with repeated exposures, peripheral neurotoxicity can develop. Specifically, n-hexane causes a neuropathy consisting of length-dependent distal sensory loss, weakness, atrophy, reduced or absent distal reflexes, and autonomic dysfunction. Among "huffers," who inhale massive quantities of n-hexane volitionally, motor and cranial nerve symptoms may predominate. Furthermore, nerve conduction studies often demonstrate reduced amplitudes with conduction velocities in the range of a primary demyelinating disorder [19]. As with arsenic, n-hexane can create a clinical picture that mimics AIDP. Chronic, low-level exposures are associated with a more typical dying-back sensorimotor neuropathy with sensory loss, distal weakness, and absent ankle reflexes [20,21]. Chronic occupational and recreational exposures also are associated with degeneration of distal corticospinal and dorsal column pathway and impairment of color vision [22].

The classic neuropathologic finding in n-hexane neuropathy is giant axonal swellings, which consist of neurofilamentous aggregates that accumulate secondary to abnormalities of axonal transport. The slow conduction velocities found on nerve conduction studies are believed to represent secondary myelin sheath damage from these focal axonal swellings [17,23–27].

Cessation of exposure is the primary means of treatment, and in one large case series, all 102 patients who had identified cases of n-hexane intoxication recovered completely without other intervention [28].

Amiodarone

Amiodarone is a di-iodinated benzofuran derivative used for refractory or life-threatening ventricular arrhythmias. Amiodarone is associated with several neurotoxic effects, including peripheral neuropathy, action tremor, myopathy, optic neuropathy, basal ganglia dysfunction, encephalopathy, and pseudotumor cerebri.

The neuropathy associated with chronic amiodarone use varies in various reports. The clinical presentation may be a symmetric, subacute to chronic sensorimotor polyneuropathy with distal predominance [29–37]. Other investigators have reported a rapidly evolving motor-predominant neuropathy that can be difficult to distinguish from AIDP [38].

Reports of nerve conduction studies vary from a sensory-predominant axonopathy with reduced amplitudes to a demyelinating picture with prominent conduction slowing [39]. The findings in sural nerve biopsies also vary, with some specimens demonstrating axonal loss and others showing almost pure demyelination [40]. Amiodarone is highly lipophilic and forms intralysosomal lipid complexes, leading to inclusions in multiple tissues. These inclusions are seen in neural structures, suggesting a possible mechanism of toxicity.

There is no specific treatment for amiodarone-induced neuropathy other than lowering or discontinuing the drug. Recovery can be slow after removal of the exposure, because amiodarone has a long half-life (25–100 days).

Motor and motor greater than sensory neuropathy, without conduction slowing

Some neurotoxicants are known to produce a motor-predominant neuropathy without conduction slowing, including certain organophosphates, vincristine and other vinca alkaloids, nitrofurantoin, cimetidine, dapsone, and possibly lead.

Organophosphates

Unlike most chemicals that cause neuropathy, organophosphates have been used widely because they are poisonous, rather than in spite of it. The neurotoxic properties of organophosphate compounds have led to their use as insecticides and "nerve" gases. Less toxic forms also have been used in hydraulic fluids, lubricants, fuel additives, plastic modifiers, and flame retardants. Today, most cases of acute neurotoxicity are in the setting of intentional ingestion of insecticides as a suicide attempt.

One of the most remarkable illustrations of large-scale organophosphate poisoning was the jake leg epidemic of 1930. Jamaica ginger, or jake, was an alcohol-based patent medicine that was popular among poor city-dwellers trying to circumvent Prohibition laws. To fool Prohibition chemists into thinking the medicine had a higher percentage of solids, one supplier contaminated Jamaica ginger with triorthocresyl phosphate (TOCP), an organophosphate that was believed harmless. By the time the source of the contamination was identified and removed, tens of thousands of Americans had developed disabling neuropathy [41–43].

Organophosphates exert their primary neurotoxic effect by inactivating acetylcholinesterase. This leads to an accumulation of acetylcholine in muscarinic and nicotinic receptors. Symptoms of cholinergic excess include bradycardia, salivation, nausea, bronchospasm, miosis, diarrhea, sweating, central nervous system dysfunction, muscle weakness, and fasciculations. After 1 to 4 days, an intermediate syndrome develops, characterized by weakness of proximal limb, neck, extraocular, bulbar, and respiratory muscles. This syndrome resembles myasthenia gravis and most likely represents a depolarizing blockade of neuromuscular transmission. A subacute motor greater than sensory neuropathy develops as the symptoms of the acute and intermediate syndromes resolve. Organophosphate-induced delayed neurotoxicity (OPIDN), as it has been called, occurs 7 to 21 days after exposure and occurs only with certain exposure to certain organophosphates. Weakness follows a length-dependent pattern, with early foot drop and weakness of hand intrinsic muscles followed by more proximal weakness. Some patients go on to develop spasticity and upper motor neuron signs, indicative of superimposed distal corticospinal tract dysfunction [44]. TOCP, the agent implicated in jake leg, is a unique organophosphate that causes OPIDN without causing overt cholinergic symptoms first [45,46].

OPIDN is a distal axonopathy that affects the peripheral nerves and the long tracts in the spinal cord. Nerve conduction studies show evidence of sensorimotor neuropathy without conduction slowing [47,48]. The pathophysiology of OPIDN is believed the result of organophosphate-induced modification of a neuronal membrane protein called neuropathy target esterase, although the exact mechanism is unknown [49,50].

Vincristine

Vincristine is a vinca alkaloid chemotherapeutic agent used for treatment of solid tumors, lymphoma, and leukemia. Peripheral neuropathy is the dose-limiting side effect of all vinca alkaloids, with vincristine the most neurotoxic [51]. The mechanism of vincristine neuropathy is believed related to impairment of the function of microtubules involved in axonal transport [52].

Pain and small-fiber sensory loss predominate early, usually occurring at 4 to 5 weeks [53]. Autonomic dysfunction also may occur early, with constipation, orthostatic hypotension, and impotence. Distal symmetric weakness invariably occurs with continued exposure, and in some patients, these symptoms may develop fulminantly [54]. There also are cases of vincristine therapy leading to a severe acute neuropathy by unmasking a subclinical inherited neuropathy, such as Charcot-Marie-Tooth disease type 1 or hereditary neuropathy with liability to pressure palsies [55–57]. Patients who have these neuropathies may be susceptible to developing severe weakness with low or even single doses of vincristine.

In vincristine neuropathy, the EMG demonstrates axonal neuropathy, with decreased sensory and motor amplitudes on nerve conduction studies. The presence of motor involvement on electrodiagnostic testing correlates with the degree of clinical weakness.

Muscle weakness usually recovers rapidly after the drug is discontinued. Up to two thirds of patients continue to have residual sensory symptoms and absent deep tendon reflexes, however. Electrodiagnostic measures of neuropathy may persist indefinitely, with low or absent sensory nerve action potentials.

Sensory neuropathy or neuronopathy, without conduction slowing

Cisplatin, pyridoxine, thallium, metronidazole, ethyl alcohol, nitrofurantoin, and thalidomide are shown to induce a pure sensory neuropathy or neuronopathy without conduction slowing.

Cisplatin

Cisplatin is a chemotherapeutic agent used for ovarian and small cell lung cancers that causes a cumulative dose-limiting axonal sensory neuropathy. The primary site of damage is the dorsal root ganglion (sensory neuronopathy), but the large myelinated sensory axons also may be affected [58,59]. Manifestations include numbness, paresthesias, and occasionally pain in the distal extremities, with loss of deep tendon reflexes and position sense. The most important condition to consider in the differential diagnosis is paraneoplastic sensory neuronopathy, which can present identically. Paraneoplastic neuropathies may be associated with autoantibodies in the serum and may continue to progress despite discontinuation of the cisplatin. In cisplatin neuropathy, nerve conduction studies show decreased sensory nerve action potential amplitudes and prolonged sensory latencies.

The toxicity of cisplatin can persist long after the medication is discontinued. In one study of patients who had been treated with cisplatin 13 or more years prior, 38% were found to have nonsymptomatic neuropathy, 28% symptomatic neuropathy, and 6% disabling polyneuropathy [60].

The mechanism of cisplatin neurotoxicity is unknown, but it is believed to relate to disruption of fast axonal transport and induction of apoptosis in dorsal root ganglion cells [61,62].

Pyridoxine

Pyridoxine, or vitamin B_6, is an essential vitamin that has neuroprotective effects when used to treat isoniazid overdose, Gyromitra mushroom or false morel (monomethylhydrazine) poisoning, and hydrazine exposure [63]. Pyridoxine also is a potent neurotoxicant, however, with low-dose, chronic exposure and with acute massive exposure. Pyridoxine toxicity produces a pure sensory neuropathy, with numbness and loss of position sense but no dysfunction of motor nerves or the central nervous system [64]. In most cases, the neuropathy is slowly reversible with discontinuation of the pyridoxine, but large acute doses may be associated with permanent profound sensory loss and pseudoathetosis [65].

Thallium

Thallium is a neurotoxic metal that has been used in the manufacture of optical lenses, semiconductors, scintillation counters, some fireworks, insecticides, and rodenticides [66]. The most common causes of thallium poisoning are homicidal, suicidal, or accidental ingestion of rat poison, although the number of cases has declined substantially since thallium was banned in the United States as a rodent poison in 1972 [67–70].

Thallium causes a predominantly small-fiber neuropathy, with painful dysesthesias in the distal lower extremities. Dysautonomia often is present and may precede neuropathy [71]. Reflexes often are preserved, a feature that helps localize the lesion to the small-fiber nerve and differentiate thallium poisoning from AIDP and other toxic neuropathies. Although most cases of thallium poisoning cause sensory symptoms only, there also are reports of motor manifestations [72].

Early signs of systemic toxicity include gastrointestinal symptoms, cardiac and respiratory failure, encephalopathy, and renal insufficiency [73]. The most pathognomonic manifestation of thallium poisoning is alopecia, which appears 15 to 39 days after intoxication and, therefore, is not useful in the acute setting [74]. Mees' lines (white stria of the nails) also may develop as a late sign.

Early in the course of the disease, there may be involvement only of the small nerve fibers. At this point, nerve conduction studies may be normal or show only mild abnormalities, such as absent plantar sensory responses. In more severe cases, evidence of axonal loss is found on electrodiagnostic testing and sural nerve biopsy [75,76].

The exact mechanism of thallium toxicity is unknown. Thallium enters cells through potassium channels and may compete with potassium in intracellular reactions and interfere with energy metabolism in the Kreb's cycle, oxidative phosphorylation, and glycolysis [77].

Sensory greater than motor (sensorimotor) neuropathy, with conduction slowing

Saxitoxin and tetrodotoxin, although not pharmaceutic agents, are biologic neurotoxicants that produce a sensory greater than motor neuropathy with conduction slowing.

Saxitoxin

Saxitoxin, otherwise known as red tide, is the neurotoxicant implicated in paralytic shellfish poisoning. The most common source of saxitoxin poisoning is the consumption of bivalve mollusks, in particular those harvested in the months of May, June, and July [78,79]. Clinical manifestations include gastrointestinal symptoms, cerebellar ataxia, and a sensorimotor neuropathy, which may be severe enough to cause respiratory depression.

Saxitoxin exerts its effects by blocking sodium channels, reducing the local currents associated with propagation of the action potential [80]. Nerve conduction studies show prolonged distal sensory and motor latencies with slowed conduction velocities and moderately diminished response amplitudes [81].

Tetrodotoxin

Tetrodotoxin is a poison derived from puffer fish, where it is found in various concentrations in the liver, ovaries, intestines, and skin [82]. Fugu, or puffer fish fillet, is a delicacy in Japan, where it is the most common cause of fatal food poisoning [83]. Clinical manifestations depend on the dose of the exposure, but neurologic symptoms and signs may range from perioral numbness to flaccid paralysis, dilated pupils, and respiratory failure without loss of consciousness. Symptoms may begin within 1 hour after ingestion of the contaminated fish and generally abate after 5 days [84].

Like saxitoxin, tetrodotoxin causes blockade of voltage-sensitive sodium channels, leading to conduction failure. Nerve conduction studies show prolongation of sensory and motor latencies, prolongation of F waves, slowing of conduction velocities, and reduced sensory and motor amplitudes [85].

Sensory greater than motor (sensorimotor) neuropathy, without conduction slowing

The majority of peripheral neurotoxicants produce a length-dependent sensorimotor neuropathy without conduction slowing. Some examples of neurotoxicants known to fit this pattern include acrylamide, amitriptyline, arsenic (chronic), carbon monoxide, ethambutol, ethyl alcohol, ethylene oxide, gold, hydralazine, isoniazid, lithium, elemental mercury, metronidazole, nitrofurantoin, nitrous oxide, paclitaxel, perhexiline, phenytoin, thallium, and vincristine.

Acrylamide

Acrylamide is a vinyl polymer used to synthesize polyacrylamide, which has many applications as a soil conditioner, flocculator, and waterproofing agent and in the cosmetic, paper, and textile industries. Although polyacrylamide is nontoxic, it can be contaminated with the toxic acrylamide, especially when it is used as a flocculator [86,87].

Acrylamide causes a typical axonal neuropathy with weakness, sensory loss, and areflexia involving primarily large axons. Systemic symptoms include irritant dermatitis, palmar erythema, and encephalopathy. Nerve conduction abnormalities generally are mild and show low amplitude sensory responses, and, to a lesser extent, low amplitude motor responses without significant conduction slowing [88]. Subclinical neuropathy also is detected in patients who have low-level industrial exposures [89,90].

The pathologic hallmark of acrylamide neurotoxicity, like that of n-hexane, is giant axonal swellings. Classically, acrylamide is believed to exert its toxicity through disruption of anterograde and retrograde axonal transport [91]. Some studies suggest, however, that the nerve terminal may be the primary site of neurotoxicity rather than the axon itself [92,93].

Nitrofurantoin

Nitrofurantoin is an antibacterial agent specific for urinary tract infections. Nitrofurantoin is implicated in the development of axonal sensorimotor neuropathy, with sensory-predominant (common) and motor-predominant (less common and typically developing after onset of the sensory neuropathy) neuropathies reported. Patients who have pre-existing renal dysfunction or diabetes mellitus are at greater risk for developing nitrofurantoin-induced neuropathy, but neuropathy also is described in otherwise healthy patients taking standard doses of this medication. [94,95]. The pathologic changes in nitrofurantoin-induced neuropathy are those of acute, severe axonal degeneration [95]. It is hypothesized that nitrofurantoin exerts its toxic effects through dose-dependent depletion of glutathione [96].

Phenytoin

Peripheral neuropathy long has been recognized as a side effect of chronic phenytoin use, especially at higher doses [97,98]. Although it is not well studied in prospective trials, most reports of phenytoin toxicity suggest that it probably does not live up to its reputation as a serious peripheral neurotoxicant. With standard doses and close monitoring of levels, phenytoin-induced neuropathy is rare. When present, patients usually are asymptomatic and the neuropathy can be detected only by physical examination or electrophysiologic studies [99–101].

Mononeuritis multiplex

Rarely, neurotoxicants can present with a clinical picture suggestive of multiple mononeuropathies, rather than a symmetric, length-dependent peripheral neuropathy. Examples include trichloroethylene, dapsone, lead, and L-tryptophan.

Trichloroethylene

Trichloroethylene is a chlorinated hydrocarbon that has been used as a cleaner, solvent, degreasing agent, and surgical anesthetic. It is unusual among neurotoxicants in that it is associated with a cranial mononeuritis multiplex with little evidence of sensory or sensorimotor neuropathy [102]. Patients develop ptosis, extraocular muscle dysfunction, facial and bulbar weakness, and signs of trigeminal dysfunction [103]. Like other neurotoxicants, trichloroethylene also is a systemic poison. It is shown to cause irritant dermatitis, cirrhosis, and cardiac failure [104].

In association with a trichloroethylene cranial mononeuritis multiplex, facial motor nerve distal latencies and blink reflex R1 latencies are prolonged. Blink reflexes also are used to suggest the presence of a subclinical trigeminal neuropathy in patients who have chronic, low-dose exposure to trichloroethylene through contaminated well water [105,106].

It is controversial whether or not trichloroethylene is directly toxic to nerves or if neurologic symptoms actually are the result of toxicity from dichloroacetylene, a metabolite of trichloroethylene that is formed only in certain conditions, such as high heat or extreme alkalinity [107]. It also is hypothesized that trichloroethylene does not actually cause a toxic neuropathy but rather triggers the reactivation of a latent herpes virus [108]. Necropsy examination of one patient showed degeneration of the brainstem nuclei and tracts, the trigeminal nerve, and cranial sensory roots [103].

Dapsone

Dapsone is an antiparasitic and antimycobacterial agent used to treat leprosy, toxoplasmosis, malaria, and the skin condition, dermatitis herpetiformis. Most descriptions of dapsone neuropathy are those of a motor-predominant neuropathy, often with an asymmetric presentation, suggesting a mononeuritis multiplex [109–112]. Mixed sensorimotor neuropathy and mild, sensory neuropathies also are described [113,114].

Neuropathy generally is seen only in patients who have been taking dapsone for several years, with most cases developing within 5 years of initiation. Ironically, dapsone has been used widely to treat leprosy, an infectious cause of peripheral neuropathy. In spite of this, most cases in the literature occur when patients are taking dapsone for dermatitis herpetiformis. Slow acetylators of dapsone likely are at additional risk for developing neuropathy [110,115].

Electrophysiologic and pathologic studies suggest a distal motor axonopathy without features of demyelination [116]. Most patients recover completely over the course of many months after the drug is withdrawn [115].

Methodology used to establish causation

The most important tenet of establishing a neurotoxic cause of any neurologic problem is that the opportunity for exposure does not prove that the symptoms were caused by the exposure. Given the widespread prevalence of peripheral neuropathy, a patient who works with industrial chemicals or takes a medication known to cause neuropathy still could develop neuropathy from a different cause. In fact, in many situations, the alternative explanation is more likely. Knowledge of the biologic effects of the toxicant and the circumstances of the exposure can help differentiate causation from mere association.

Most clinicians apply general scientific principals in the formulation of differential diagnosis without giving thought to the process, but formal criteria exist for evaluating the role of a suspected toxin in a specific case [117]. The purported effect of the toxicant needs to be biologically plausible. The relative risk of neuropathy varies significantly between neurotoxicants, and large epidemiologic studies, in particular cohort or case control studies, that demonstrate a strong association between the toxicant and neuropathy confer more support for the hypothesis than isolated case reports or cross-sectional studies. The existence of a well-studied animal model also can be helpful in identifying potential mechanisms of neurotoxicity.

The circumstances of the exposure can provide additional information. For instance, the temporal nature of the exposure is important in establishing causation. Obviously, the neuropathy cannot precede the exposure. Conversely, a neuropathy that develops months or years after a single acute exposure is not consistent with causation.

In almost all toxic neuropathies, there should be a dose-response relationship between the level of toxicant exposure and the severity of the neuropathy. For many toxicants, biologic markers can be measured in the blood, urine, or hair. Established reference levels can be used to suggest whether or not the degree of exposure is substantial enough to account for a patient's symptoms. Resolution of the neuropathy and normalization of the biologic markers after removal of the exposure provide some of the strongest evidence of causation. Some toxic neuropathies, however, continue to progress for a few weeks after removal of exposure before stabilizing and eventually improving, a phenomenon known as "coasting."

The most difficult task in establishing causation is eliminating other causes from the differential diagnosis. Although a patient's symptoms, signs, and electrodiagnostic findings may be "consistent with" a toxic neuropathy, it is likely that the same findings are "consistent with" several other causes also. Eliminating all competing causes from the differential diagnosis requires a working knowledge of systemic, genetic, inflammatory, infectious, and nutritional causes of neuropathy and other neurotoxicants that could produce a similar form of neuropathy.

Industrial, environmental, and pharmacologic causes of neuropathy are uncommon, and may account for only a small fraction of neuropathies in which no underlying cause is identified with routine tests. Most likely, physicians who attribute a neuropathy to a toxic cause as a diagnosis of exclusion simply are not generating an accurate or complete differential diagnosis. Nevertheless, it is important to become familiar with the most common and representative neurotoxicants, because toxic neuropathies are among the most treatable forms of peripheral nervous system dysfunction.

References

[1] Schaumburg HH, Spencer PS. Recognizing neurotoxic disease. Neurology 1987;37:276–8.

[2] Albers JW. Clinical neurophysiology of generalized polyneuropathy. J Clin Neurophysiol 1993;10:149–66.

[3] Feldman RG, Niles CA, Kelly-Hayes M, et al. Peripheral neuropathy in arsenic smelter workers. Neurology 1979;29:939–44.

[4] Kreiss K, Zack MM, Landrigan PJ, et al. Neurologic evaluation of a population exposed to arsenic in Alaskan well water. Arch Environ Health 1983;38:116–21.

[5] Mukherjee SC, Rahman MM, Chowdhury UK, et al. Neuropathy in arsenic toxicity from groundwater arsenic contamination in West Bengal, India. J Environ Sci Health [A] 2003; 38:165–83.

[6] Greenberg SA. Acute demyelinating polyneuropathy with arsenic ingestion. Muscle Nerve 1996;19:1611–3.
[7] Jenkins RB. Inorganic arsenic and the nervous system. Brain 1966;89:479–98.
[8] Chhuttani PN, Chawla LS, Sharma TD. Arsenical neuropathy. Neurology 1967;17:269–74.
[9] Ghariani M, Adrien ML, Raucoules M, et al [Subacute arsenic poisoning]. Ann Fr Anesth Reanim 1991;10:304–7 [in French].
[10] Donofrio PD, Wilbourn AJ, Albers JW, et al. Acute arsenic intoxication presenting as Guillain-Barre-like syndrome. Muscle Nerve 1987;10:114–20.
[11] Bromberg MB, Albers JW. Patterns of sensory nerve conduction abnormalities in demyelinating and axonal peripheral nerve disorders. Muscle Nerve 1993;16:262–6.
[12] Landrigan PJ. Arsenic—state of the art. Am J Ind Med 1981;2:5–14.
[13] Valenzuela OL, Borja-Aburto VH, Garcia-Vargas GG, et al. Urinary trivalent methylated arsenic species in a population chronically exposed to inorganic arsenic. Environ Health Perspect 2005;113:250–4.
[14] Wax PM, Thornton CA. Recovery from severe arsenic-induced peripheral neuropathy with 2,3-dimercapto-1-propanesulphonic acid. J Toxicol Clin Toxicol 2000;38:777–80.
[15] Heyman A, Pfeiffer JB Jr, Willett RW, et al. Peripheral neuropathy caused by arsenical intoxication; a study of 41 cases with observations on the effects of BAL (2, 3, dimercaptopropanol). N Engl J Med 1956;254:401–9.
[16] Kuwabara S, Kai MR, Nagase H, et al. n-Hexane neuropathy caused by addictive inhalation: clinical and electrophysiological features. Eur Neurol 1999;41:163–7.
[17] Kuwabara S, Nakajima M, Tsuboi Y, et al. Multifocal conduction block in n-hexane neuropathy. Muscle Nerve 1993;16:1416–7.
[18] Krasavage WJ, O'Donoghue JL, DiVincenzo GD, et al. The relative neurotoxicity of methyl-n-butyl ketone, n-hexane and their metabolites. Toxicol Appl Pharmacol 1980; 52:433–41.
[19] Smith AG, Albers JW. n-Hexane neuropathy due to rubber cement sniffing. Muscle Nerve 1997;20:1445–50.
[20] Paulson GW, Waylonis GW. Polyneuropathy due to n-hexane. Arch Intern Med 1976;136: 880–2.
[21] Ruff RL, Petito CK, Acheson LS. Neuropathy associated with chronic low level exposure to n-hexane. Clin Toxicol 1981;18:515–9.
[22] Issever H, Malat G, Sabuncu HH, et al. Impairment of colour vision in patients with n-hexane exposure-dependent toxic polyneuropathy. Occup Med (Lond) 2002;52:183–6.
[23] Korobkin R, Asbury AK, Sumner AJ, et al. Glue-sniffing neuropathy. Arch Neurol 1975; 32:158–62.
[24] Spencer PS, Schaumburg HH. Organic solvent neurotoxicity. Facts and research needs. Scand J Work Environ Health 1985;11(Suppl 1):53–60.
[25] Griffin JW. Hexacarbon neurotoxicity. Neurobehav Toxicol Teratol 1981;3:437–44.
[26] Yokoyama K, Feldman RG, Sax DS, et al. Relation of distribution of conduction velocities to nerve biopsy findings in n-hexane poisoning. Muscle Nerve 1990;13:314–20.
[27] Chang CM, Yu CW, Fong KY, et al. N-hexane neuropathy in offset printers. J Neurol Neurosurg Psychiatry 1993;56:538–42.
[28] Kuang S, Huang H, Liu H, et al. [A clinical analysis of 102 cases of chronic n-hexane intoxication]. Zhonghua Nei Ke Za Zhi 2001;40:329–31 [in Chinese].
[29] Besser R, Treese N, Bohl J, et al. [Clinical, neurophysiologic and biopsy findings in neurotoxic amiodarone syndrome]. Med Klin 1994;89:367–72 [in German].
[30] Meier C, Kauer B, Muller U, et al. Neuromyopathy during chronic amiodarone treatment. A case report. J Neurol 1979;220:231–9.
[31] Lemaire JF, Autret A, Biziere K, et al. Amiodaron neuropathy: further arguments for human drug-induced neurolipidosis. Eur Neurol 1982;21:65–8.
[32] Martinez-Arizala A, Sobol SM, McCarty GE, et al. Amiodarone neuropathy. Neurology 1983;33:643–5.

[33] Charness ME, Morady F, Scheinman MM. Frequent neurologic toxicity associated with amiodarone therapy. Neurology 1984;34:669–71.
[34] Pellissier JF, Pouget J, Cros D, et al. Peripheral neuropathy induced by amiodarone chlorhydrate. A clinicopathological study. J Neurol Sci 1984;63:251–66.
[35] Anderson NE, Lynch NM, O'Brien KP. Disabling neurological complications of amiodarone. Aust N Z J Med 1985;15:300–4.
[36] Abarbanel JM, Osiman A, Frisher S, et al. Peripheral neuropathy and cerebellar syndrome associated with amiodarone therapy. Isr J Med Sci 1987;23:893–5.
[37] Fernando Roth R, Itabashi H, Louie J, et al. Amiodarone toxicity: myopathy and neuropathy. Am Heart J 1990;119:1223–5.
[38] Pulipaka ULD, Omalu B. Amiodarone-induced neuromyopathy: three cases and a review of the literature. J Clin Neuromusc Dis 2002;3:97–105.
[39] Palakurthy PR, Iyer V, Meckler RJ. Unusual neurotoxicity associated with amiodarone therapy. Arch Intern Med 1987;147:881–4.
[40] Jacobs JM, Costa-Jussa FR. The pathology of amiodarone neurotoxicity. II. Peripheral neuropathy in man. Brain 1985;108(Pt 3):753–69.
[41] Morgan JP. The Jamaica ginger paralysis. JAMA 1982;248:1864–7.
[42] Morgan JP, Penovich P. Jamaica ginger paralysis. Forty-seven-year follow-up. Arch Neurol 1978;35:530–2.
[43] Woolf AD. Ginger Jake and the blues: a tragic song of poisoning. Vet Hum Toxicol 1995; 37:252–4.
[44] Eyer P. Neuropsychopathological changes by organophosphorus compounds—a review. Hum Exp Toxicol 1995;14:857–64.
[45] Konno N. [Neurotoxicity of organophosphorus and dithiocarbamate compounds]. Nippon Eiseigaku Zasshi 2003;57:645–54 [in Japanese].
[46] Barrett DS, Oehme FW. The effect of a single oral dose of tri-o-cresyl phosphate on neurotoxic esterase and acetylcholinesterase activities in the central nervous system, erythrocytes and plasma. Vet Hum Toxicol 1994;36:1–4.
[47] Senanayake N, Johnson MK. Acute polyneuropathy after poisoning by a new organophosphate insecticide. N Engl J Med 1982;306:155–7.
[48] Van den Neucker K, Vanderstraeten G, De Muynck M, et al. The neurophysiologic examination in organophosphate ester poisoning. Case report and review of the literature. Electromyogr Clin Neurophysiol 1991;31:507–11.
[49] McConnell R, Delgado-Tellez E, Cuadra R, et al. Organophosphate neuropathy due to methamidophos: biochemical and neurophysiological markers. Arch Toxicol 1999;73: 296–300.
[50] Akassoglou K, Malester B, Xu J, et al. Brain-specific deletion of neuropathy target esterase/swisscheese results in neurodegeneration. Proc Natl Acad Sci U S A 2004; 101:5075–80.
[51] Pace A, Bove L, Nistico C, et al. Vinorelbine neurotoxicity: clinical and neurophysiological findings in 23 patients. J Neurol Neurosurg Psychiatry 1996;61:409–11.
[52] Topp KS, Tanner KD, Levine JD. Damage to the cytoskeleton of large diameter sensory neurons and myelinated axons in vincristine-induced painful peripheral neuropathy in the rat. J Comp Neurol 2000;424:563–76.
[53] Nozaki-Taguchi N, Chaplan SR, Higuera ES, et al. Vincristine-induced allodynia in the rat. Pain 2001;93:69–76.
[54] Moudgil SS, Riggs JE. Fulminant peripheral neuropathy with severe quadriparesis associated with vincristine therapy. Ann Pharmacother 2000;34):1136–8.
[55] Chauvenet AR, Shashi V, Selsky C, et al. Vincristine-induced neuropathy as the initial presentation of charcot-marie-tooth disease in acute lymphoblastic leukemia: a Pediatric Oncology Group study. J Pediatr Hematol Oncol 2003;25:316–20.
[56] Mercuri E, Poulton J, Buck J, et al. Vincristine treatment revealing asymptomatic hereditary motor sensory neuropathy type 1A. Arch Dis Child 1999;81:442–3.

[57] Orejana-Garcia AM, Pascual-Huerta J, Perez-Melero A. Charcot-Marie-Tooth disease and vincristine. J Am Podiatr Med Assoc 2003;93:229–33.
[58] Roelofs RI, Hrushesky W, Rogin J, et al. Peripheral sensory neuropathy and cisplatin chemotherapy. Neurology 1984;34:934–8.
[59] Thompson SW, Davis LE, Kornfeld M, et al. Cisplatin neuropathy. Clinical, electrophysiologic, morphologic, and toxicologic studies. Cancer 1984;54:1269–75.
[60] Strumberg D, Brugge S, Korn MW, et al. Evaluation of long-term toxicity in patients after cisplatin-based chemotherapy for non-seminomatous testicular cancer. Ann Oncol 2002; 13:229–36.
[61] Russell JW, Windebank AJ, McNiven MA, et al. Effect of cisplatin and ACTH4–9 on neural transport in cisplatin induced neurotoxicity. Brain Res 1995;676:258–67.
[62] McDonald ES, Windebank AJ. Cisplatin-induced apoptosis of DRG neurons involves bax redistribution and cytochrome c release but not fas receptor signaling. Neurobiol Dis 2002; 9:220–33.
[63] Lheureux P, Penaloza A, Gris M. Pyridoxine in clinical toxicology: a review. Eur J Emerg Med 2005;12:78–85.
[64] Schaumburg H, Kaplan J, Windebank A, et al. Sensory neuropathy from pyridoxine abuse. A new megavitamin syndrome. N Engl J Med 1983;309:445–8.
[65] Albin RL, Albers JW, Greenberg HS, et al. Acute sensory neuropathy-neuronopathy from pyridoxine overdose. Neurology 1987;37:1729–32.
[66] Moore D, House I, Dixon A. Thallium poisoning. Diagnosis may be elusive but alopecia is the clue. BMJ 1993;306:1527–9.
[67] Rangel-Guerra R, Martinez HR, Villarreal HJ. [Thallium poisoning. Experience with 50 patients]. Gac Med Mex 1990;126:487–94 [in Spanish].
[68] Meggs WJ, Hoffman RS, Shih RD, et al. Thallium poisoning from maliciously contaminated food. J Toxicol Clin Toxicol 1994;32:723–30.
[69] Kubis N, Talamon C, Smadja D, et al. [Peripheral neuropathy caused by thallium poisoning]. Rev Neurol (Paris) 1997;153:599–601.
[70] Desenclos JC, Wilder MH, Coppenger GW, et al. Thallium poisoning: an outbreak in Florida, 1988. South Med J 1992;85:1203–6.
[71] Herrero F, Fernandez E, Gomez J, et al. Thallium poisoning presenting with abdominal colic, paresthesia, and irritability. J Toxicol Clin Toxicol 1995;33:261–4.
[72] Andersen O. Clinical evidence and therapeutic indications in neurotoxicology, exemplified by thallotoxicosis. Acta Neurol Scand Suppl 1984;100:185–92.
[73] Sharma AN, Nelson LS, Hoffman RS. Cerebrospinal fluid analysis in fatal thallium poisoning: evidence for delayed distribution into the central nervous system. Am J Forensic Med Pathol 2004;25:156–8.
[74] Pau PW. Management of thallium poisoning. Hong Kong Med J 2000;6:316–8.
[75] Kuo HC, Huang CC, Tsai YT, et al. Acute painful neuropathy in thallium poisoning. Neurology 2005;65:302–4.
[76] Dumitru D, Kalantri A. Electrophysiologic investigation of thallium poisoning. Muscle Nerve 1990;13:433–7.
[77] Hoffman RS. Thallium toxicity and the role of Prussian blue in therapy. Toxicol Rev 2003; 22:29–40.
[78] Lehane L. Paralytic shellfish poisoning: a potential public health problem. Med J Aust 2001;175:29–31.
[79] Wu JY, Zheng L, Wang JH. Contamination of shellfish from Shanghai seafood markets with paralytic shellfish poisoning and diarrhetic shellfish poisoning toxins determined by mouse bioassay and HPLC. Food Addit Contam 2005;22:647–51.
[80] de Carvalho M, Jacinto J, Ramos N, et al. Paralytic shellfish poisoning: clinical and electrophysiological observations. J Neurol 1998;245:551–4.
[81] Long RR, Sargent JC, Hammer K. Paralytic shellfish poisoning: a case report and serial electrophysiologic observations. Neurology 1990;40:1310–2.

[82] Isbister GK, Kiernan MC. Neurotoxic marine poisoning. Lancet Neurol 2005;4:219–28.
[83] Kanchanapongkul J. Puffer fish poisoning: clinical features and management experience in 25 cases. J Med Assoc Thai 2001;84:385–9.
[84] Isbister GK, Son J, Wang F, et al. Puffer fish poisoning: a potentially life-threatening condition. Med J Aust 2002;177:650–3.
[85] Oda K, Araki K, Totoki T, et al. Nerve conduction study of human tetrodotoxication. Neurology 1989;39:743–5.
[86] Friedman M. Chemistry, biochemistry, and safety of acrylamide. A review. J Agric Food Chem 2003;51:4504–26.
[87] Mulloy KB. Two case reports of neurological disease in coal mine preparation plant workers. Am J Ind Med 1996;30:56–61.
[88] Kjuus H, Goffeng LO, Heier MS, et al. Effects on the peripheral nervous system of tunnel workers exposed to acrylamide and N-methylolacrylamide. Scand J Work Environ Health 2004;30:21–9.
[89] Myers JE, Macun I. Acrylamide neuropathy in a South African factory: an epidemiologic investigation. Am J Ind Med 1991;19:487–93.
[90] Deng H, He F, Zhang S, Calleman CJ, et al. Quantitative measurements of vibration threshold in healthy adults and acrylamide workers. Int Arch Occup Environ Health 1993;65:53–6.
[91] Harris CH, Gulati AK, Friedman MA, et al. Toxic neurofilamentous axonopathies and fast axonal transport. V. Reduced bidirectional vesicle transport in cultured neurons by acrylamide and glycidamide. J Toxicol Environ Health 1994;42:343–56.
[92] LoPachin RM, Ross JF, Lehning EJ. Nerve terminals as the primary site of acrylamide action: a hypothesis. Neurotoxicology 2002;23:43–59.
[93] LoPachin RM. Acrylamide neurotoxicity: neurological, morhological and molecular endpoints in animal models. Adv Exp Med Biol 2005;561:21–37.
[94] Jacknowitz AI, Le Frock JL, Prince RA. Nitrofurantoin polyneuropathy: report of two cases. Am J Hosp Pharm 1977;34:759–62.
[95] Yiannikas C, Pollard JD, McLeod JG. Nitrofurantoin neuropathy. Aust N Z J Med 1981; 11:400–5.
[96] Spielberg SP, Gordon GB. Nitrofurantoin cytotoxicity. In vitro assessment of risk based on glutathione metabolism. J Clin Invest 1981;67:37–41.
[97] Lovelace RE, Horwitz SJ. Peripheral neuropathy in long-term diphenylhydantoin therapy. Trans Am Neurol Assoc 1967;92:262–4.
[98] Eisen AA, Woods JF, Sherwin AL. Peripheral nerve function in long-term therapy with diphenylhydantoin. A clinical and electrophysiologic correlation. Neurology 1974;24: 411–7.
[99] Shorvon SD, Reynolds EH. Anticonvulsant peripheral neuropathy: a clinical and electrophysiological study of patients on single drug treatment with phenytoin, carbamazepine or barbiturates. J Neurol Neurosurg Psychiatry 1982;45:620–6.
[100] Taylor JW, Murphy MJ, Rivey MP. Clinical and electrophysiologic evaluation of peripheral nerve function in chronic phenytoin therapy. Epilepsia 1985;26:416–20.
[101] Swift TR, Gross JA, Ward LC, et al. Peripheral neuropathy in epileptic patients. Neurology 1981;31:826–31.
[102] Bauer M, Rabens SF. Trichloroethylene toxicity. Int J Dermatol 1977;16:113–6.
[103] Buxton PH, Hayward M. Polyneuritis cranialis associated with industrial trichloroethylene poisoning. J Neurol Neurosurg Psychiatry 1967;30:511–8.
[104] Annau Z. The neurobehavioral toxicity of trichloroethylene. Neurobehav Toxicol Teratol 1981;3:417–24.
[105] Feldman RG. Facial nerve latency studies in man: effects of trichlorethylene intoxication. Electromyography 1970;10:93–100.
[106] Feldman RG, Chirico-Post J, Proctor SP. Blink reflex latency after exposure to trichloroethylene in well water. Arch Environ Health 1988;43:143–8.

[107] Laureno R. Trichloroethylene does not cause trigeminal neuropathy. Muscle Nerve 1993; 16:217.
[108] Cavanagh JB, Buxton PH. Trichloroethylene cranial neuropathy: is it really a toxic neuropathy or does it activate latent herpes virus? J Neurol Neurosurg Psychiatry 1989;52: 297–303.
[109] Rhodes LE, Coleman MD, Lewis-Jones MS. Dapsone-induced motor peripheral neuropathy in pemphigus foliaceus. Clin Exp Dermatol 1995;20:155–6.
[110] Rosen I, Sornas R. Peripheral motor neuropathy caused by excessive intake of dapsone (Avlosulfon). Arch Psychiatr Nervenkr 1982;232:63–9.
[111] Koller WC, Gehlmann LK, Malkinson FD, et al. Dapsone-induced peripheral neuropathy. Arch Neurol 1977;34:644–6.
[112] Gutmann L, Martin JD, Welton W. Dapsone motor neuropathy—an axonal disease. Neurology 1976;26(6 PT 1):514–6.
[113] Mery L, Dega H, Prost C, Dubertret L. [Dapsone-induced sensory peripheral neuropathy]. Ann Dermatol Venereol 2003;130:447–9 [in French].
[114] Ahrens EM, Meckler RJ, Callen JP. Dapsone-induced peripheral neuropathy. Int J Dermatol 1986;25:314–6.
[115] Waldinger TP, Siegle RJ, Weber W, et al. Dapsone-induced peripheral neuropathy. Case report and review. Arch Dermatol 1984;120:356–9.
[116] Sirsat AM, Lalitha VS, Pandya SS. Dapsone neuropathy–report of three cases and pathologic features of a motor nerve. Int J Lepr Other Mycobact Dis 1987;55:23–9.
[117] Hill AB. The environment and disease: association or causation? Proc R Soc Med 1965;58: 295–300.

ELSEVIER
SAUNDERS

Neurol Clin 25 (2007) 277–301

NEUROLOGIC
CLINICS

Autonomic Peripheral Neuropathy

Roy Freeman, MD

Department of Neurology, Harvard Medical School, Center for Autonomic and Peripheral Nerve Disorders, Beth Israel Deaconess Medical Center, One Deaconess Road, Boston, MA 02215, USA

Most generalized peripheral polyneuropathies are accompanied by clinical or subclinical autonomic dysfunction. There is a group of peripheral neuropathies in which the small or unmyelinated fibers are selectively targeted [1]. In these neuropathies, autonomic dysfunction is the most prominent manifestation. The autonomic nervous system innervates viscera, vascular smooth muscle, endocrine and exocrine glands, the immune system, and soft tissues, and the associated signs and symptoms include impairment of cardiovascular, gastrointestinal, urogenital, thermoregulatory, pseudomotor, and pupillomotor autonomic function. A list of common peripheral neuropathies with autonomic manifestations is found in Box 1.

Diabetic autonomic neuropathy

Diabetes mellitus is the most common cause of autonomic neuropathy in the developed world [2,3]. This topic has been covered in detail in several recent reviews [4,5]. Diabetic cardiovascular autonomic neuropathy often manifests initially as an increased resting heart rate caused by a cardiac vagal neuropathy. As the autonomic neuropathy progresses, cardiac sympathetic fibers are involved and the resting tachycardia is replaced with a slowed, and ultimately fixed, heart rate [6–8]. Orthostatic hypotension occurs in diabetes as a consequence of efferent sympathetic vasomotor denervation, causing reduced vasoconstriction of the splanchnic and other peripheral vascular beds [9]. There is an increase in overall mortality and sudden death in patients with diabetic autonomic neuropathy [10–17]. In a meta-analysis of 15 studies, a significant association between cardiovascular autonomic neuropathy and subsequent mortality was observed. There was a pooled relative risk of 2.14 (95% confidence interval 1.83–2.51; $P < 0.0001$). The relative risk was stronger for studies for which two or

E-mail address: rfreeman@bidmc.harvard.edu

0733-8619/07/$ - see front matter
doi:10.1016/j.ncl.2007.01.001

Box 1. Autonomic peripheral neuropathies

Diabetes
Amyloidosis
Guillain-Barré syndrome
Acute and subacute autonomic neuropathies
Immune-mediated and paraneoplastic neuropathies
- Paraneoplastic neuropathies
- Connective tissue diseases
- Sjögren's syndrome
- Systemic lupus erythematosus
- Rheumatoid arthritis
- Mixed connective tissue disease

Hereditary neuropathies
- Hereditary sensory and autonomic neuropathies
- Fabry's disease
- Allgrove syndrome
- Navajo Indian neuropathy
- Tangier disease
- Multiple endocrine neoplasia, type 2b

Infectious diseases
- Chagas disease
- HIV neuropathy
- Botulism
- Leprosy
- Diphtheria

Toxic neuropathies
- Organic solvents
- Acrylamide
- Heavy metals
- Vacor
- Vincristine
- Cisplatinum
- Taxol
- Doxorubicin
- Cytosine arabinoside
- Perhexiline maleate
- Amiodarone
- Pentamidine
- Gold
- Podophyllin
- Marine toxins

more measures were used to define cardiac autonomic neuropathy. The stronger association observed in studies defining cardiac autonomic neuropathy by the presence of two or more abnormalities may be caused by more severe autonomic dysfunction in these subjects or a higher frequency of other comorbid complications that contributed to their higher mortality risk [18].

Symptoms of bladder dysfunction are observed in up to 50% of patients who have diabetes [19–21]. The earliest manifestation is impaired bladder sensation that increases the threshold for initiating the micturition reflex. A decrease in detrusor activity follows, which causes incomplete bladder emptying, an increased postvoid residual, decreased peak urinary flow rate, bladder overdistension, and ultimately, urinary retention and overflow incontinence [22,23].

Erectile failure affects up to 75% of men who have diabetes and may be the earliest symptom of diabetic autonomic neuropathy [24–28]. Vascular and psychogenic causes also may contribute to this symptom. In vitro studies of isolated corpus cavernosum tissue from men who have diabetes suggest that the erectile failure is caused by impairment in autonomic and endothelial-dependent nitric oxide–mediated relaxation of corpus cavernosum smooth muscle [29]. Ejaculatory failure caused by sympathetic nervous system dysfunction may precede the appearance of erectile dysfunction, although erectile failure can occur with retained ability to ejaculate and experience orgasm. There are few studies of genital autonomic neuropathy in women who have diabetes [30]. Reduced vaginal lubrication is a commonly reported symptom [31].

Autonomic dysfunction occurs throughout the gastrointestinal tract and produces several specific clinical syndromes [32,33]. Diabetic gastroparesis—delayed gastric emptying of solids or liquids—is present in up to 50% of individuals who have diabetes [34–36]. Gastroparesis may manifest as nausea, postprandial vomiting, bloating, belching, loss of appetite, and early satiety. Many patients, however, are asymptomatic despite impaired gastric motility [33]. Gastroparesis often impairs the establishment of adequate glycemic control. Dysfunction of the vagus nerve and intrinsic enteric autonomic nerves may play a role in this disorder. Recent studies have implicated hyperglycemia as a cause of reversible impairment in gastric and small intestinal motility during fasting and after food intake [37,38].

Constipation is the most frequently reported gastrointestinal autonomic symptom and is found in up to 60% of persons who have diabetes [39–41]. Diabetic diarrhea and other lower gastrointestinal tract symptoms also may occur. The diarrhea is profuse and watery and typically occurs at night. The diarrhea can last for hours or days and frequently alternates with constipation. In individuals who have type 2 diabetes, metformin therapy is a common cause of diarrhea [42]. Fecal incontinence caused by anal sphincter incompetence or reduced rectal sensation is often exacerbated by diarrhea [43,44].

Diabetic autonomic neuropathy initially results in a loss of thermoregulatory sweating in a glove and stocking distribution that can extend to the upper aspects of the limbs and anterior abdomen, conforming to the well-recognized length dependency of diabetic neuropathy [45]. Hyperhidrosis also may accompany diabetic autonomic neuropathy. Gustatory sweating, an abnormal production of sweating that appears over the face, head, neck, shoulders, and chest after eating even nonspicy foods, is observed occasionally. The pathophysiology of this phenomenon, which suggests aberrant reinnervation, is not fully elucidated [46].

Preliminary evidence indicates that impaired glucose tolerance is associated with and may be the direct cause of a peripheral neuropathy that predominantly affects small nerve fibers. The prevalence of this association is unknown. There are few community-based epidemiologic studies of this disorder, and the evidence is mainly derived from studies in tertiary care centers. Sudomotor abnormalities are a prominent manifestation of this neuropathy [47–51]. An open label diet and exercise program based on the Diabetes Prevention Program improved the metabolic parameters (including weight, lipids, and 2-hour glucose levels) and measures of small fiber structure and function. After 1 year of treatment there was a significant improvement in proximal intraepidermal nerve fiber density. The change in intraepidermal nerve fiber density correlated with pain scores. There also was a significant improvement in foot sweat volume measured by quantitative sudomotor axon reflex test (QSART) [49].

Amyloid neuropathy

Amyloidosis is caused by the deposition of insoluble fibrillar proteins in a beta-pleated sheet configuration within the extracellular space of various tissues and organs. Various amyloidogenic proteins have been associated with amyloidosis. The current classification of the systemic amyloidoses is based on the biochemistry of the precursor protein [52,53]. Although the fibril precursor proteins differ, there are strong similarities between the clinical presentations and pathology of the neuropathies associated with the different amyloidoses. Autonomic dysfunction frequently accompanies the polyneuropathy of primary ([AL] immunoglobulin light chain associated) and hereditary amyloidosis (familial amyloid polyneuropathy [FAP]) but in contrast is not common in secondary (amyloid A protein-associated) amyloidosis [52,53].

Patients who have amyloid neuropathy typically present with distal sensory symptoms, such as numbness, pain, paresthesias, and dysesthesias, although the autonomic manifestations occasionally may be the presenting feature of the neuropathy. On examination, there are signs of a sensorimotor polyneuropathy that predominantly involves the small fibers that mediate nociceptive and thermal sensation. Touch-pressure, position, and vibration perception are typically less severely impaired, particularly in patients who have FAP. Weakness is not a prominent feature and usually occurs later in the course of the disease. Painless, trophic ulcers may occur because of sensory loss and autonomic dysfunction. Characteristic autonomic signs and symptoms include postural hypotension, early satiety, diarrhea, constipation, fecal incontinence, disturbances in bladder function, pupillary abnormalities, and erectile failure. These autonomic manifestations are similar to those described with diabetic autonomic neuropathy. Sick sinus syndrome and A-V conduction deficits also are frequently present. Tests results for assessing cardiac vagal function are often abnormal [54].

Amyloid neuropathy is characterized pathologically by the deposition of insoluble beta-fibrillar proteins in the epi-, peri-, and endoneurium, the perineuronal tissues, and the neural vasculature. Ischemic, infiltrative, inflammatory, and toxic-metabolic factors have been implicated in the pathogenesis of the peripheral neuropathy, which remains unresolved [54].

The pathogenesis of amyloid peripheral neuropathy is unresolved [54]. Proposed pathogenic processes include ischemia caused by obliteration of small arteries and arterioles of nerves by amyloid deposits [55–57], infiltration and compression of peripheral nerves, dorsal nerve root ganglia, or autonomic ganglia by amyloid [56–58], inflammation, and toxic-metabolic factors, including oxidative stress [59,60].

Amyloidosis can be diagnosed by subcutaneous fat pad aspiration, gingival biopsy, or biopsy of rectal (and other gastrointestinal tract) mucosa. Nerve biopsy may be less sensitive because of the focal distribution of the amyloid deposits [61]. Amyloid deposits have a homogeneous, eosinophilic appearance on light microscopy and reveal a characteristic yellow-green birefringence when viewed under polarized light with Congo red staining.

Primary (AL) amyloidosis is the most common form of amyloidosis in the Western world. This disorder is a plasma cell dyscrasia in which a monoclonal population of bone marrow cells produces monoclonal immunoglobulin light chains or light-chain fragments that deposit as amyloid [62]. Symptoms typically appear in the sixth or seventh decade. Patients usually present with weight loss and fatigue. Peripheral neuropathy, which may be the presenting feature of the disease or an incidental finding, is present in up to 20% of patients who have AL [58]. Autonomic involvement of the cardiovascular, gastrointestinal, and urogenital systems is common [52,58,63]. Other systemic features include hepatomegaly, macroglossia, cutaneous ecchymoses, cardiomyopathy, and nephrotic range proteinuria. Immunofixation electrophoresis of serum or urine detects immunoglobulins or light chains in 90% of patients who have AL amyloidosis [62].

The median survival of patients who have AL amyloid neuropathy ranges from 13 to 35 months, with a 3-year survival rate of 38% to 50%. The prognosis for patients who have heart failure is considerably worse [64,65]. Treatment with melphalan and prednisone improves survival, particularly when associated with a reduction in serum or urine monoclonal protein [64,65]. Stem cell transplantation in carefully selected patients may improve survival further [66].

FAP is a manifestation of hereditary generalized amyloidosis. This disorder was first reported in Portugal in 1952 [67]. The hereditary amyloidoses are autosomal dominantly inherited diseases in which the amyloid precursor is a mutant protein. Mutant transthyretin (TTR), previously called prealbumin, a 14-kDa protein that serves as the transport protein for thyroxine and retinol-binding protein, is the most common cause of hereditary amyloidosis. It is encoded by a single gene on chromosome 18. The most commonly observed mutation is a substitution of methionine for valine at position 30 (Met-Val 30) [68,69]. This disorder, which encompasses what was previously called FAP I (Portuguese or Andrade amyloidosis) [67] and FAP II (Indiana-Swiss or Rukavina amyloidosis) [70,71], has been associated with more than 100 single or double mutations or deletions of the TTR gene [72].

TTR amyloidosis typically presents in the third to fifth decade. Characteristic features include prominent dysautonomia that accompanies a painful sensorimotor neuropathy, carpal tunnel syndrome, vitreous opacities, nephropathy, and cardiomyopathy. Sensory neuropathy and gastrointestinal symptoms are the most frequent initial symptoms. Death occurs 5 to 15 years after the appearance of symptoms [53,72]. The clinical phenotype is variable, however, and depends on the position and nature of the amino acid substitution. Variant presentations include late onset [73], isolated carpal tunnel syndrome, and a distal sensory or sensorimotor neuropathy without autonomic dysfunction [70,71]. Clusters of hereditary amyloidosis caused by mutant TTR have been found in Portugal, Japan, Sweden, United States, Spain, Finland, Ireland, France, and Germany [53,72].

A late-onset, seemingly sporadic FAP (TTR Met 30) has been documented in Portugal and Japan. Patients in the sixth decade or older typically present with lower extremity paresthesias. The autonomic features are mild and not incapacitating. This disorder has an autosomal dominant pattern of inheritance with low penetrance. There is a high male/female ratio (10.7:1) [73].

FAP is also rarely caused by mutations in other proteins besides TTR. FAP rarely may be caused by mutations in the genes encoding for apolipoprotein-A1, fibrinogen Aα, lysozyme, and gelsolin [52]. A recent report documented that almost 10% of patients with sporadic amyloidosis, presumed to be primary (AL) amyloidosis, actually had hereditary amyloidosis. In more than half of these patients, neuropathy was the dominant clinical presentation. These results suggest that hereditary amyloidosis may occur more frequently than previously suspected. Given the different prognoses and therapies for the two conditions, these findings emphasize the importance of genetic testing in patients with amyloidosis who do not have a pathologically confirmed diagnosis of AL disease. A low-grade monoclonal gammopathy was present in 24% of patients who were found later to have hereditary amyloidosis [74].

Because most of the mutated amyloidogenic TTR is secreted by the liver, orthotopic liver transplant is the most effective treatment for hereditary amyloidosis. Liver transplant removes the principal source of variant TTR and reduces circulating TTR by up to 90%. In appropriately selected patients, liver transplant improves neurophysiologic measures, nerve morphology, and survival [75,76]. Although the extent of the benefits of liver transplantation on the sensorimotor peripheral neuropathy is unresolved [76,77], the features of an established autonomic neuropathy do not seem to improve significantly with this intervention [76,78,79]. Similarly, conduction system abnormalities and arrhythmias seem to progress despite liver transplantation [79]. Pharmacotherapeutic interventions that inhibit amyloidogenesis eventually may replace liver transplant [80].

Acute and subacute autonomic neuropathies

Guillain-Barré syndrome

Guillain-Barré syndrome (acute inflammatory demyelinating polyradiculoneuropathy) is a monophasic illness of immune etiology that presents as an acutely evolving sensorimotor polyneuropathy of varying severity. Autonomic manifestations such as sinus tachycardia, sinus pauses and other tachy- and bradyarrhythmias, blood pressure lability, bowel and bladder dysfunction, pupillomotor disturbances, sudomotor dysfunction, and vasomotor abnormalities frequently accompany Guillain-Barré syndrome [81,82]. Autonomic manifestations, which occasionally may be the presenting feature of Guillain-Barré syndrome [83], may be more prominent in patients with respiratory failure, severe motor deficits, and the axonal variant of Guillain-Barré syndrome [84–86]. The autonomic features can result in significant mortality and morbidity in some patients, although they are usually overshadowed by the motor features of the disorder.

Acute and subacute autonomic neuropathies

Autonomic manifestations may be the sole or predominant feature of an acute or subacute peripheral neuropathy [87]. Although acute or subacute autonomic neuropathy is usually immune-mediated or paraneoplastic, the differential diagnosis includes botulism, porphyria [88], and some toxic neuropathies (see later discussion). The hallmark of these autonomic neuropathies is the acute or subacute presentation, in varying combinations, of orthostatic hypotension, anhidrosis, constipation, bladder atony, impotence, secretomotor paralysis, and blurring of vision associated with tonic pupils. Mild sensorimotor manifestations may accompany the autonomic manifestations but are not the predominant aspect of the presentation. The autonomic features of this disorder may involve the sympathetic and parasympathetic divisions of the autonomic nervous system (pandysautonomia) [89] or the sympathetic or parasympathetic nervous system alone (also called cholinergic dysautonomia) [90]. Only 40% of cases recover fully to premorbid status. Autonomic testing in the recovery phase of illness in these patients often shows evidence of persisting subclinical autonomic dysfunction [87].

Acute dysautonomia has been described in association with infectious mononucleosis or Epstein Barr virus [91,92], streptococcus [93], Coxsackie B virus [94], rubella [95], and herpes simplex virus [96] infections in addition to other nondiagnosed viral syndromes. Associations with malignancies [97,98] (see later discussion) and connective tissue diseases have been described in other cases [99,100]. Lending further support to the likelihood that some of these cases are immune mediated, a positive therapeutic response to intravenous immunoglobulin has been reported in uncontrolled case studies [101,102].

An acute case of subacute autonomic neuropathy may occur in association with connective tissue disease, including Sjögren's syndrome [103], rheumatoid arthritis [104], systemic lupus erythematosus [99,100], and mixed connective tissue disease. No specific autoantibodies have been associated with the dysautonomia in connective tissue diseases.

Immune-mediated and paraneoplastic autonomic neuropathies (specific autoantibody-associated autonomic neuropathies)

Autonomic dysfunction has been associated with the presence of specific autoantibodies (Box 2). The subacute appearance of autonomic symptoms, including orthostatic hypotension, pupillomotor dysfunction, sudomotor dysfunction, constipation, urinary retention, impotence, and xerophthalmia, has been associated with the presence of anti-Hu antibodies (also known as Type 1 antineuronal nuclear antibody, ANNA-1) in patients with malignancies, especially small-cell lung cancer. Other associated malignancies include non–small-cell lung cancer and malignancies of the gastrointestinal tract, prostate, breast, bladder, kidney, pancreas, testicle, and ovary [105–108]. Dysautonomia may be an isolated manifestation of a paraneoplastic disorder or part of a generalized paraneoplastic syndrome that includes a sensory neuronopathy, limbic and brainstem encephalitis, encephalomyelitis,

Box 2. Specific antibodies associated with autonomic neuropathies

Anti-Hu antibodies (Type 1 anti-neuronal nuclear antibody, ANNA-1)
Purkinje cell antibodies Type 2 (PCA-2)
Collapsing response mediator protein-5 (CRMP-5)
Neuronal nicotinic acetylcholine receptor antibodies
P/Q-type Ca2 + channel antibodies
Acetylcholine receptor antibodies

cerebellar degeneration, and a sensorimotor peripheral neuropathy. Other autoantibodies that are associated with a paraneoplastic autonomic neuropathy include Purkinje cell cytoplasmic antibodies Type 2 (PCA-2) [109] and antibodies to the neuron cytoplasmic protein, collapsin response-mediator protein-5 (CRMP-5) [110].

Patients who have autoantibodies to ganglionic acetylcholine receptors typically present with a subacute autonomic neuropathy with progression to panautonomic failure [111]. Based on studies in animals, these antibodies impair ganglionic synaptic transmission by depleting acetylcholine receptors on the ganglionic neuron [112]. The typical clinical findings in autoimmune autonomic neuropathy include dry eyes and mouth, fixed heart rate, impaired pupillary response to light and accommodation, gastrointestinal dysmotility, and urinary retention [111,113,114]. Orthostatic hypotension can be the most incapacitating feature, with frequent syncopal episodes and restrictions on activities of daily living. Laboratory studies reveal substantially reduced levels of plasma catecholamines [112]. Some [115], but not all [116], patients respond to plasmapheresis and immune modulation. Malignancies associated with these antibodies include small-cell lung carcinoma, thymoma, bladder carcinoma, and rectal carcinoma. These antibodies may be present in patients with the clinical phenotype of pure autonomic failure [117]. When cholinergic features are prominent, the diagnosis of an immune-mediated autonomic neuropathy should be entertained [113].

Celiac disease (gluten-sensitive enteropathy) is the most common manifestation of gluten sensitivity; however, diverse manifestations may accompany the disorder [118,119]. Several recent reports have drawn attention to the association between gluten sensitivity with elevated antigliadin antibodies and neurologic disorders [118,119], although given the high percentage of antigliadin antibodies in the general population (6%–12%), the etiologic significance of this association is uncertain in most patients [120,121]. We have documented that 2.4% of patients referred for autonomic testing had biopsy-proven celiac disease and dysautonomia [122], a frequency of celiac disease similar to that reported in idiopathic peripheral neuropathy [119]. In these patients, nausea, which was postural in nature, was the primary symptom for referral. Other reported autonomic symptoms included lightheadedness, palpitations, fatigue, presyncope, and syncope. Autonomic test results revealed abnormalities in sympathetic and parasympathetic nervous system function [122]. Esophageal dysmotility and subclinical abnormalities of cardiovascular reflexes, which were present in 19% of patients, also have been reported in patients who have celiac disease [123].

Hereditary autonomic neuropathies

The hereditary autonomic neuropathies are a heterogeneous group of disorders, some of which have significant involvement of autonomic fibers (see Box 1) [124–127]. Autonomic features are most prominent in the hereditary sensory and autonomic neuropathies (HSAN) and Fabry's disease [124–127]. Other hereditary autonomic neuropathies include Allgrove syndrome [128], Tangier disease [129–131], a sensory and autonomic neuropathy with arthropathy that is present in Navajo children [132,133], and multiple endocrine neoplasia, type 2b [134]. HSANs are characterized by prominent sensory loss without motor involvement and by often striking dysautonomia. The axon reflex-mediated vasomotor response (the flare) after intradermal histamine is absent in all HSAN.

Hereditary sensory and autonomic neuropathy type I

HSAN type I is an autosomal dominant, hereditary sensory radiculoneuropathy that presents in the second decade. Patients who have this disorder present with distal pain that is associated with sensory loss that predominantly involves nociceptive and thermal perception while relatively sparing touch-pressure sensation and proprioception. The sensory loss progresses gradually and is accompanied by anhidrosis, trophic ulcers, acral injuries, stress fractures, and osteomyelitis [125,126]. HSAN type I has been associated with a mutation in the SPTLC1 gene on chromosome 9q22.1-q22.3 that encodes for subunit 1 of serine palmitoyltransferase—the rate limiting enzyme for the synthesis of the sphingolipids, ceramide, and sphingomyelin [135,136]. A variant of this disorder, associated with chronic cough and gastroesophageal reflux, has been mapped to a locus on chromosome 3p22-p24 [137].

Hereditary sensory and autonomic neuropathy type II

HSAN type II (congenital sensory neuropathy or Morvan's disease) is an autosomal recessive or sporadic disorder that presents in infancy or early childhood. This disorder is associated with profound sensory loss that involves large and small fiber modalities (pain and temperature perception and proprioception). Marked hypotonia and decreased deep tendon reflexes are common [127]. Trophic changes are present in the upper and lower extremities. Painless fractures may occur. Autonomic features include episodic hyperhidrosis, tonic pupils, constipation, and apneic episodes [125,126]. Tearing may be delayed but is eventually normal. Sural nerve biopsy reveals depletion of large and small myelinated fibers but only slightly decreased number of unmyelinated fibers. This disorder has been associated with a mutation on a gene, HSN2, with a locus that maps to chromosome 12p13.33 [138].

Hereditary sensory and autonomic neuropathy type III

Autonomic manifestations are prominent in HSAN type III (Riley-Day syndrome or familial dysautonomia). This autosomal recessive disorder is seen primarily in Ashkenazi Jewish children. The incidence of familial dysautonomia is 1 in 3700 live births among Ashkenazi Jews, and the carrier frequency is 1 in 32 individuals [139,140]. The defective gene that causes familial dysautonomia has been mapped to the long arm of chromosome 9 (9q31) [141]. Most (99.5%) patients who have familial dysautonomia have a single, splicing mutation in the I-kappa B kinase associated protein (*IKBKAP*) gene that results in tissue-specific expression of a truncated IKAP protein [142].

HSAN III presents in infancy. The clinical features of this disease include insensitivity to pain and temperature stimuli but sparing visceral pain, absence of tears (alacrima), hypoactive corneal and tendon reflexes, and absence of lingual fungiform papillae. Poor suck and feeding, esophageal reflux with vomiting and aspiration, and swallowing dyscoordination may be the first clinical manifestations [140,143]. Autonomic disturbances may be prominent at any point in the disease. Autonomic manifestations include episodic hyperhidrosis, vasomotor instability with defective temperature homeostasis, breath-holding episodes, protracted episodes of vomiting, postural hypotension, hypertensive crises, and supersensitivity to cholinergic and adrenergic agents.

Hereditary sensory and autonomic neuropathy type IV

HSAN type IV (congenital insensitivity to pain with anhidrosis, anhidrotic sensory neuropathy), the second most common HSAN, is an autosomal recessive disorder that manifests in the first months of life with insensitivity to pain, anhidrosis, episodes of unexplained fever, and mental and motor developmental retardation [127]. The skin appears thick, hyperkeratotic, and callused because of the anhidrosis. Virtual absence of unmyelinated fibers has been noted in peripheral nerves [144,145]. Skin biopsy morphology of patients who have HSAN IV reveals deficient C and A delta fibers in the epidermis and absent or hypoplastic dermal sweat glands without innervation [146,147]. Intradermal injection or iontophoresis of cholinergic agonists, such as acetylcholine or methacholine, does not produce direct sweat gland–stimulated or axon reflex–mediated sweating [148]. Frame-shift, splice, and missense mutations have been documented in the NTRK1 (TRKA) gene located on chromosome 1 (1q21-q22). This gene encodes for neurotrophic tyrosine kinase receptor type I, which is autophosphorylated in response to nerve growth factor [149].

Hereditary sensory and autonomic neuropathy type V

This rare disorder presents in infancy with loss of pain perception that leads to acral ulcers, painless fractures, and other trophic injuries. Sudomotor abnormalities are present [150]. A mutation in the NTRK1 gene also may be responsible for this neuropathy [151].

Fabry's disease

Fabry's disease, or angiokeratoma corporis diffusum, is an X-linked, recessively inherited disorder that is associated with deficiency of the enzyme alpha-galactosidase A (ceramide trihexosidase). The enzyme deficiency results in the accumulation of ceramide trihexoside and other neutral glycosphingolipids in homozygotes. There is extensive lipid deposition in various tissues, including the skin, nervous system, vascular endothelium, kidney, cardiovascular system, and eye [152]. The neurologic manifestations of this disorder are caused by the deposition of glycolipids in autonomic and dorsal root ganglia, perineurial cells, and unmyelinated and myelinated axons [153–155].

The autonomic manifestations include hypo- or anhidrosis, reduced saliva and tear formation, impaired cutaneous flare response to scratch and histamine, and disordered intestinal motility. Gastrointestinal symptoms may be as severe as their sensory complaints. The generalized presentation of the anhidrosis has suggested that sweat gland dysfunction, perhaps caused by intracytoplasmic inclusions in the eccrine glands, may play a role in the anhidrosis [156]. Sural nerve biopsies studies have demonstrated degeneration and loss of unmyelinated fibers [153–155]. Skin biopsies show decreased intraepidermal small nerve fibers [157]. Fabry's disease can be diagnosed by assaying the enzyme alpha-galactosidase A in leukocytes or skin fibroblasts [158].

Enzyme replacement therapy leads to a modest improvement in the clinical manifestations of the small-fiber neuropathy associated with this disorder. QSART testing may even normalize in some patients; however, no evidence indicates that these functional changes are associated with improvement in intraepidermal innervation [159,160].

Allgrove's syndrome

Allgrove's syndrome is an autosomal recessive disorder characterized by achalasia, alacrima, autonomic impairment, and adrenocorticotropin hormone (ACTH) insensitivity and progressive neurologic dysfunction. Affected individuals have between two and four of these relatively common symptoms occurring in varying combinations. Because these are relatively common clinical conditions, individuals with this syndrome may be undiagnosed [128]. The pattern of inheritance is autosomal recessive. Most cases of Allgrove's syndrome have no family history. A locus on chromosome 12q13 has been identified using genetic linkage analysis in a small number of families [128]. The disorder rarely may be unrecognized until adulthood [161].

Other hereditary autonomic neuropathies

Autonomic neuropathies are associated with several other hereditary disorders, including Tangier disease [129–131], a sensory and autonomic neuropathy with arthropathy that is present in Navajo children [132,133], and multiple endocrine neoplasia, type 2b [134].

Autonomic neuropathy caused by infectious diseases

The peripheral neuropathies associated with several infectious diseases have prominent accompanying autonomic manifestations.

Botulism

Botulism is an acute neuromuscular disorder caused by the binding of a neurotoxin from the anaerobic bacterium, *Clostridium botulinum*, to the presynaptic nerve terminal, preventing acetylcholine release [162]. The illness begins with gastrointestinal manifestations, followed by autonomic symptoms and a descending paralysis that spreads from the extraocular and bulbar muscles to the limbs [163–166]. Autonomic symptoms result from cholinergic dysfunction and include constipation, blurred vision, urinary hesitancy and retention, and dry mouth and eyes. Dilated pupils, with poor response to light and accommodation, are characteristic autonomic signs. Orthostatic hypotension also may be present. Autonomic symptoms may occur in botulism, even in the absence of the characteristic motor and cranial nerve abnormalities [163–165]. Among toxigenic strains of *C botulinum*, types A, B, and E account for most human cases [162].

Bowel and bladder symptoms often persist after resolution of the infection. Diagnosis is based on the clinical and electrophysiologic findings and is verified by demonstrating neurotoxin in the serum, stool, or contaminated food or by culturing *C botulinum* from the stool. Botulism may manifest as a subacute cholinergic disturbance without associated clinical or electromyographic evidence of motor-endplate pathology [167,168]. Treatment involves eliminating sources of toxin. Intravenous trivalent equine antitoxin can prevent progression and reduce mortality, which remains at approximately 5% to 15%. Case studies of patients with the subacute onset of cholinergic disturbance without associated clinical or electromyographic evidence of motor-endplate pathology [167] underscore that dysautonomia may occur in botulism without the typical motor abnormalities [168].

HIV infection

Autonomic dysfunction may occur in patients with HIV infection. Although autonomic dysfunction seems to occur more frequently and with greater severity in patients who have AIDS, several reports suggest that seropositive patients and patients in the early stages of infection exhibit evidence of dysautonomia. The severity of autonomic dysfunction seems to constitute a continuum from the early to later stages of HIV infection [169–172]. In addition to direct virus effects and virus host interactions, toxins, medications, vitamin deficiency, and malnutrition may play a role in the manifestations of this syndrome in the later stages of illness. The symptoms of dysautonomia have included orthostatic hypotension, syncope, presyncope, sweating disturbances, bladder and bowel dysfunction, and impotence [169]. Autonomic testing reveals sympathetic and parasympathetic nervous system abnormalities [169,173].

Chagas' disease

Chagas' disease, which is caused by a parasitic infection by the protozoan *Trypanosoma cruzi*, is found predominantly in Latin America. Because of immigration patterns, there is an increasing incidence of Chagas' disease in the United States, and the autonomic manifestations of this disease should be considered in the differential diagnosis of dysautonomia in nonendemic areas. Vectorial transmission is the most common mode of infection in Latin America, whereas in nonendemic areas, transmission via blood transfusions is more common [174].

Clinical manifestations occur in two stages, the acute and chronic phases of the disease, which are separated by an indeterminate phase. Acute infection is characterized by fevers, myalgias, and sweating. Congestive heart failure may be present. Autonomic abnormalities occur in the chronic phase of the disease and are characterized by severe gastrointestinal and cardiovascular dysfunction. Gastrointestinal complaints include dysphagia, sialorrhea and constipation; reduced bowel motility, megaesophagus, and megacolon are the most frequent gastrointestinal findings. These abnormalities are caused by denervation of the intrinsic enteric neurons of the submucosal (Meissner) and myenteric (Auerbach) plexuses [175–177]. Cardiovascular manifestations include impaired blood pressure response to standing, resting bradycardia, conduction system abnormalities, arrhythmias, cardiomegaly, and cardiac failure [178–183]. The pathogenesis of the autonomic dysfunction is unresolved and may be caused by direct neural injury during the acute illness, an immune-mediated response, or both.

Leprosy

Autonomic dysfunction is observed in patients with leprous neuropathy caused by infection by the acid-fast bacillus *Mycobacterium leprae*. Focal anhidrosis, which is the best documented autonomic abnormality, occurs in association with impaired pain and temperature perception in the cooler regions of the body. These are the earliest neurologic manifestations of leprosy and correlate with the loss of cutaneous innervation [184]. More generalized autonomic symptoms, such as syncope, gustatory sweating, and erectile dysfunction, also may occur [185].

Diphtheria

A toxin-mediated sensorimotor neuropathy occurs some weeks after pharyngeal or cutaneous diphtheria. Early palatal paralysis in the disease is probably a direct effect of diphtheria toxin but can occur at any time between the first and seventh weeks after infection [186,187]. Accommodation paralysis, with preserved light responses, is an early manifestation in 10% to 50% of cases [186]. The sparing of the light reflex is a clinical feature that distinguishes diphtheritic from botulism-related pupillary changes. Temporary loss of bladder or bowel control has been reported. Resting tachycardia and an often serious myocarditis are other features. Abnormalities on tests of cardiac vagal function have been documented [187,188].

Toxic neuropathies

Several industrial and environmental toxins and medications can cause autonomic neuropathy (see Box 1). Autonomic neuropathy has been reported in individuals exposed to organic solvents [189,190], arsenic [191], mercury [192], other heavy metals [193], industrial-use acrylamide [194], thallium [192,195], and the rat poison, Vacor (N-3-pyridylmethyl-N'-paranitrophenyl urea) [196].

Autonomic neuropathy also may follow treatment with cytotoxic agents used in cancer chemotherapy. Clinically evident dysautonomia occurs most consistently with the vinca-alkaloid, vincristine [197,198]. Autonomic abnormalities are also observed in patients treated with cisplatin [199–202] and paclitaxel [203–206]. There are interindividual differences in susceptibility to chemotherapy-induced peripheral neuropathies; however, patients with pre-existing peripheral nerve injury caused by diabetes mellitus, ethanol, and inherited and other peripheral neuropathies may show a greater predisposition to the development of chemotherapy-induced neurotoxicity. Other medications that may cause autonomic dysfunction include the anti-arrhythmic agent, amiodarone [207], the coronary vasodilator, perhexiline [208], and pentamidine [209].

Marine toxins may affect ion transport, induce channels or pores in neural and muscular cellular membranes, alter intracellular membranes of organelles, and release mediators of inflammation. The box jellyfish, particularly *Chironex fleckeri*, which is in the Indo-Pacific region, is the world's most venomous marine animal and causes severe sympathetic and parasympathetic nervous system dysfunction in exposed patients [210]. Ciguatera poisoning is the most prevalent marine toxic exposure. Ciguatoxins are potent heat stable, non-protein, lipophilic sodium channel activator toxins that bind to the voltage sensitive sodium channel. The toxin is stored in the viscera of fish that have eaten the photosynthetic dinoflagellate and is progressively concentrated upwards along the food chain. The initial manifestations are characteristically sensory and include paresthesias, dysesthesias, and pain. Autonomic features may be prominent, including hypersalivation, bradycardia, hypotension, mydriasis, and meiosis [210–212]. Intravenous mannitol may reverse the acute sensory and autonomic features of ciguatera toxicity [212].

References

[1] Freeman R. Autonomic peripheral neuropathy. Lancet 2005;365(9466):1259–70.
[2] Hilsted J, Low PA. Diabetic autonomic neuropathy. In: Low PA, editor. Clinical autonomic disorders. Philadelphia: Lipincott-Raven; 1997. p. 487–508.
[3] Freeman R. The peripheral nervous system and diabetes. In: Kahn CR, Weir GC, King GL, editors. Joslin's diabetes mellitus. Philadelphia: Lippincott Williams & Wilkins; 2004. p. 951–68.
[4] Vinik AI, Freeman R, Erbas T. Diabetic autonomic neuropathy. Semin Neurol 2003;23(4): 365–72.
[5] Vinik AI, Maser RE, Mitchell BD, et al. Diabetic autonomic neuropathy. Diabetes Care 2003;26(5):1553–79.
[6] Lloyd-Mostyn RH, Watkins PJ. Defective innervation of heart in diabetic autonomic neuropathy. BMJ 1975;3:15–7.
[7] Bennett T, Hosking DJ, Hampton JR. Cardiovascular control in diabetes mellitus. BMJ 1975;2:585–7.
[8] Ewing DJ, Campbell IW, Clarke BF. Heart rate changes in diabetes mellitus. Lancet 1981;1:183–6.
[9] Low PA, Walsh JC, Huang CY, et al. The sympathetic nervous system in diabetic neuropathy: a clinical and pathological study. Brain 1975;98:341–56.
[10] Ewing DJ, Campbell IW, Clarke BF. The natural history of diabetic autonomic neuropathy. Q J Med 1980;49:95–108.
[11] O'Brien IA, McFadden JP, Corrall RJ. The influence of autonomic neuropathy on mortality in insulin-dependent diabetes. Q J Med 1991;79:495–502.
[12] Navarro X, Kennedy WR, Loewenson RB, et al. Influence of pancreas transplantation on cardiorespiratory reflexes, nerve conduction, and mortality in diabetes mellitus. Diabetes 1990;39:802–6.
[13] Rathmann W, Ziegler D, Jahnke M, et al. Mortality in diabetic patients with cardiovascular autonomic neuropathy. Diabet Med 1993;10(9):820–4.
[14] Sampson MJ, Wilson S, Karagiannis P, et al. Progression of diabetic autonomic neuropathy over a decade in insulin-dependent diabetics. Q J Med 1990;75:635–46.
[15] Chen HS, Hwu CM, Kuo BI, et al. Abnormal cardiovascular reflex tests are predictors of mortality in type 2 diabetes mellitus. Diabet Med 2001;18(4):268–73.
[16] Gerritsen J, Dekker JM, TenVoorde BJ, et al. Impaired autonomic function is associated with increased mortality, especially in subjects with diabetes, hypertension, or a history of cardiovascular disease: the Hoorn Study. Diabetes Care 2001;24(10):1793–8.
[17] Maser RE, Pfeifer MA, Dorman JS, et al. Diabetic autonomic neuropathy and cardiovascular risk: Pittsburgh Epidemiology of Diabetes Complications Study III. Arch Intern Med 1990;150:1218–22.
[18] Maser RE, Mitchell BD, Vinik AI, et al. The association between cardiovascular autonomic neuropathy and mortality in individuals with diabetes: a meta-analysis. Diabetes Care 2003;26(6):1895–901.
[19] Frimodt-Moller C, Mortensen S. Treatment of diabetic cystopathy. Ann Intern Med 1980; 92:327–8.
[20] Ellenberg M. Development of urinary bladder dysfunction in diabetes mellitus. Ann Intern Med 1980;92:321–3.
[21] Ioanid CP, Noica N. Incidence and diagnostic aspects of the bladder disorders in diabetics. Eur Urol 1981;7:211–4.
[22] Kaplan SA, Blaivas JG. Diabetic cystopathy [review]. J Diabet Complications 1988;2(3): 133–9.
[23] Kaplan SA, Te AE, Blaivas JG. Urodynamic findings in patients with diabetic cystopathy [see comments]. J Urol 1995;153(2):342–4.

[24] McCulloch DK, Campbell IW, Wu FC, et al. The prevalence of diabetic impotence. Diabetologia 1980;18:279–83.
[25] Ellenberg M. Impotence in diabetes: the neurologic factor. Ann Intern Med 1971;75(2): 213–9.
[26] Kaiser FE, Korenman SG. Impotence in diabetic men. Am J Med 1988;85(Suppl 5A): 147–52.
[27] Hakim LS, Goldstein I. Diabetic sexual dysfunction [review]. Endocrinol Metab Clin North Am 1996;25(2):379–400.
[28] Bacon CG, Hu FB, Giovannucci E, et al. Association of type and duration of diabetes with erectile dysfunction in a large cohort of men. Diabetes Care 2002;25(8):1458–63.
[29] de Tejada IS, Goldstein I, Azadzoi K, et al. Impaired neurogenic and endothelium-mediated relaxation of penile smooth muscle from diabetic men with impotence. N Engl J Med 1989;320:1025–30.
[30] Ellenberg M. Sexual function in diabetic patients. Ann Intern Med 1980;92:331–3.
[31] Enzlin P, Mathieu C, Van den BA, et al. Sexual dysfunction in women with type 1 diabetes: a controlled study. Diabetes Care 2002;25(4):672–7.
[32] Wegener M, Borsch G, Schaffstein J, et al. Gastrointestinal transit disorders in patients with insulin-treated diabetes mellitus. Dig Dis 1990;8:23–36.
[33] Horowitz M, Harding PE, Maddox AF, et al. Gastric and oesophageal emptying in patients with Type 2 (non-insulin-dependent) diabetes mellitus. Diabetologia 1989;32:151–9.
[34] Enck P, Frieling T. Pathophysiology of diabetic gastroparesis. Diabetes 1997;46(Suppl 2): S77–81.
[35] Kong MF, Horowitz M, Jones KL, et al. Natural history of diabetic gastroparesis. Diabetes Care 1999;22(3):503–7.
[36] Jones KL, Russo A, Stevens JE, et al. Predictors of delayed gastric emptying in diabetes. Diabetes Care 2001;24(7):1264–9.
[37] Hebbard GS, Samsom M, Sun WM, et al. Hyperglycemia affects proximal gastric motor and sensory function during small intestinal triglyceride infusion. Am J Physiol 1996; 271(5 Pt 1):G814–9.
[38] Rayner CK, Samsom M, Jones KL, et al. Relationships of upper gastrointestinal motor and sensory function with glycemic control. Diabetes Care 2001;24(2):371–81.
[39] Battle WM, Snape WJ Jr, Alavi A, et al. Colonic dysfunction in diabetes mellitus. Gastroenterology 1980;79:1217–21.
[40] Feldman M, Schiller LR. Disorders of gastrointestinal motility associated with diabetes mellitus. Ann Intern Med 1983;98:378–84.
[41] Maleki D, Locke GR III, Camilleri M, et al. Gastrointestinal tract symptoms among persons with diabetes mellitus in the community. Arch Intern Med 2000 160(18):2808–16.
[42] Lysy J, Israeli E, Goldin E. The prevalence of chronic diarrhea among diabetic patients. Am J Gastroenterol 1999;94(8):2165–70.
[43] Schiller LR, Santa Ana CA, Schmulen AC, et al. Pathogenesis of fecal incontinence in diabetes mellitus: evidence for internal-anal-sphincter dysfunction. N Engl J Med 1982;307: 1666–71.
[44] Fedorak RN, Field M, Chang EB. Treatment of diabetic diarrhea with clonidine. Ann Intern Med 1985;102:197–9.
[45] Fealey RD, Low PA, Thomas JE. Thermoregulatory sweating abnormalities in diabetes mellitus. Mayo Clin Proc 1989;64(6):617–28.
[46] Shaw JE, Parker R, Hollis S, et al. Gustatory sweating in diabetes mellitus. Diabet Med 1996;13(12):1033–7.
[47] Singleton JR, Smith AG, Bromberg MB. Increased prevalence of impaired glucose tolerance in patients with painful sensory neuropathy. Diabetes Care 2001;24(8):1448–53.
[48] Smith AG, Ramachandran P, Tripp S, et al. Epidermal nerve innervation in impaired glucose tolerance and diabetes-associated neuropathy. Neurology 2001;57(9):1701–4.

[49] Smith AG, Russell J, Feldman EL, et al. Lifestyle intervention for pre-diabetic neuropathy. Diabetes Care 2006;29(6):1294–9.
[50] Sumner CJ, Sheth S, Griffin JW, et al. The spectrum of neuropathy in diabetes and impaired glucose tolerance. Neurology 2003;60(1):108–11.
[51] Novella SP, Inzucchi SE, Goldstein JM. The frequency of undiagnosed diabetes and impaired glucose tolerance in patients with idiopathic sensory neuropathy. Muscle Nerve 2001;24(9):1229–31.
[52] Falk RH, Comenzo RL, Skinner M. The systemic amyloidoses. N Engl J Med 1997; 337(13):898–909.
[53] Adams D. Hereditary and acquired amyloid neuropathies. J Neurol 2001;248(8):647–57.
[54] Kyle RA, Dyck PJ. Amyloidosis and neuropathy. In: Dyck PJ, Thomas PK, Griffin JW, et al, editors. Peripheral neuropathy. Philadelphia: WB Saunders; 1993. p. 1294–309.
[55] Kernohan JW, Woltman HW. Amyloid neuritis. Arch Neurol Psychiatry 1967;27:132–40.
[56] DeNavasguez S, Treble HA. A case of generalized amyloid disease with involvement of nerves. Brain 1938;61:116–28.
[57] Sullivan JF, Twitchel T, Gherardi GJ, et al. Amyloid polyneuropathy. Neurology 1955;5: 847–55.
[58] Rajkumar SV, Gertz MA, Kyle RA. Prognosis of patients with primary systemic amyloidosis who present with dominant neuropathy. Am J Med 1998;104(3):232–7.
[59] Ando Y, Nyhlin N, Suhr O, et al. Oxidative stress is found in amyloid deposits in systemic amyloidosis. Biochem Biophys Res Commun 1997;232(2):497–502.
[60] Ando Y, Suhr O, El Salhy M. Oxidative stress and amyloidosis. Histol Histopathol 1998; 13(3):845–50.
[61] Simmons Z, Blaivas M, Aguilera AJ, et al. Low diagnostic yield of sural nerve biopsy in patients with peripheral neuropathy and primary amyloidosis. J Neurol Sci 1993;120(1): 60–3.
[62] Falk RH, Skinner M. The systemic amyloidoses: an overview. Adv Intern Med 2000;45: 107–37.
[63] Kyle RA, Gertz MA. Systemic amyloidosis. Crit Rev Oncol Hematol 1990;10(1):49–87.
[64] Skinner M, Anderson J, Simms R, et al. Treatment of 100 patients with primary amyloidosis: a randomized trial of melphalan, prednisone, and colchicine versus colchicine only. Am J Med 1996;100(3):290–8.
[65] Kyle RA, Gertz MA, Greipp PR, et al. A trial of three regimens for primary amyloidosis: colchicine alone, melphalan and prednisone, and melphalan, prednisone, and colchicine. N Engl J Med 1997;336(17):1202–7.
[66] Gertz MA, Lacy MQ, Dispenzieri A, et al. Stem cell transplantation for the management of primary systemic amyloidosis. Am J Med 2002;113(7):549–55.
[67] Andrade C. A peculiar form of peripheral neuropathy: familiar atypical generalized amyloidosis with special involvement of the peripheral nerves. Brain 1952;75:408–26.
[68] Saraiva MJM, Costa PP, Goodman DS. Biochemical marker in familial amyloidotic polyneuropathy, Portuguese type: family studies of transthyretin (prealbumin)-methionine-30 variant. J Clin Invest 1985;76:2171–7.
[69] Hund E, Linke RP, Willig F, et al. Transthyretin-associated neuropathic amyloidosis: pathogenesis and treatment. Neurology 2001;56(4):431–5.
[70] Rukavina JG, Block WD, Jackson CE, et al. Primary systemic amyloidosis: a review and an experimental genetic and clinical study of 29 cases with particular emphasis on the familial form. Medicine 1956;35:239–334.
[71] Mahloudji M, Teasdall RD, Adamkiewicz JJ, et al. The genetic amyloidoses with particular reference to hereditary neuropathic amyloidosis, type II (Indiana or Rukavina type). Medicine (Baltimore) 1969;48(1):1–37.
[72] Ando Y, Nakamura M, Araki S. Transthyretin-related familial amyloidotic polyneuropathy. Arch Neurol 2005;62(7):1057–62.

[73] Misu K, Hattori N, Nagamatsu M, et al. Late-onset familial amyloid polyneuropathy type I (transthyretin Met30-associated familial amyloid polyneuropathy) unrelated to endemic focus in Japan: clinicopathological and genetic features. Brain 1999;122(Pt 10): 1951–62.
[74] Lachmann HJ, Booth DR, Booth SE, et al. Misdiagnosis of hereditary amyloidosis as AL (primary) amyloidosis. N Engl J Med 2002;346(23):1786–91.
[75] Holmgren G, Ericzon BG, Groth CG, et al. Clinical improvement and amyloid regression after liver transplantation in hereditary transthyretin amyloidosis. Lancet 1993;341(8853): 1113–6.
[76] Adams D, Samuel D, Goulon-Goeau C, et al. The course and prognostic factors of familial amyloid polyneuropathy after liver transplantation. Brain 2000;123(Pt 7):1495–504.
[77] Bergethon PR, Sabin TD, Lewis D, et al. Improvement in the polyneuropathy associated with familial amyloid polyneuropathy after liver transplantation. Neurology 1996;47(4): 944–51.
[78] Pomfret EA, Lewis WD, Jenkins RL, et al. Effect of orthotopic liver transplantation on the progression of familial amyloidotic polyneuropathy. Transplantation 1998;65(7): 918–25.
[79] Delahaye N, Rouzet F, Sarda L, et al. Impact of liver transplantation on cardiac autonomic denervation in familial amyloid polyneuropathy. Medicine (Baltimore) 2006;85(4):229–38.
[80] Hammarstrom P, Wiseman RL, Powers ET, et al. Prevention of transthyretin amyloid disease by changing protein misfolding energetics. Science 2003;299(5607):713–6.
[81] Tuck RR, McLeod JG. Autonomic dysfunction in Guillain-Barré syndrome. J Neurol Neurosurg Psychiatry 1981;44:983–90.
[82] Zochodne DW. Autonomic involvement in Guillain-Barré syndrome: a review. Muscle Nerve 1994;17(10):1145–55.
[83] Cortelli P, Contin M, Lugaresi A, et al. Severe dysautonomic onset of Guillain-Barré syndrome with good recovery: a clinical and autonomic follow-up study. Ital J Neurol Sci 1990; 11:159–62.
[84] Feasby TE, Gilbert JJ, Brown WF, et al. An acute axonal form of Guillain-Barré polyneuropathy. Brain 1986;109:1115–26.
[85] Winer JB, Hughes RAC. Identification of patients at risk of arrhythmia in the Guillain-Barré syndrome. Q J Med 1988;257:735–9.
[86] Ropper AH, Wijdicks EFM, Truax BT. Guillain-Barré syndrome. Philadelphia: FA Davis; 1991.
[87] Suarez GA, Fealey RD, Camilleri M, et al. Idiopathic autonomic neuropathy: clinical, neurophysiologic, and follow-up studies on 27 patients. Neurology 1994;44:1675–82.
[88] Stewart PM, Hensley WJ. An acute attack of variegate porphyria complicated by severe autonomic neuropathy. Aust N Z J Med 1981;11:82–3.
[89] Young RR, Asbury AK, Corbett JL, et al. Pure pan-dysautonomia with recovery. Brain 1975;98:613–36.
[90] Hart RG, Kanter MC. Acute autonomic neuropathy: two cases and a clinical review. Arch Intern Med 1990;150:2373–6.
[91] Yahr MD, Frontera AT. Acute autonomic neuropathy: Its occurrence in infectious mononucleosis. Arch Neurol 1975;32:132–3.
[92] Fujii N, Tabira T, Shibasaki H, et al. Acute autonomic and sensory neuropathy associated with elevated Epstein-Barr virus antibody titre [letter]. J Neurol Neurosurg Psychiatry 1982;45:656–7.
[93] Thomashefsky AJ, Horwitz SJ, Feingold MH. Acute autonomic neuropathy. Neurology 1972;22:251–5.
[94] Pavesi G, Gemignani F, Macaluso GM, et al. Acute sensory and autonomic neuropathy: possible association with coxsackie B virus infection. J Neurol Neurosurg Psychiatry 1992;55(7):613–5.

[95] Summers Q, Harris A. Autonomic neuropathy after rubella infection. Med J Aust 1987;147(7):353–5.
[96] Neville BG, Sladen GE. Acute autonomic neuropathy following primary herpes simplex infection. J Neurol Neurosurg Psychiatry 1984;47:648–50.
[97] Fagius J, Westerberg CE, Olsson Y. Acute pandysautonomia and severe sensory deficit with poor recovery: a clinical, neurophysiological and pathological case study. J Neurol Neurosurg Psychiatry 1983;46(8):725–33.
[98] van Lieshout JJ, Wieling W, van Montfrans GA, et al. Acute dysautonomia associated with Hodgkin's disease. J Neurol Neurosurg Psychiatry 1986;49:830–2 [Published erratum appears in J Neurol Neurosurg Psychiatry 1986;49(12):1461].
[99] Hoyle C, Ewing DJ, Parker AC. Acute autonomic neuropathy in association with systemic lupus erythematosus. Ann Rheum Dis 1985;44:420–4.
[100] Arruda WO, Teive HA, Ramina R, et al. Autonomic neuropathy in systemic lupus erythematosus. J Neurol Neurosurg Psychiatry 1989;52(4):539–40.
[101] Heafield MT, Gammage MD, Nightingale S, et al. Idiopathic dysautonomia treated with intravenous gammaglobulin. Lancet 1996;347(8993):28–9.
[102] Smit AA, Vermeulen M, Koelman JH, et al. Unusual recovery from acute panautonomic neuropathy after immunoglobulin therapy. Mayo Clin Proc 1997;72(4):333–5.
[103] Wright RA, Grant IA, Low PA. Autonomic neuropathy associated with sicca complex. J Auton Nerv Syst 1999;75(1):70–6.
[104] Edmonds ME, Jones TC, Saunders WA, et al. Autonomic neuropathy in rheumatoid arthritis. BMJ 1979;2:173–5.
[105] Lucchinetti CF, Kimmel DW, Lennon VA. Paraneoplastic and oncologic profiles of patients seropositive for type 1 antineuronal nuclear autoantibodies. Neurology 1998;50(3):652–7.
[106] Lennon VA, Sas DF, Busk MF, et al. Enteric neuronal autoantibodies in pseudo-obstruction with small cell lung carcinoma. Gastroenterology 1991;100:137–42.
[107] Dalmau J, Graus F, Rosenblum MK, et al. Anti-Hu–associated paraneoplastic encephalomyelitis/sensory neuronopathy: a clinical study of 71 patients. Medicine 1992;71:59–72.
[108] Camdessanche JP, Antoine JC, Honnorat J, et al. Paraneoplastic peripheral neuropathy associated with anti-Hu antibodies: a clinical and electrophysiological study of 20 patients. Brain 2002;125(Pt 1):166–75.
[109] Vernino S, Lennon VA. New Purkinje cell antibody (PCA-2): marker of lung cancer-related neurological autoimmunity. Ann Neurol 2000;47(3):297–305.
[110] Yu Z, Kryzer TJ, Griesmann GE, et al. CRMP-5 neuronal autoantibody: marker of lung cancer and thymoma-related autoimmunity. Ann Neurol 2001;49(2):146–54.
[111] Vernino S, Low PA, Fealey RD, et al. Autoantibodies to ganglionic acetylcholine receptors in autoimmune autonomic neuropathies. N Engl J Med 2000;343(12):847–55.
[112] Vernino S, Low PA, Lennon VA. Experimental autoimmune autonomic neuropathy. J Neurophysiol 2003;90(3):2053–9.
[113] Klein CM, Vernino S, Lennon VA, et al. The spectrum of autoimmune autonomic neuropathies. Ann Neurol 2003;53(6):752–8.
[114] Sandroni P, Vernino S, Klein CM, et al. Idiopathic autonomic neuropathy: comparison of cases seropositive and seronegative for ganglionic acetylcholine receptor antibody. Arch Neurol 2004;61(1):44–8.
[115] Schroeder C, Vernino S, Birkenfeld AL, et al. Plasma exchange for primary autoimmune autonomic failure. N Engl J Med 2005;353(15):1585–90.
[116] Gibbons CH, Vernino SA, Kaufmann H, et al. L-DOPS therapy for refractory orthostatic hypotension in autoimmune autonomic neuropathy. Neurology 2005;65(7):1104–6.
[117] Goldstein DS, Holmes C, Dendi R, et al. Pandysautonomia associated with impaired ganglionic neurotransmission and circulating antibody to the neuronal nicotinic receptor. Clin Auton Res 2002;12(4):281–5.

[118] Hadjivassiliou M, Grunewald RA, Davies-Jones GA. Gluten sensitivity as a neurological illness. J Neurol Neurosurg Psychiatry 2002;72(5):560–3.
[119] Chin RL, Sander HW, Brannagan TH, et al. Celiac neuropathy. Neurology 2003;60(10): 1581–5.
[120] Cross AH, Golumbek PT. Neurologic manifestations of celiac disease: proven, or just a gut feeling? Neurology 2003;60(10):1566–8.
[121] Hadjivassiliou M, Davies-Jones GA, Sanders DS, et al. Dietary treatment of gluten ataxia. J Neurol Neurosurg Psychiatry 2003;74(9):1221–4.
[122] Gibbons CH, Freeman R. Autonomic neuropathy and coeliac disease. J Neurol Neurosurg Psychiatry 2005;76(4):579–81.
[123] Usai P, Usai SP, Lai M, et al. Autonomic dysfunction and upper digestive functional disorders in untreated adult coeliac disease. Eur J Clin Invest 1997;27(12):1009–15.
[124] Axelrod FB, Pearson J. Congenital sensory neuropathies: diagnostic distinction from familial dysautonomia. Am J Dis Child 1984;138(10):947–54.
[125] Dyck PJ. Neuronal atrophy and degeneration predominantly affecting peripheral sensory and autonomic neurons. In: Dyck PJ, Thomas PK, Griffin JW, et al, editors. Peripheral neuropathy. Philadelphia: WB Saunders; 1993. p. 1065–93.
[126] Thomas PK. Autonomic involvement in inherited neuropathies. Clin Auton Res 1992;2: 51–6.
[127] Axelrod FB. Hereditary sensory and autonomic neuropathies: familial dysautonomia and other HSANs. Clin Auton Res 2002;12(Suppl 1):12–4.
[128] Houlden H, Smith S, de Carvalho M, et al. Clinical and genetic characterization of families with triple A (Allgrove) syndrome. Brain 2002;125(Pt 12):2681–90.
[129] Herbert PN. Abetalipoproteinemia, hypobetalipoproteineima, and Tangier disease. In: Dyck PJ, Thomas PK, Lambert EH, et al, editors. Peripheral neuropathy. Philadelphia: WB Saunders; 1984. p. 1728–44.
[130] Dyck PJ, Ellefson RD, Yao JK. Adult-onset of Tangier disease: I. Morphometric and pathologic studies suggesting delayed degradation of neutral lipids after fiber degeneration. J Neuropathol Exp Neurol 1978;37:119–37.
[131] Low PA, Dyck PJ, Okazaki H, et al. The splanchnic autonomic outflow in amyloid neuropathy and Tangier disease. Neurology 1981;31:461–3.
[132] Appenzeller O, Kornfeld M, Snyder R. Acromutilating, paralyzing neuropathy with corneal ulceration in Navajo children. Arch Neurol 1976;33:733–8.
[133] Johnsen SD, Johnson PC, Stein SR. Familial sensory autonomic neuropathy with arthropathy in Navajo children. Neurology 1993;43(6):1120–5.
[134] Dyck PJ, Carney JA, Sizemore GW, et al. Multiple endocrine neoplasia, type 2b: phenotype recognition; neurological features and their pathological basis. Ann Neurol 1979;6(4): 302–14.
[135] Bejaoui K, Wu C, Scheffler MD, et al. SPTLC1 is mutated in hereditary sensory neuropathy, type 1. Nat Genet 2001;27(3):261–2.
[136] Dawkins JL, Hulme DJ, Brahmbhatt SB, et al. Mutations in SPTLC1, encoding serine palmitoyltransferase, long chain base subunit-1, cause hereditary sensory neuropathy type I. Nat Genet 2001;27(3):309–12.
[137] Kok C, Kennerson ML, Spring PJ, et al. A locus for hereditary sensory neuropathy with cough and gastroesophageal reflux on chromosome 3p22-p24. Am J Hum Genet 2003; 73(3):632–7.
[138] Lafreniere RG, MacDonald ML, Dube MP, et al. Identification of a novel gene (HSN2) causing hereditary sensory and autonomic neuropathy type II through the Study of Canadian Genetic Isolates. Am J Hum Genet 2004;74(5):1064–73.
[139] Maayan C, Kaplan E, Shachar S, et al. Incidence of familial dysautonomia in Israel 1977–1981. Clin Genet 1987;32(2):106–8.
[140] Axelrod FB. Familial dysautonomia. Muscle Nerve 2004;29(3):352–63.

[141] Blumenfeld A, Slaugenhaupt SA, Axelrod FB, et al. Localization of the gene for familial dysautonomia on chromosome 9 and definition of DNA markers for genetic diagnosis. Nat Genet 1993;4(2):160–4.
[142] Slaugenhaupt SA, Blumenfeld A, Gill SP, et al. Tissue-specific expression of a splicing mutation in the IKBKAP gene causes familial dysautonomia. Am J Hum Genet 2001;68(3): 598–605.
[143] Axelrod FB, Iyer K, Fish I, et al. Progressive sensory loss in familial dysautonomia. Pediatrics 1981;67(4):517–22.
[144] Goebel HH, Vogel P, Gabriel M. Neuropathologic and morphometric studies in hereditary motor and sensory neuropathy type II with neurofilament accumulation. Ital J Neurol Sci 1986;7:325–32.
[145] Swanson AG, Buchan GC, Alvord EC. Anatomic changes in congenital insensitivity to pain: absence of small primary sensory neurons in ganglia, roots and Lissauer's tract. Arch Neurol 1965;12:12–24.
[146] Nolano M, Crisci C, Santoro L, et al. Absent innervation of skin and sweat glands in congenital insensitivity to pain with anhidrosis. Clin Neurophysiol 2000;111(9):1596–601.
[147] Langer J, Goebel HH, Veit S. Eccrine sweat glands are not innervated in hereditary sensory neuropathy type IV: an electron-microscopic study. Acta Neuropathol (Berl) 1981;54(3): 199–202.
[148] Indo Y. Genetics of congenital insensitivity to pain with anhidrosis (CIPA) or hereditary sensory and autonomic neuropathy type IV: clinical, biological and molecular aspects of mutations in TRKA(NTRK1) gene encoding the receptor tyrosine kinase for nerve growth factor. Clin Auton Res 2002;12(Suppl 1):I20–32.
[149] Indo Y, Tsuruta M, Hayashida Y, et al. Mutations in the TRKA/NGF receptor gene in patients with congenital insensitivity to pain with anhidrosis. Nat Genet 1996;13(4):485–8.
[150] Low PA, Burke WJ, McLeod JG. Congenital sensory neuropathy with selective loss of small myelinated fibers. Ann Neurol 1978;3:179–82.
[151] Houlden H, King RH, Hashemi-Nejad A, et al. A novel TRKA (NTRK1) mutation associated with hereditary sensory and autonomic neuropathy type V. Ann Neurol 2001;49(4): 521–5.
[152] Brady RO. Fabry disease. In: Dyck PJ, Thomas PK, Griffin JW, et al, editors. Peripheral neuropathy. Philadelphia: WB Saunders; 1993. p. 1169–78.
[153] Ohnishi A, Dyck PJ. Loss of small peripheral sensory neurons in Fabry disease: histologic and morphometric evaluation of cutaneous nerves, spinal ganglia, and posterior columns. Arch Neurol 1974;31:120–7.
[154] Sima AAF, Robertson DM. Involvement of peripheral nerve and muscle in Fabry's disease. Ann Neurol 1978;35:291–301.
[155] Kocen RS, Thomas PK. Peripheral nerve involvement in Fabry's disease. Arch Neurol 1970;22:81–8.
[156] Kang WH, Chun SI, Lee S. Generalized anhidrosis associated with Fabry's disease. J Am Acad Derm 1987;17:883–7.
[157] Scott LJ, Griffin JW, Luciano C, et al. Quantitative analysis of epidermal innervation in Fabry disease. Neurology 1999;52(6):1249–54.
[158] Cable WJ, Kolodny EH, Adams RD. Fabry disease: impaired autonomic function. Neurology 1982;32:498–502.
[159] Schiffmann R, Hauer P, Freeman B, et al. Enzyme replacement therapy and intraepidermal innervation density in Fabry disease. Muscle Nerve 2006;34(1):53–6.
[160] Schiffmann R, Floeter MK, Dambrosia JM, et al. Enzyme replacement therapy improves peripheral nerve and sweat function in Fabry disease. Muscle Nerve 2003;28(6):703–10.
[161] Kimber J, McLean BN, Prevett M, et al. Allgrove or 4 "A" syndrome: an autosomal recessive syndrome causing multisystem neurological disease. J Neurol Neurosurg Psychiatry 2003;74(5):654–7.

[162] Merson MH, Hughes JM, Dowell VR, et al. Current trends in botulism in the United States. JAMA 1974;229:1305–8.
[163] Hughes JM, Blumenthal JR, Merson MH, et al. Clinical features of types A and B food-borne botulism. Ann Intern Med 1981;95:442–5.
[164] Koenig MG, Spickard A, Cardella MA, et al. Clinical and laboratory observations on type E botulism in man. Medicine 1964;43:517–45.
[165] Koenig MG, Drutz DJ, Mushlin AI, et al. Type B botulism in man. Am J Med 1967;42: 208–19.
[166] Merz B, Bigalke H, Stoll G, et al. Botulism type B presenting as pure autonomic dysfunction. Clin Auton Res 2003;13(5):337–8.
[167] Jenzer G, Mumenthaler M, Ludin HP, et al. Autonomic dysfunction in botulism B: a clinical report. Neurology 1975;25:150–3.
[168] Vita G, Girlanda P, Puglisi RM, et al. Cardiovascular-reflex testing and single-fiber electromyography in botulism: a longitudinal study. Arch Neurol 1987;44(2):202–6.
[169] Freeman R, Roberts MS, Friedman LS, et al. Autonomic function and human immunodeficiency virus infection. Neurology 1990;40(4):575–80.
[170] Rüttimann S, Hilti P, Spinas GA, et al. High frequency of human immunodeficiency virus-associated autonomic neuropathy and more severe involvement in advanced stages of human immunodeficiency virus disease [see comments]. Arch Intern Med 1991;151(12): 2441–3.
[171] Gastaut JL, Pouget J, Valentin P, et al. Study of sensory involvement and dysautonomia in HIV infected patients: a prospective study of 55 cases [in French]. Neurophysiol Clin 1992; 22(5):417–30.
[172] Villa A, Foresti V, Confalonieri F. Autonomic nervous system dysfunction associated with HIV infection in intravenous heroin users. AIDS 1992;6(1):85–9.
[173] Cohen JA, Laudenslager M. Autonomic nervous system involvement in patients with human immunodeficiency virus infection. Neurology 1989;39(8):1111–2.
[174] Schmunis GA. Trypanosoma cruzi, the etiologic agent of Chagas' disease: status in the blood supply in endemic and nonendemic countries. Transfusion 1991;31(6):547–57.
[175] Meneghelli UG. Chagas' disease: a model of denervation in the study of digestive tract motility. Braz J Med Biol Res 1985;18(3):255–64.
[176] Dantas RO, Godoy RA, Oliveira RB, et al. Cholinergic innervation of the lower esophageal sphincter in Chagas' disease. Braz J Med Biol Res 1987;20(5):527–32.
[177] Santos SL, Barcelos IK, Mesquita MA. Total and segmental colonic transit time in constipated patients with Chagas' disease without megaesophagus or megacolon. Braz J Med Biol Res 2000;33(1):43–9.
[178] Neto JA, Gallo L Jr, Manco JC, et al. Postural reflexes in chronic Chagas's heart disease: heart rate and arterial pressure responses. Cardiology 1975;60(6):343–57.
[179] Marin Neto JA, Gallo L Jr, Manco JC, et al. Mechanisms of tachycardia on standing: studies in normal individuals and in chronic Chagas' heart patients. Cardiovasc Res 1980;14(9): 541–50.
[180] Amorim DS, Manco JC, Gallo L Jr, et al. Chagas' heart disease as an experimental model for studies of cardiac autonomic function in man. Mayo Clin Proc 1982;57(Suppl):48–60.
[181] Sousa AC, Marin-Neto JA, Maciel BC, et al. Cardiac parasympathetic impairment in gastrointestinal Chagas' disease. Lancet 1987;1(8539):985.
[182] Iosa D, Dequattro V, De-Ping Lee D, et al. Pathogenesis of cardiac neuro-myopathy in Chagas' disease and the role of the autonomic nervous system. J Auton Nerv Syst 1990; 30:S83–8.
[183] Ribeiro AL, Moraes RS, Ribeiro JP, et al. Parasympathetic dysautonomia precedes left ventricular systolic dysfunction in Chagas disease. Am Heart J 2001;141(2):260–5.
[184] Facer P, Mathur R, Pandya SS, et al. Correlation of quantitative tests of nerve and target organ dysfunction with skin immunohistology in leprosy. Brain 1998;121(Pt 12):2239–47.

[185] Shah PK, Malhotra YK, Lakhotia M, et al. Cardiovascular dysautonomia in patients with lepromatous leprosy. Indian J Lepr 1990;62(1):91–7.
[186] McDonald WI, Kocen RS. Diphtheritic neuropathy. In: Dyck PJ, Thomas PK, Lambert EH, et al, editors. Peripheral neuropathy. Philadelphia: WB Saunders; 1984. p. 2010–7.
[187] Piradov MA, Pirogov VN, Popova LM, et al. Diphtheritic polyneuropathy: clinical analysis of severe forms. Arch Neurol 2001;58(9):1438–42.
[188] Idiaquez J. Autonomic dysfunction in diphtheritic neuropathy. J Neurol Neurosurg Psychiatry 1992;55:159–61.
[189] Matikainen E, Juntunen J. Autonomic nervous system dysfunction in workers exposed to organic solvents. J Neurol Neurosurg Psychiatry 1985;48(10):1021–4.
[190] Murata K, Araki S, Yokoyama K, et al. Autonomic and peripheral nervous system dysfunction in workers exposed to mixed organic solvents. Int Arch Occup Environ Health 1991;63(5):335–40.
[191] LeQuesne PM, McLeod JG. Peripheral neuropathy following a single exposure to arsenic. J Neurol Sci 1977;32:437–51.
[192] Windebank AJ, McCall JT, Dyck PJ. Metal neuropathy. In: Dyck PJ, Thomas PK, Lambert EH, et al, editors. Peripheral neuropathy. Philadelphia: WB Saunders; 1984. p. 2133–61.
[193] Murata K, Araki S. Autonomic nervous system dysfunction in workers exposed to lead, zinc, and copper in relation to peripheral nerve conduction: a study of R-R interval variability. Am J Ind Med 1991;20(5):663–71.
[194] Auld RB, Bedwell SF. Peripheral neuropathy with sympathetic overactivity from industrial contact with acrylamide. Can Med Assoc J 1967;96:652–4.
[195] Nordentoft T, Andersen EB, Mogensen PH. Initial sensorimotor and delayed autonomic neuropathy in acute thallium poisoning. Neurotoxicology 1998;19(3):421–6.
[196] LeWitt PA. The neurotoxicity of the rat poison vacor: a clinical study of 12 cases. N Engl J Med 1980;302:73–7.
[197] Hancock BW, Naysmith A. Vincristine-induced autonomic neuropathy. BMJ 1975;3:207.
[198] Legha SS. Vincristine neurotoxicity: pathophysiology and management. Med Toxicol 1986;1(6):421–7.
[199] Rosenfeld CS, Broder LE. Cisplatin-induced autonomic neuropathy. Cancer Treat Rep 1984;68:659–60.
[200] Hansen SW. Autonomic neuropathy after treatment with cisplatin, vinblastine, and bleomycin for germ cell cancer [see comments]. BMJ 1990;300:511–2.
[201] Richardson P, Cantwell BM. Autonomic neuropathy after cisplatin based chemotherapy [letter; comment]. BMJ 1990;300:1466–7.
[202] Cohen SC, Mollman JE. Cisplatin-induced gastric paresis. J Neurooncol 1987;5:237–40.
[203] Ekholm EM, Salminen EK, Huikuri HV, et al. Impairment of heart rate variability during paclitaxel therapy. Cancer 2000;88(9):2149–53.
[204] Ekholm E, Rantanen V, Antila K, et al. Paclitaxel changes sympathetic control of blood pressure. Eur J Cancer 1997;33(9):1419–24.
[205] Rowinsky EK, Chaudhry V, Cornblath DR, et al. Neurotoxicity of taxol. J Natl Cancer Inst Monogr 1993;15:107–15.
[206] Jerian SM, Sarosy GA, Link CJ Jr, et al. Incapacitating autonomic neuropathy precipitated by taxol. Gynecol Oncol 1993;51(2):277–80.
[207] Manolis AS, Tordjman T, Mack KD, et al. Atypical pulmonary and neurologic complications of amiodarone in the same patient: report of a case and review of the literature. Arch Intern Med 1987;147:1805–9.
[208] Fraser DM, Campbell IW, Miller HC. Peripheral and autonomic neuropathy after treatment with perhexiline maleate. BMJ 1977;2:675–6.
[209] Siddiqui MA, Ford PA. Acute severe autonomic insufficiency during pentamidine therapy [letter]. South Med J 1995;88(10):1087–8.

[210] Burnett JW, Weinrich D, Williamson JA, et al. Autonomic neurotoxicity of jellyfish and marine animal venoms. Clin Auton Res 1998;8(2):125–30.
[211] Geller RJ, Benowitz NL. Orthostatic hypotension in ciguatera fish poisoning. Arch Intern Med 1992;152(10):2131–3.
[212] Pearn J. Neurology of ciguatera. J Neurol Neurosurg Psychiatry 2001;70(1):4–8.

ELSEVIER
SAUNDERS

Neurol Clin 25 (2007) 303–317

NEUROLOGIC
CLINICS

Diabetic Neuropathies: Unanswered Questions

Yadollah Harati, MD, FACP

Baylor Neuropathy Center and Muscle and Nerve Pathology Laboratory, Department of Neurology, Baylor College of Medicine, 6550 Fannin Street, #1801, Houston, TX 77030, USA

Diabetic neuropathies are the most common types of neuropathies worldwide. Although there has been significant progress in the understanding of the clinical aspects of these conditions, many questions remain unanswered or difficult to answer in terms of causation, risk factors and genetic susceptibility, effective treatments and restoration of nerve functions, and pain management. The major handicap in studying diabetic neuropathies is the lack of a suitable animal model that addresses both acute and chronic events leading to diabetic neuropathy. Unfortunately and despite numerous drug trials, other than strict glycemic control, which is often difficult to maintain, there are no other treatment to slow the progression or delay the development of diabetic neuropathy. This article attempts, in a limited and selected fashion, to highlight a few unanswered or controversial questions regarding diabetic neuropathies.

What are the risk factors for the development and progression of diabetic peripheral neuropathies?

The duration of diabetes and degree of metabolic control are the two major predictors of the development of neuropathy and determinant of its severity. Other factors, such as patient's age, height, and presence of proliferative retinopathy, nephropathy, and cardiovascular diseases, also have been implicated (Box 1) [1]. Longer duration of diabetes also increases the possibility of developing more than one form of diabetic neuropathy. This factor is exemplified by a threefold increase in the prevalence of sympathetic and parasympathetic neuropathies in patients with diabetic neuropathy 10 years after the initial diagnosis of neuropathy [2]. The role of

E-mail address: yharati@bcm.edu

0733-8619/07/$ - see front matter
doi:10.1016/j.ncl.2007.01.002

Box 1. Risk factors for diabetic neuropathy

- Poor glycemic control
- Longer duration of diabetes
- Older age
- Male sex
- Height
- Alcohol
- Hypertension
- Nicotine use
- Hyperlipidemia
- APOE genotype
- Aldose reductase gene hyperactivity
- Angiotensin-converting enzyme genotype

excessive alcohol consumption as an independent risk factor for the development of diabetic neuropathy also has been emphasized [3], but the role for smoking is less clear. Smoking is not only a major dose-dependent risk factor for atherosclerosis and cardiovascular diseases but also may serve as an independent risk factor for cardiovascular autonomic dysfunction [4] and peripheral neuropathy [1,5,6]. Smoking and agents contained in nicotine induce an increase in insulin resistance, an abnormal state in which an impairment of cellular insulin signaling results in an overt resistance to the physiologic effects of insulin in terms of disposal of glucose and suppression of gluconeogenesis. This state leads to a combination of hyperinsulinemia and hyperglycemia, endothelial cell dysfunction, and hypertension and microvascular complications [7]. It is not clear whether cessation of smoking results in the improvement or slower progression of these complications, but it is prudent that patients be encouraged to do so.

Genetic factors also may play a role in individual susceptibility to diabetic neuropathy. APO-E genotype has been proposed as a risk factor for the *severity* of neuropathy in patients who have diabetes [8]. Having an E3/4 and 4/4 APOE genotype is the equivalent of having 15 extra years of age or diabetes duration. The APOE-4, however, does not function as susceptibility gene for the *development* of diabetic neuropathy in type II diabetes [9]. APOE genotype may influence the severity of neuropathy by several mechanisms, including acceleration of atherosclerosis, impairment of cytoskeletal stabilization, changes in cell adhesion, or use of growth factors [10]. This possible risk factor requires further longitudinal studies with large numbers of patients who have diabetes in different stages of disease to establish its potential clinical use.

Aldose reductase gene (AKR1B1) polymorphisms also have been implicated in the rate of decline in neuropathic function in diabetes and the early development of neuropathy and albuminuria in type II diabetes [11,12]. Aldose reductase is the rate-limiting enzyme of the polyol pathway of glucose metabolism expressed in many tissues and is implicated in the pathogenesis of diabetic microvascular complications. It catalyzes the NADPH-dependent reduction of glucose to sorbitol, which leads to intracellular accumulation of sorbitol and various metabolic imbalances, including enhanced oxidative stress. A recent longitudinal genetic association study of a cohort of 262 adolescent patients with type I diabetes followed for a median of 7 years revealed that the rate of decline in quantitative sensory and autonomic testing was strongly associated with AKR1B1 polymorphism [13]. Further and larger studies regarding different neuropathy subtypes and aldose reductase genes are required to clarify the role of aldose reductase gene polymorphism as a predictor for the development and severity of neuropathy and its use in clinical practice.

The presence of the D allele of the angiotensin I converting enzyme (ACE) is reported to be associated with increased risk of peripheral neuropathy in women with type II diabetes but not in men [14]. The role of angiotensin II, which is pro-inflammatory and pro-oxidant, in the development of vascular complications of type II diabetes has been implicated in several studies. By catalyzing the conversion of angiotensin I to angiotensin II, ACE facilitates this process. ACE inhibitors are shown to be effective in delaying the progression of microvascular complications, including nephropathy and retinopathy, and improving nerve conduction velocity, temperature discrimination threshold, and vibration perception in patients who have diabetes [15]. The D allele of the ACE gene has also been associated with higher ACE activity and macrovascular and microvascular complications and progression of nephropathy. Exactly why there should be a gender difference in the ACE genotype in determining the risk of neuropathy is not clear; however, modulation of ACE activity by estrogens at the level of transcription resulting in a relatively higher ACE level may play a role [16]. If female carriers of the D allele of ACE are at greater risk for diabetic neuropathy, an earlier treatment with ACE inhibitors or angiotensin receptor blockers may reduce the risk of neuropathy.

Although familial clustering for diabetic nephropathy and retinopathy has been demonstrated, such a familial clustering has not been observed in diabetic neuropathy [17,18].

Can a unified hypothesis for the pathogenesis of diabetic neuropathy be formulated?

Several mechanisms for the pathogenesis of diabetic neuropathy have been proposed, but none has achieved general acceptance. In general, they are divided into two major subgroups: (1) abnormalities that suggest a metabolic etiology and (2) abnormalities that suggest a vascular etiology (Box 2). For several of these hypotheses there is strong experimental support,

Box 2. Proposed abnormalities implicated in the pathogenesis of diabetic neuropathy

Abnormalities that suggest a vascular etiology
- Advanced glycation of vessel wall
- Basement membrane thickening and reduplication
- Endothelial cell swelling and pericyte degeneration
- Occlusive platelet thrombi
- Closed capillaries
- Multifocal ischemic proximal nerve lesions
- Epineurial vessel atherosclerosis
- Increased oxygen free radical activities
- Reduced endothelial nitric oxide activity
- Nerve hypoxia

Abnormalities that suggest a metabolic etiology
- Accumulation of sorbitol
- Reduction in the rate of synthesis and transport of intra-axonal proteins
- Reduction in nerve sodium-potassium-ATPase
- Enhanced protein kinase C activity
- Reduced amino acid incorporation into dorsal root ganglion
- Reduced incorporation into myelin of glycolipids and amino acids
- Reduced nerve L-carnitine level
- Abnormal inositol lipid metabolism
- Impaired essential fatty acid and prostaglandin metabolism
- Excessive glycogen accumulation
- Increased nonenzymatic peripheral nerve protein glycation
- Increased oxygen free radical activity
- Increased diacylglycerol –protein kinase C-beta signal transduction
- Nerve hypoxia

Other abnormalities
- Increased nerve edema
- Increased blood-nerve permeability
- Impaired endogenous neurotrophic or vascular growth factors
- Insulin deficiency

but the precise detail of each mechanism and—more importantly—their possible interrelationships remain unanswered.

Among these abnormalities, the formation of advanced glycation end products (AGEs) may serve as a unifying bridge between the two major hypotheses and explain many of the diabetic complications. AGEs are formed as a result of irreversible binding of high levels of glucose—and possibly fructose—to various proteins both intracellularly and extracellularly (glycated proteins). This is a relatively slow process that results in alteration of proteins physicochemical properties and their interaction with other molecules. The accumulation of glycated proteins in areas such as endothelial cells basement membrane or elastic lamina leads to vascular dysfunction. In patients who have diabetes and aged normal individuals there is an abundance of accumulated glycated proteins in the inner elastic layers of arteries. Binding of glucose to proteins also occurs with DNA and various crucial enzymes, such as antioxidants, matrix metalloproteinases and their tissue inhibitors, transforming growth factor-β, and extracellular signal-regulated kinases, among others. Bindng leads to ineffectiveness, deficiency, or dysfunction of these enzymes. Formation of AGE in the peripheral nerves and intra-axonal structures further interferes with axonal transport and nerve function. The intensity of AGE accumulation in the microvessels, endoneurium, and perineurium of nerve biopsies of patients who have diabetic neuropathy has been shown to correlate with the severity of axonal loss [19].

The glycated proteins, especially elastin and collagen, also bind to transition metals, which accumulate within the subendothelium and prevent access of endothelium-derived relaxing factor to smooth muscles. Reversal of this binding by administration of transition metal chelators (ie, desferrioxamine and trientin) in diabetic rats results in improved nerve function [20]. Impaired blood vessel relaxation leads to reduced nerve blood flow and nerve hypoxia or other nutritional deficiencies [21] and, ultimately, nerve degeneration. Reduced nerve perfusion and oxygenation in human diabetic neuropathy has been demonstrated. The accumulation of AGEs in the vessel wall also results in increasing macrophage recognition and uptake, stimulation of macrophage-derived and other growth factors, and increased vessel wall low-density lipoproteins, which lead to smooth muscle proliferation, atherogenesis, and further nerve hypoxia. Binding of glucose to the proteins of antioxidant enzymes, such as glutathione, catalase, and superoxide dismutase, results in further damage by rendering these enzymes ineffective in removing harmful free radical species. The excess free radical species damage cellular proteins, mitochondria, nuclear and mitochondrial DNA, and membranes. The interaction between AGEs, their receptor, and their primary effectors (activated NF-kappa B and interleukin-6) is also of interest because receptor AGE and its effectors have been co-localized in the sural nerve microvessels of patients who have diabetes [22]. Receptor AGE is thought to play a role in internalization and clearance of AGE. The various effects of glycation in the pathogenesis of diabetic neuropathy are depicted in Fig. 1.

If the accumulation of AGE is responsible for the initiation of cascades of metabolic, physiologic, and structural abnormalities in various tissues, including the peripheral nerve, would the inhibition of AGE formation

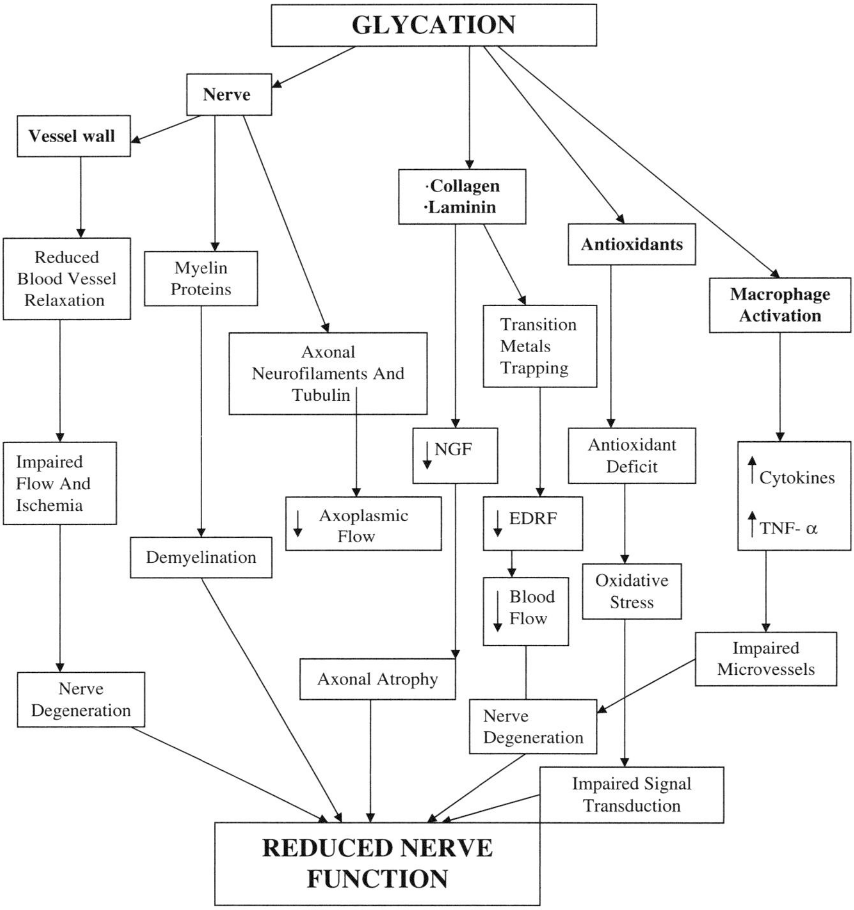

Fig. 1. Protein glycation as the pathogenesis of diabetic neuropathy.

prevent or ameliorate these complications? The answer to this question is far from clear. Although some agents effectively inhibit formation of AGE (including aminoguanidine, 2, 3-diaminophenazone, tenilsetam, and pyridoxamine) and in experimental animals cause improvement of vascular and nerve conduction abnormalities, their effect in human complications (eg, nephropathy) has been disappointing and they have not been tested in human diabetic neuropathy.

Regardless of how vascular abnormalities begin in diabetes, a substantial body of data implicates the dysfunction of nerves' blood vessels in the development of metabolic, functional, and structural nerve abnormalities. Patients who have diabetic neuropathy and reduced nerve oxygen tension and impaired nerve blood flow fail to raise nerve conduction velocities immediately after exercise, which suggests poor blood flow [23]. Patients who have diabetes and lower limb vascular insufficiency tend to have a more severe neuropathy than patients without ischemia [24]. Although these and other observations strongly suggest that a microvascular-induced nerve ischemia hypoxia can serve as an all-encompassing explanation for the pathogenesis of diabetic neuropathy, many unanswered questions remain. The structural microvascular and electrophysiologic abnormalities seen in diabetic neuropathy are late occurrence, and the earliest adverse effects of hyperglycemia are generally metabolic and result from direct exposure of nerve to glucose, where, unlike in other tissues, its uptake and transfer do not require insulin. The initial metabolic phase, which is potentially amenable to therapeutic intervention, is progressively replaced by a structural phase that becomes increasingly unresponsive to such interventions.

Is it "diabetic neuropathy" or "neuropathy in a diabetic patient"?

This question has become increasingly relevant because there has been an alarming worldwide rise in the prevalence of diabetes mellitus in recent years, with further increases predicted for the next decades. This rise is attributed to increased obesity, especially among younger individuals. Currently, diabetes affects approximately 20.8 million people in the United States [25], and it is predicted that approximately 220 million people worldwide will be afflicted by the year 2010. Earlier observations and more recent population-based cohort studies have shown that 66% of patients who have type I diabetes and 59% of patients who have type II diabetes develop objective neuropathy [26]. These results, when applied to the US population with diabetes, suggest that as many as 11 million people in this country may have some degree of one or more diabetic peripheral neuropathies. Because diabetes is such a common disorder, however, it may coincide with other conditions that cause peripheral neuropathies. The mere association of neuropathic symptoms with diabetes is not sufficient for diagnosis of diabetic neuropathy, and other causes of peripheral neuropathy always must be excluded. This approach is particularly relevant when the neuropathy is rapidly progressive, there is prominent motor abnormality or cranial nerve involvement, or there are disproportionate large fiber abnormalities. If there is involvement of the entire lower limbs without neuropathy of the distal upper limbs, it is unlikely that the process would be related to diabetic neuropathy and other causes should be investigated. It has been estimated that approximately one third of patients who have diabetes have a neuropathy unrelated to diabetes [20]. In The Rochester Diabetic Neuropathy Study [26], 10% of patients who have diabetes and distal sensory neuropathy had other possible causes of neuropathy. Gorson and Ropper [27] recently showed that this number is significantly higher, because 55% of their 103 consecutive patients with diabetes and distal sensory neuropathy had apparent additional causes for neuropathy. Chronic alcohol use, neurotoxic medications, low serum vitamin B_{12} or B_6, hypertriglyceridemia, and monoclonal proteins and paraproteinemia were the frequent findings. Patients who had additional causes for neuropathy more often had sensory symptoms and findings in the hands, and their neuropathy was more severe. In agreement with previous studies, 9% of Gorson and Ropper patients had electrophysiologic features of demyelination and 6% had conduction blocks [28]. It is possible that an immune-mediated neuropathy be an additional cause for neuropathy, responding to the appropriate treatment and necessitating further diagnostic evaluation. Similarly, with the high prevalence of diabetes it is likely that patients with diabetic neuropathy *and* chronic immune-mediated demyelinating polyneuropathy would be encountered in the neurology practice. Such a coincidence has led to the exaggerated conclusion that diabetic neuropathy itself is an immune-mediated disorder. Considering the current prevalence of diabetes in the United States and the crude overall estimates of prevalence of chronic immune-mediated demyelinating polyneuropathy at 0.81 to 1.9 per 100,000 population [29–31], approximately 1600 to 3800 patients are expected to have both conditions. These numbers would be even significantly higher for patients in the 70- to 79-year-old age group or male patients if the respective prevalences of 6.7 and 9.5 per 100,000 population for chronic immune-mediated demyelinating polyneuropathy in these groups are considered [31]. A clear answer to the question of immune-mediated diabetic neuropathy must await prospective studies in which a comprehensive and systematic evaluation of large numbers of patients is performed.

Does glucose modulate pain perception in diabetic neuropathy?

This important question has received scant attention despite the clinical observations that pain intensity in diabetic neuropathy fluctuates diurnally and in response to meals and that such variations may influence pain management or pain evaluation in drug trials. Research has suggested that, at least in experimental animals, glucose or serum insulin level plays an important mediating factor in the painful symptoms [32,33] and there may be a direct hyperalgesic effect of hyperglycemia on the dorsal root ganglia [34]. In humans, the idea that glucose may be an important contributing factor in painful diabetic neuropathy has been suggested in several clinical studies. In a randomized, single-blind study, Morley and coworkers [35] demonstrated in nondiabetic humans that a 50-g infusion of glucose resulted in increased pain detection and reduced tolerance thresholds to electric stimuli. Patients who had hyperglycemic type II diabetes were shown to be hyperalgesic when compared with nondiabetic control patients [35]. Research also has shown that recovery from painful diabetic neuropathy is more likely to occur if patients are maintained in good diabetic control, which is particularly true if the onset of painful symptoms is acute or subacute but is less evident when the onset is insidious and is followed by sensory loss.

Because infusion of glucose in healthy subjects results in a marked stimulation of insulin secretion, it is difficult to attribute the hyperalgesic effects of glucose infusion observed by Morley and colleagues solely to hyperglycemia alone. In contrast to the study by Morley and colleagues, infusion of glucose in eight healthy young adults had no effect on heat-induced pain threshold in another double-blind study [36] and in a small study of five patients who had type I diabetes. Thye-Ronn and colleagues [37] also demonstrated no effect of short-term hyperglycemia in ten patients who had nonneuropathic type I diabetes after the infusion of glucose on the heat-pain threshold but not on pressure-pain threshold. These studies and others [38] raised some doubt as to the reported effect of hyperglycemia on increased pain perception. It is known that glucose or sucrose administered orally to neonates provides effective analgesia for painful procedures. This effect can be decreased by opioid receptors antagonists. Whether there is a direct enhancing effect of glucose on the opioid receptors or an indirect effect via the release of endogenous opioids after the oral glucose administration remains to be investigated. In one study that used an in vitro expression system for mu-opioid receptors, no direct interaction between these receptors and glucose could be demonstrated [39]. In another study, 3 to 4 weeks' consumption of 32% sucrose in rats resulted in an increased morphine antinociceptive effect [40].

These conflicting studies indicate that the suggested relation between hyperglycemia and pain perception, the glucose and diverse functions of opioid receptors, and the effects of pharmacologic agents on these interrelationships are far from clear but worthy of further investigation.

Types I and II diabetes have different pathogenesis. Is there a difference between neuropathy of types I and II diabetes?

Type I diabetes is a multifactorial autoimmune disease that results in severe insulin deficiency that is influenced by environmental and genetic factors. Type II diabetes is a nonimmune disorder with varying degrees of insulin resistance and impaired insulin secretion usually associated with obesity. Despite the differences in causation of both types of diabetes, it has traditionally been assumed that the neuropathy of types I and II diabetes is the consequence of hyperglycemia and the same pathogenetic factors. Although this assumption is to a large extent true, there are structural and electrophysiologic differences between these two types of neuropathies, at least in experimental animals. In obese, hyperglycemic BBZ rats, which have no insulin deficiency and serve as a model for diabetes with insulin resistance (type II), a slowly progressive nerve conduction deficit, severe reduction in Na + /K ± ATPase activity, moderate myelinated fiber atrophy, and relatively severe segmental demyelination and Wallerian degeneration are observed. On the other hand, in type I diabetic BB/WOR rats with acute onset of hyperglycemia caused by an immune-mediated destruction of insulin producing cells, there is axonal swelling in paranodal regions, distal to proximal axonal atrophy, excessive myelin wrinkling, and impaired axonal regeneration [41]. Insulin deficiency and C-peptide impairment that occur in human type I diabetes and only in advanced type II diabetes play an important role in the abnormal protein interactions, perturbation of gene regulatory mechanisms, and impaired neurotrophic factors, which collectively contribute to the development of diabetic complications, including neuropathy [42]. These observations suggest that there should be some appreciable differences between the two types of diabetes in terms of type, severity, or progression of neuropathy. Population-based studies, however, have demonstrated modest differences only in the degree of the severity of neuropathy between the two types of diabetes. The Rochester Diabetic Neuropathy Study [26], which prospectively studied 380 of 870 patients who had diabetes in Rochester, Minnesota, revealed that 278 patients (73.2%) had type II diabetes, whereas 102 patients (26.8%) had type I diabetes. Fifty-nine percent of patients who had type II and 66% of patients who had type I had some forms of neuropathy (Table 1).

Symptomatic degrees of polyneuropathy occurred with similar frequency in types I and II diabetes (15% versus 13%), but more severe stages of neuropathy with distal sensory and autonomic dysfunction occurred more frequently in type I (6%) than II (1%) diabetes.

Is there an effective therapeutic measure for eradication of pain in diabetic neuropathy?

Only approximately 10% of all diabetic neuropathies are painful; however, the distressing nature of symptoms and difficulties in their treatment have given rise to the false impression that diabetic neuropathy is usually a painful condition. Persons who have diabetes with painless neuropathies are rarely referred to neurologists and often are cared for by their primary care physicians or endocrinologists. Pain control in diabetic neuropathy is often difficult and disappointing, with the best agents available providing only 30% more pain relief above placebo and eradication of pain remaining a longing for patients and physicians alike. Persistent pain exerts a substantial impact on the quality and enjoyment of life and causes significant disturbances in sleep. Because there is a possible effect of hyperglycemia in

Table 1
The Rochester Diabetic Neuropathy Study

	Type I (%)	Type II (%)
Polyneuropathy	54	45
Asymptomatic carpal tunnel syndrome	22	29
Symptomatic carpal tunnel syndrome	11	6
Visceral autonomic neuropathy	7	5
Other variants	3	3

reducing the pain threshold, a better control of blood glucose and prevention of wide fluctuation of blood glucose level may aid in alleviating the pain. Arriving at an appropriate drug and dosage may require several attempts and must strike a balance between pain relief and side effects. Some patients with similar painful symptoms respond to one class of drug, whereas others respond to a different group of medications. This difference should be emphasized to patients before initiating treatment. Genetic differences in pain-mediating pathways may explain this phenomenon. Patients should be told about the possibility of spontaneous resolution of pain because a simple reassurance that pain is not permanent is usually sufficient to ensure cooperation in coping with the pain. Patients who are seen by neurologists already have tried simple analgesics, but the use of nonsteroidal anti-inflammatory drugs should be discouraged because of their potential nephrotoxicity. To avoid early and unacceptable side effects, the principle of "start low, go slow" in initiating drug therapy should be followed for all classes of drugs, especially tricyclic antidepressants. Many treatment failures can be attributed to insufficient dosing or intolerance caused by rapid dose escalations. Drugs from several different pharmacologic classes have been shown to be safe and effective in alleviating neuropathic pain, but none has caused elimination of pain. These drugs include tricyclic antidepressants, anticonvulsants, sodium-channel blockers, opioids and non-narcotic analgesics, and topical agents. In practice, combinations of these drugs often are used; however, no data from clinical trials provide guidance regarding which combination to choose.

To compare efficacy among the different agents, the number needed to treat (NNT) is given whenever possible. The NNT is an estimate of the total number of patients who must be treated to obtain one patient with at least 50% pain relief [43]. In other words, the lower the NNT value, the more effective the drug. Tricyclics, which reduce pain independent from their effect on mood, have an NNT between 2 and 3. Most studies have shown that doses of tricyclics of 75 to 150 mg (less for elderly patients) are required for pain suppression. At such high dosage levels, sedation, confusion, anticholinergic effects (eg, constipation, dry mouth, urinary retention), and orthostatic hypotension are common side effects, particularly in elderly patients and patients who have clinical or nonapparent diabetic autonomic neuropathy. In such cases, if a patient seems to respond to amitriptyline, a trial of nortriptyline, a major metabolite of amitriptyline with a lesser propensity to cause orthostatic hypotension, may be worthwhile. Because of the weaker serotonergic activity of nortriptyline, however, it may be less effective for pain relief. Venlafaxine, with an NNT of 5 to 6.9, is an inhibitor of norepinephrine and serotonin reuptake with fewer side effects than tricyclics. At a dose of 150 to 225 mg/day, it is less effective than imipramin (NNT of 1.3–3.0) [44]. Duloxetin, a newly introduced dual reuptake inhibitor of 5-HT and norepinephrine, has a moderate effect on pain (60–120 mg/day) with an NNT of 5.2 [45]. The most frequent side effects include nausea, somnolence, dizziness, constipation, dry mouth, and reduced appetite. Other antidepressants are either ineffective or have minimal effect.

Anticonvulsants are considered second-line agents but are frequently given to all patients who have diabetic neuropathies, even patients who have painless sensory symptoms, a practice that should be discouraged. There is also a misunderstanding among some patients who have diabetic neuropathy that these agents treat the neuropathy itself. They should be appropriately educated that these agents are designed to modulate the pain without favorably influencing the course of the underlying neuropathy. The efficacy of carbamazepine (1000–1600 mg/day) is equivalent to tricyclic antidepressants (NNT of 3), but intolerable side effects limit its use. Its analog, oxcarbazepine, at a dose of 1200 mg or more daily, may be modestly effective [46]. Gabapentin, with an unknown mechanism of action, is used for many types of pain, but a median effective dose ranges from 900 to 1600 mg/day; even 3600 mg is needed for effective pain relief in diabetic neuropathy. Its NNT is 4. At a high dose there may be unacceptable side effects, including dizziness, sedation, confusion, mild gastrointestinal symptoms, gait problems, weight gain, and increased pedal edema. The latter two side effects may pose particular problems—diagnostically and therapeutically—among older patients who have diabetes. Pregabalin, which is structurally similar to gabapentin, has been shown in several trials to be consistently effective, with an average NNT of 3.9. The side-effect profile is essentially the same as gabapentin. Topiramate had a marginal effect with NNT of 7.4. This drug also decreases insulin resistance, lowers blood pressure, and has a favorable impact on lipid metabolism. Lamotrigine, which acts by blocking sodium channels and inhibiting the presynaptic release of glutamate, results in moderate (NNT of 4) pain relief at 200 to 400 mg/day. A recent study showed even fewer and inconsistent beneficial effects, however [47].

In patients who have not responded to tricyclics or anticonvulsants, tramadol may provide significant pain relief. This drug has at least two complementary modes of action: (1) low affinity (one-tenth of codeine) binding to mu-opioid receptors and (2) inhibition of reuptake of synaptic norepinephrine and serotonin. This combined mode of action makes it desirable for the treatment of painful diabetic neuropathy. In clinical trials, doses of 200 to 400 mg/day have proved effective with an NNT of 3.4. The drug is generally well tolerated, but transient nausea and constipation occur in approximately 20% of patients [48]. Tramadol has been reported to have little potential for abuse but should not be used in patients with a history of substance abuse.

Mexiletin, the oral analog of lidocaine, is generally ineffective, and gastrointestinal side effects make its use problematic. High-dose dextromethorphan, a low-affinity NMDA antagonist, provides partial pain relief but is associated with significant sedation and ataxia. The use of narcotics in painful diabetic neuropathy is generally discouraged because of the potential for drug dependency and their modest effect on neuropathic pain. In severe cases that are refractory to other treatments, however, narcotics may be used under guidelines established for chronic narcotic drug use.

Topical use of capsaicin-containing creams in the treatment of painful diabetic neuropathy may be modestly and temporarily effective, but most patients find the initial irritation after topical application too unpleasant and discomforting to continue the treatment.

Alpha-lipoic acid, an antioxidant with hypoglycemic effects, has been shown to be effective in an oral dose of 600 mg once daily for reducing stabbing and burning pain [49]. The drug has an overall favorable safety profile. The effect of drug is usually evident within 1 to 2 weeks after treatment.

Nonpharmacologic approaches, such as transcutaneous nerve stimulation, high-frequency muscle stimulation, frequency-modulated electromagnetic nerve stimulation, monochromatic infrared energy and biofeedback, and psychological support have been tried with minimum sustained benefit.

The use of surgical decompression of multiple peripheral nerves as an alternative approach to treatment of painful diabetic neuropathy is a contentious issue that cannot be supported, despite public interest and promotional statements by the proponents of this procedure. No prospectively conducted randomized controlled trials using standard definitions for neuropathy and outcome measures have been conducted to allow recommending this procedure [50].

Summary

Despite several novel analgesic drugs, the pharmacologic or nonpharmacologic treatment of chronic painful diabetic neuropathy remains a challenge, and the current state of treatment remains unsatisfactory and far from being able to eradicate pain. Ultimately, an effective treatment may include a combination of pain relief and improvement and slowing the progression of the underlying diabetic neuropathy.

References

[1] Tesfaye S, Stevens LK, Stephenson JM, et al. and the EURODIAB IDDM Study Group. Prevalence of diabetic peripheral neuropathy and its relation to glycaemic control and potential risk factors: the EURODIAB IDDM Complications Study. Diabetologia 1996;39(11): 1377–84.

[2] Dyck PJ, Davies JL, Wilson DM, et al. Risk factors for severity of diabetic polyneuropathy: intensive longitudinal assessment of the Rochester Diabetic Neuropathy Study cohort. Diabetes Care 1999;22(9):1479–86.

[3] Swade TF, Emanuele NV. Alcohol and diabetes. Compr Ther 1997;23(2):135–40.

[4] Anan F, Takahashi N, Shinohara T, et al. Smoking is associated with insulin resistance cardiovascular autonomic dysfunction in type 2 diabetic patients. Eur J Clin Invest 36(7):459–65.

[5] Mitchell BD, Hawthorne VM, Vinik AI. Cigarette smoking and neuropathy in di tients. Diabetes Care 1990;13(4):434–7.

[6] Sands ML, Shetterly SM, Franklin GM, et al. Incidence of distal symme neuropathy in NIDDM: the San Luis Valley Diabetes Study. Diabetes C 322–9.

[7] Groop PH, Forsblom C, Thomas MC, et al. Mechanisms of disease: Pathway-selective insulin resistance and microvascular complications of diabetes. Nat Clin Pract Endocrinol Metab 2005;1:100–10.

[8] Bedlack RS, Edelman D, Gibbs JW III, et al. APOE genotype is a risk factor for neuropathy severity in diabetic patients. Neurology 2003;60(6):1022–4.

[9] Zhou Z, Hoke A, Cornblath DR, et al. APOE epsilon4 is not a susceptibility gene in idiopathic or diabetic sensory neuropathy. Neurology 2005;64(1):139–41.

[10] Bedlack RS, Strittmatter WJ, Morgenlander JC. Apolipoprotein E and neuromuscular disease: a critical review of the literature. Arch Neurol 2000;57(11):1561–5.

[11] Sivenius K, Pihlajamaki J, Partanen J, et al. Aldose reductase gene polymorphisms and peripheral nerve function in patients with type 2 diabetes. Diabetes Care 2004;27(8): 2021–6.

[12] Sivenius K, Niskanen L, Voutilainen-Kaumisto R, et al. Aldose reductase gene polymorphisms and susceptibility to microvascular complications in type 2 diabetes. Diabet Med 2004;21(12):1325–33.

[13] Thamotharampillai K, Chan AK, Bennetts B, et al. Decline in neurophysiological function after 7 years in an adolescent diabetic cohort and the role of aldose reductase gene polymorphisms. Diabetes Care 2006;29(9):2053–7.

[14] Stephens JW, Dhamrait SS, Acharya J, et al. A common variant in the ACE gene is associated with peripheral neuropathy in women with type 2 diabetes mellitus. J Diabetes Complications 2006;20(5):317–21.

[15] Malik RA. Can diabetic neuropathy be prevented by angiotensin-converting enzyme inhibitors? Ann Med 2000;32(1):1–5.

[16] Sanada M, Higashi Y, Nakagawa K, et al. Relationship between the angiotensin-converting enzyme genotype and the forearm vasodilator response to estrogen replacement therapy in postmenopausal women.

[17] Seaqist ER, Goetz FC, Rich S, et al. Familial clustering of diabetic kidney disease. Evidence for genetic susceptibility to diabetic nephropathy. N Engl J Med 1989;320(18):1161–5.

[18] Clustering of long-term complications in families with diabetes in the diabetes control and complications trial. The Diabetes Control and Complications Trial Research Group. Diabetes 1997;46(11):1829–39.

[19] Misur I, Zarkovic K, Barada A, et al. Advanced glycation endproducts in peripheral nerve in type 2 diabetes with neuropathy. Acta Diabetol 2004;41(4):158–66.

[20] Lozeron P, Nahum L, Lacroix C, et al. Symptomatic diabetic and non-diabetic neuropathies in a series of 100 diabetic patients. J Neurol 2002;249(5):569–75.

[21] Eaton JW, Qian M. Molecular bases of cellular iron toxicity. Free Radic Biol Med 2002; 32(9):833–40.

[22] Bierhaus A, Haslbeck KM, Humpert PM, et al. Loss of pain perception in diabetes is dependent on a receptor of the immunoglobulin superfamily. J Clin Invest 2004;114(12):1741–51.

[23] Tesfaye S, Harris ND, Wilson RM, et al. Exercise-induced conduction velocity increment: a marker of impaired peripheral nerve blood flow in diabetic neuropathy. Diabetologia 1992;35(2):155–9.

[24] Ram Z, Sadeh M, Walden R, et al. Vascular insufficiency quantitatively aggravates diabetic neuropathy. Arch Neurol 1991;48(12):1239–42.

...tional Diabetes Information Clearinghouse. National Diabetes Statistics. NIH Publica- ...o. 06-3892.2005.

... Kratz KM, Karnes JL, et al. The prevalence by staged severity of various types of ...opathy, retinopathy, and nephropathy in a population-based cohort: the Ro- ... Neuropathy Study. Neurology 1993;43(4):817–24.

... r AH. Additional causes for distal sensory polyneuropathy in diabetic ... rosurg Psychiatry 2006;77(3):354–8.

... h DR, Avila OL, et al. Conduction block in diabetic neuropathy. ... 58–62.

[29] Kusumi M, Nakashima K, Nakayama H, et al. Epidemiology of inflammatory neurological and inflammatory neuromuscular diseases in Tottori Prefecture, Japan. Psychiatry Clin Neurosci 1995;49(3):169–74.

[30] Lunn MP, Manji H, Choudhary PP, et al. Chronic inflammatory demyelinating polyradiculoneuropathy: a prevalence study in south east England. J Neurol Neurosurg Psychiatry 1999;66(5):677–80.

[31] McLeod JG, Pollard JD, Macaskill P, et al. Prevalence of chronic inflammatory demyelinating polyneuropathy in New South Wales, Australia. Ann Neurol 1999;46(6):910–3.

[32] Lee JH, Cox DJ, Mook DG, et al. Effect of hyperglycemia on pain threshold in alloxan-diabetic rats. Pain 1990;40(1):105–7.

[33] Holder MD, Bolger GT. Chronic sweet intake lowers pain thresholds without changing brain mu- or delta-opiate receptors. Behav Neural Biol 1988;50(3):335–43.

[34] Dobrestov M, Hastings SL, Stimers JR, et al. Mechanical hyperalgesia in rats with chronic perfusion of lumbar dorsal root ganglion with hyperglycemic solution. J Neurosci Methods 2001;110(1–2):9–15.

[35] Morley GK, Mooradian AD, Levine AS, et al. Mechanism of pain in diabetic peripheral neuropathy. Effect of glucose on pain perception in humans. Am J Med 1984;77(1):79–82.

[36] Chan AW, MacFarlane IA, Bowsher DR, et al. Does acute hyperglycaemia influence heat pain thresholds? J Neurol Neurosurg Psychiatry 1988;51(5):688–90.

[37] Thye-Ronn P, Sindrup SH, Arendt-Nielsen L, et al. Effect of short-term hyperglycemia per se on nociceptive and non-nociceptive thresholds. Pain 1994;56(1):43–9.

[38] Chan AW, MacFarlane IA, Bowsher DR. Short term fluctuations in blood glucose concentrations do not alter pain perception in diabetic-patients with and without painful peripheral neuropathy. Diabetes Res 1990;14(1):15–9.

[39] Kracke GR, Uthoff KA, Tobias JD. Sugar solution analgesia: the effects of glucose on expressed mu opioid receptors. Anesth Analg 2005;101(1):64–8.

[40] D'Anci KE, Kanarek RB, Marks-Kaufman R. Beyond sweet taste: saccharin, sucrose, and polycose differ in their effects upon morphine-induced analgesia. Pharmacol Biochem Behav 1997;56(3):341–5.

[41] Sima AA, Zhang W, XU G, et al. A comparison of diabetic polyneuropathy in type II diabetic BBZDR/Wor rats and in type I diabetic BB/Wor rats. Diabetologia 2002;43(6):786–93.

[42] Sima AA. Pathological mechanisms involved in diabetic neuropathy: can we slow the process? Curr Opin Investig Drugs 2006;7(4):324–37.

[43] Sindrup SH, Jensen TS. Pharmacologic treatment of pain in polyneuropathy. Neurology 2000;55(7):915–20.

[44] Sindrup SH, Bach FW, Madsen C, et al. Venlafaxine versus imipramine in painful polyneuropathy: a randomized, controlled trial. Neurology 2003;60(8):1284–9.

[45] Wernicke JF, Pritchett YL, D'Souza DN, et al. A randomized controlled trial of duloxetine in diabetic peripheral neuropathic pain. Neurology 2006;67(8):1411–20.

[46] Grosskopf J, Mazzola J, Wan Y, et al. A randomized, placebo-controlled study of oxcarbazepine in painful diabetic neuropathy. Acta Neurol Scand 2006;114(3):177–80.

[47] Vinik AI, Tuchman M, Safirstein B, et al. Lamotrigine for treatment of pain associated with diabetic neuropathy: Results of two randomized, double-blind, placebo-controlled studies. Pain 2006; Dec 8 [Epub ahead of print].

[48] Harati Y, Gooch C, Swenson M, et al. Double-blind randomized trial of tramadol for the treatment of the pain of diabetic neuropathy. Neurology 1998;50(6):1842–6.

[49] Ziegler D, Ametov A, Barinov A, et al. Oral treatment with alpha-lipoic acid improves symptomatic diabetic polyneuropathy: the SYDNEY 2 trial. Diabetes Care 2006;29(11):2365–70.

[50] Chaudry V, Stevens JC, Kincaid J, et al. Practice Advisory: utility of surgical decompression for treatment of diabetic neuropathy: report of the Therapeutics and Technology Assessment Subcommittee of the American Academy of Neurology. Neurology 2006;66(12): 1805–8.

ELSEVIER
SAUNDERS

NEUROLOGIC CLINICS

Neurol Clin 25 (2007) 319–329

Index

Note: Page numbers of article titles are in **boldface** type.

A

doi:10.1016/S0733-8619(07)00024-2

G

H

M

O

P

T